Cancer Epidemiology Among Asian Americans

Anna H. Wu • Daniel O. Stram
Editors

Cancer Epidemiology Among Asian Americans

Springer

Editors
Anna H. Wu
Department of Preventive Medicine
Keck School of Medicine of USC
University of Southern California
Los Angeles, CA, USA

Daniel O. Stram
Department of Preventive Medicine
Keck School of Medicine of USC
University of Southern California
Los Angeles, CA, USA

ISBN 978-3-319-82270-9 ISBN 978-3-319-41118-7 (eBook)
DOI 10.1007/978-3-319-41118-7

Softcover reprint of the hardcover 1st edition 2016

Printed on acid-free paper

This Springer imprint is published by Springer Nature
The registered company is Springer International Publishing AG Switzerland

Preface

There are profound differences between countries, ethnic groups, and races in risks of virtually all common cancers; variations in cancer rates by population may reflect the influence of genetic, environmental, or behavioral risk factors and such variations have long motivated speculation about the causes of cancer. Our knowledge about whether the causes of the observed differences in cancer risk are modifiable is greatly enhanced by consideration of migration studies. When rates of a particular disease change rapidly among migrants, then this is supporting evidence that risk of that disease may be at least partly environmentally or behaviorally driven, rather than solely due to differences in the genetic background and therefore not amenable to intervention. This is especially true when risks in migrants approach those seen in the host country.

The most rapidly developing countries in the world today are in Asia, and Asians constitute the fastest growing immigrant populations in the USA. Asian Americans represent a heterogeneous population that includes Asian Indians, Chinese, Filipino, Japanese, Kampuchean (Cambodian), Korean, Vietnamese, and other Southeast Asians. Cancer is the leading cause of death for Asian American men and women. Studies of cancer in Asian Americans can reveal important clues to disease etiology since increases or decreases in cancer rates in Asian Americans can help to identify environmental and lifestyle causes of cancer. This book describes the current state of knowledge about the epidemiology of cancer risks in Asian Americans with specific references to changes in behavior and exposures due to the process of acculturation in the USA. The usual approaches to analytic investigation of epidemiology of complex diseases in US populations, i.e., case–control and cohort studies, have only sometimes or recently included Asian Americans to any large degree. Part of the rationale for this book is to be as thorough as possible in bringing to light what has been learned from these traditional approaches despite the often lack of data on Asian Americans. In addition, an overall theme of the book is the judicious use of ecologic comparisons as a source of information about the Asian American cancer experience, the risk factors underlying that experience, and the relevancy of the Asian American cancer experience to the rest of the Americas and the world, particularly as a source of information about the effects of continued globalization and acculturation on cancer risks.

The first section includes four chapters. Chapter "Resources and Methods for Studying Cancer among Asian Americans" summarizes the resources in the US and established study methods to conduct such studies in Asian Americans. Chapters "Cancer Incidence and Mortality Patterns among Chinese Americans" and "Cancer Incidence and Mortality among Filipinos in the United States and the Philippines: Patterns and Trends" provide a review of the specific cancer patterns in the two largest Asian American groups in the USA. Chapter "Cancer Screening among Asian Americans" examines the utilization of cancer screening tests among selected Asian American ethnic groups and describes the research on factors that are associated with screening. The second section includes eight chapters. Upon migration to the USA, there are increases in the incidence of cancers that are typically associated with westernization and decreases in the incidence of cancers that are linked to an infectious origin and other lifestyle factors that are prevalent in Asia. Chapters "Lung Cancer Among Asian Americans," "Colorectal Cancer among Asian Americans," "Prostate Cancer Among Asian Americans," "Breast Cancer among Asian Americans," and "Endometrial Cancer among Asian Americans" cover the cancer sites (lung, colorectum, prostate, breast, and endometrium) that are traditionally associated with Western lifestyles. Reasons that are favored to explain the increases in these cancers in Asian Americans are explored, including increased prevalence of the higher risk profiles in Asian Americans, timing of exposure to particular risk factors, and the magnitude of risk associations in Asian Americans. Chapters "Liver Cancer Among Asian Americans," "Gastric Cancer Among Asian Americans," and "Cervical Cancer Among Asian Americans" cover cancer sites that are historically very common in Asia; while the incidence rates of these cancers decline in Asian Americans, their rates remain relatively high. In these chapters, reasons that may explain the decline in the incidence of these cancers upon migration are discussed, paying attention to the prevalence of changing risk factors, the importance of timing of exposures, and other cofactors important in the etiology of these cancers. Whenever possible, genetic determinants and gene–environment relationships associated with specific cancers were included in the discussion. As will be evident, most of the information on Asian Americans is based largely on studies conducted in Japanese Americans. While Chinese and Filipino Americans were included in some analytic epidemiologic studies, few studies focused on their risk factors specifically. Even less has been done in the other Asian American groups. As the population of the other Asian ethnicities increases in the USA, there is a need to include other Asian ethnic groups in etiologic studies despite the challenges of small sample sizes, language, and other barriers.

In summary, this book aims to provide important and up-to-date information on cancer trends and risk factor patterns among the large and growing Asian American population in the USA. The chapters place an emphasis on the most common cancers diagnosed in Asian Americans, examining risk factor patterns, but also pointing to the gaps in knowledge as we often had to rely on results from studies conducted in Asia.

Los Angeles, CA Anna H. Wu, Ph.D.
Daniel O. Stram, Ph.D.

Contents

Resources and Methods for Studying Cancer Among Asian Americans .. 1
Ann S. Hamilton, Anna H. Wu, and Daniel O. Stram

Cancer Incidence and Mortality Patterns Among Chinese Americans 19
Lihua Liu, Dennis Deapen, and Anna H. Wu

Cancer Incidence and Mortality Among Filipinos in the USA and the Philippines: Patterns and Trends 47
Scarlett Lin Gomez, Meg A. McKinley, Caroline A. Thompson, Rita Leung, Iona Cheng, Anne-Michelle Noone, Latha Palaniappan, Mark Cullen, Christina A. Clarke, Theresa H.M. Keegan, and Sally L. Glaser

Cancer Screening Among Asian Americans 81
Annette E. Maxwell, Victoria M. Taylor, and Roshan Bastani

Lung Cancer Among Asian Americans 107
S. Lani Park, Daniel O. Stram, Mindy C. De Rouen, Scarlett Lin Gomez, Anna H. Wu, and Iona Cheng

Colorectal Cancer Among Asian Americans 137
Song-Yi Park and Loïc Le Marchand

Prostate Cancer Among Asian Americans 161
Shannon M. Conroy, Song-Yi Park, Scarlett Lin Gomez, and Iona Cheng

Breast Cancer Among Asian Americans 187
Anna H. Wu, Eunjung Lee, and Daniel O. Stram

Endometrial Cancer Among Asian Americans 219
Veronica Wendy Setiawan

Liver Cancer Among Asian Americans 233
Channa R. Jayasekera and Mindie H. Nguyen

Gastric Cancer Among Asian Americans 249
Afsaneh Barzi, Dongyun Yang, and Anna H. Wu

Cervical Cancer Among Asian Americans 271
Patti E. Gravitt, Ruby H.N. Nguyen, and Grace X. Ma

Index 287

Editors and List of Contributors

Editors

Daniel O. Stram, Ph.D. Department of Preventive Medicine, Keck School of Medicine of USC, University of Southern California, Los Angeles, CA, USA

Anna H. Wu, Ph.D. Department of Preventive Medicine, Keck School of Medicine of USC, University of Southern California, Los Angeles, CA, USA

List of Contributors

Afsaneh Barzi University of Southern California, Norris Comprehensive Cancer Center, Los Angeles, CA, USA

Roshan Bastani Jonsson Comprehensive Cancer Center, UCLA Kaiser Permanente Center for Health Equity, Fielding School of Public Health, University of California at Los Angeles, Los Angeles, CA, USA

Iona Cheng Cancer Prevention Institute of California, Fremont, CA, USA

Christina A. Clarke Cancer Prevention Institute of California, Fremont, CA, USA

Stanford Cancer Institute, Stanford, CA, USA

Shannon M. Conroy Cancer Prevention Institute of California, Fremont, CA, USA

Mark Cullen School of Medicine, Stanford University, Stanford, CA, USA

Dennis Deapen Los Angeles Cancer Surveillance Program, Department of Preventive Medicine, Keck School of Medicine of USC, University of Southern California, Los Angeles, CA, USA

Eunjung Lee Department of Preventive Medicine, Keck School of Medicine of USC, University of Southern California, Los Angeles, CA, USA

Sally L. Glaser Cancer Prevention Institute of California, Fremont, CA, USA

Stanford Cancer Institute, Stanford, CA, USA

Scarlett Lin Gomez Cancer Prevention Institute of California, Fremont, CA, USA

Stanford Cancer Institute, Stanford, CA, USA

Patti E. Gravitt Department of Pathology, University of New Mexico Health Sciences Center, Albuquerque, NM, USA

Department of Global Health, George Washington University, Milken Institute School of Public Health, Washington, DC, USA

Ann S. Hamilton Department of Preventive Medicine, Keck School of Medicine of USC, University of Southern California, Los Angeles, CA, USA

Channa R. Jayasekera The Barry S Levin Department of Transplantation, California Pacific Medical Center, San Francisco, CA, USA

Theresa H.M. Keegan Stanford Cancer Institute, Stanford, CA, USA

Division of Hematology and Oncology, Department of Internal Medicine, University of California Davis School of Medicine, Sacramento, CA, USA

Rita Leung Cancer Prevention Institute of California, Fremont, CA, USA

Lihua Liu Los Angeles Cancer Surveillance Program, Department of Preventive Medicine, Keck School of Medicine of USC, University of Southern California, Los Angeles, CA, USA

Grace X. Ma Lewis Katz School of Medicine, Temple University, Philadelphia, PA, USA

Loïc Le Marchand Epidemiology Program, University of Hawaii Cancer Center, Honolulu, HI, USA

Annette E. Maxwell Jonsson Comprehensive Cancer Center, UCLA Kaiser Permanente Center for Health Equity, Fielding School of Public Health, University of California at Los Angeles, Los Angeles, CA, USA

Meg A. McKinley Cancer Prevention Institute of California, Fremont, CA, USA

Mindie H. Nguyen Division of Gastroenterology and Hepatology, Stanford University Medical Center, Stanford, CA, USA

Ruby H.N. Nguyen Division of Epidemiology and Community Health, School of Public Health, University of Minnesota, Minneapolis, MN, USA

Anne-Michelle Noone Division of Cancer Control and Population Sciences, National Cancer Institute, Bethesda, MD, USA

Latha Palaniappan Palo Alto Medical Foundation Research Institute, Palo Alto, CA, USA

School of Medicine, Stanford University, Stanford, CA, USA

S. Lani Park Department of Preventive Medicine, Keck School of Medicine of USC, University of Southern California, Los Angeles, CA, USA

Song-Yi Park Epidemiology Program, University of Hawaii Cancer Center, Honolulu, HI, USA

Mindy C. De Rouen Cancer Prevention Institute of California, Fremont, CA, USA

Veronica Wendy Setiawan Department of Preventive Medicine, Keck School of Medicine of USC, University of Southern California, Los Angeles, CA, USA

Daniel O. Stram Department of Preventive Medicine, Keck School of Medicine of USC, University of Southern California, Los Angeles, CA, USA

Victoria M. Taylor Division of Public Health Sciences, Fred Hutchinson Cancer Research Center, Department of Health Services, University of Washington, Seattle, WA, USA

Caroline A. Thompson Graduate School of Public Health, San Diego State University, San Diego, CA, USA

Palo Alto Medical Foundation Research Institute, Palo Alto, CA, USA

Anna H. Wu Department of Preventive Medicine, Keck School of Medicine of USC, University of Southern California, Los Angeles, CA, USA

Dongyun Yang University of Southern California, Norris Comprehensive Cancer Center,, Los Angeles, CA, USA

Resources and Methods for Studying Cancer Among Asian Americans

Ann S. Hamilton, Anna H. Wu, and Daniel O. Stram

Abstract Asian Americans are a diverse group and have a long history of migration to the United States (USA). Large differences in cancer rates between countries of origin and the USA, as well as diversity in lifestyle and environmental exposures, provide an opportunity to identify and study risk factors for specific cancers that can provide insights into cancer etiology and methods of prevention. The migration experience has created a type of natural experiment in which populations with a common genetic background have been exposed to different risk factors in a new environment and provides the opportunity to determine if risk factor changes can be linked to changes in their cancer rates. Multiple data sources are available to study cancer in Asian Americans, including US Census data to provide denominators for rates, cancer registries to assess cancer incidence, as well as observational studies in which personal risk factor information is obtained. Study designs which have been used include the ecologic, cross-sectional, case series, case-control, and cohort studies. Limitations and caveats in using these resources and study designs are described.

Keywords Asian Americans • Cancer • Risk factors • Cancer registry • Study designs • Migration

Introduction

Asian Americans are extraordinarily diverse with respect to country of origin, time since immigration, socioeconomic status, languages and dialects spoken, religion, diet, and other characteristics, many of which may affect health. There has been a long history of migration from Asia to the United States (USA) in substantial numbers and from countries with differing cancer incidence rates, both higher and lower than found in the USA. If cancer rates differ between Asians in their country of origin, migrants, and their counterparts born in the USA, these differences provide important clues to determine environmental and lifestyle risk factors for cancer,

A.S. Hamilton, Ph.D. (✉) • A.H. Wu • D.O. Stram
Department of Preventive Medicine, Keck School of Medicine of USC,
University of Southern California, Los Angeles, CA, USA
e-mail: ahamilt@med.usc.edu

A.H. Wu, D.O. Stram (eds.), *Cancer Epidemiology Among Asian Americans*,
DOI 10.1007/978-3-319-41118-7_1

since these comparison groups generally have a similar genetic background. On the other hand, if cancer rates do not differ between migrants and nonmigrants, this may be due to similar environmental factors in both locations or alternatively due to host/genetic factors.

Asian Americans are defined by the US Census Bureau as individuals with origins in "any of the original people of the Far East, Southeast Asia, or the Indian Subcontinent." Modern Asian immigration to the USA began in the 1880s, when first Chinese and later Japanese, Filipino, and Korean workers were recruited to work on plantations and farms in Hawaii and California (See Chaps. 2 and 3 for details on migration history of Chinese and Filipinos). Various Exclusion Acts limited other forms of immigration by Asians until 1965, when discrimination based on country of origin was prohibited. Asian immigration to the USA has increased steadily since then.

Here, we describe the composition and numbers of Asian Americans in the USA today, sources of data used to assess cancer rates among the various Asian subgroups both in the USA and in their countries of origin, and discuss methodological issues, study designs, and potential biases that should be assessed when studying the role of migration on changing cancer risk factors.

Asian-American Population Characteristics (2000–2010)

Coding for specific Asian ethnic groups was added to the US Census over time beginning in 1870 for Chinese which included all east Asians, 1890 for Japanese; 1920 for Hindu (South Asia Indian), Korean, and Filipino; and 1980 for Vietnamese and Pacific Islander groups. In the past three censuses (1990, 2000, 2010), the racial categories were the same except that the option for listing multiple races was not provided until 2000. In 2010, the US Census obtained a person's race according to the form shown in Fig. 1 [1]. In addition to the specific Asian groups listed as check boxes in the questionnaire (Asian Indian, Chinese, Filipino, Japanese, Korean, and Vietnamese), there was a box for "Other Asian" allowing the person to write in other groups. From this text field, additional Asian groups were identified, including Bangladeshi, Bhutanese, Kampuchean (Cambodian), Hmong, Indonesian, Iwo Jima, Laotian, Malaysian, Mongolian, Nepalese, Okinawan, Pakistani, Singaporean, Sri Lankan, Thai, and other Asian, not specified. In 2010, over 17 million people listed at least one Asian race, and of them, 15.3 % or 2.6 million listed more than one race [1]. The total Asian population, including those listing more than one race, comprised 5.6 % of the US population. The US population grew by 9.7 % between 2000 and 2010; however, the Asian population grew faster during this decade than any other racial group, rising by 43 % for those who reported an Asian race alone and by 46 % when including those reporting an Asian race in combination with another race.

Among the detailed Asian ethnic subgroups in 2010, the Chinese population was the largest (Table 1); Filipinos were the next most prevalent, followed by Asian Indians, Vietnamese, Koreans, and Japanese. The Asian ethnic subgroups with the

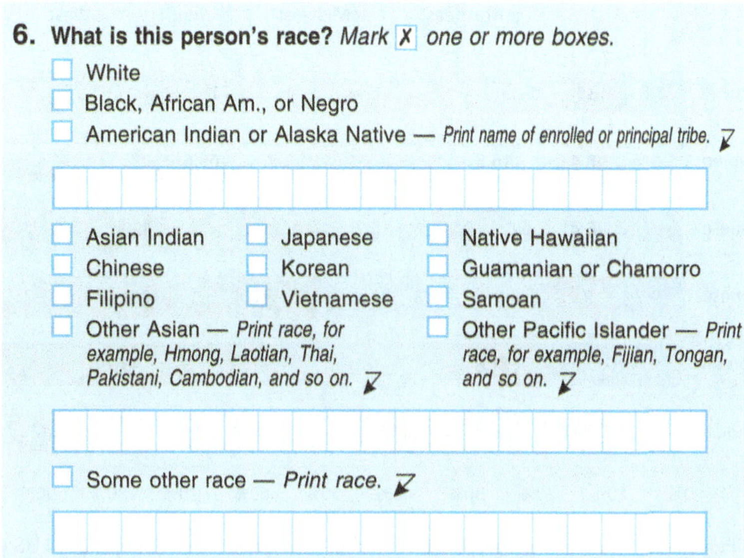

6. What is this person's race? *Mark* X *one or more boxes.*

- ☐ White
- ☐ Black, African Am., or Negro
- ☐ American Indian or Alaska Native — *Print name of enrolled or principal tribe.*
- ☐ Asian Indian
- ☐ Chinese
- ☐ Filipino
- ☐ Other Asian — *Print race, for example, Hmong, Laotian, Thai, Pakistani, Cambodian, and so on.*
- ☐ Japanese
- ☐ Korean
- ☐ Vietnamese
- ☐ Native Hawaiian
- ☐ Guamanian or Chamorro
- ☐ Samoan
- ☐ Other Pacific Islander — *Print race, for example, Fijian, Tongan, and so on.*
- ☐ Some other race — *Print race.*

Fig. 1 Reproduction of the question on race from the 2010 Census [1]

Table 1 Total 2010 US population by detailed Asian subgroup [1]

	Asian alone	Asian in combination
Chinese	3,535,382	474,732
Filipino	2,649,973	766,867
Asian Indian	2,918,807	264,256
Vietnamese	1,632,717	104,716
Korean	1,463,474	243,348
Japanese	841,824	462,462

highest proportion of people naming an Asian race in combination with another race were Japanese (35.4 %) and Filipinos (22.4 %). Among the 2.6 million Asian in combination with another race population, 1.6 million named the White race as a second racial group [1].

The increasing Asian-American population over the last decade is reflected in the timing of when foreign-born Asians have come to the USA. Over 30 % of foreign-born males and females have arrived in the USA between 2000 and 2009, and another 5–6 % have arrived since 2010. Over 56 % of the Asians in the USA were foreign born in 2010, including those who were Asian alone or in combination with another race, about 30 % of Asian Americans were in the 35–54 age group, with relatively low percentages in the over 65 age group.

In 2010, the highest proportion of the total Asian population (i.e., Asian alone + Asian in combination with another race) lived in the West (46.2 %), followed by the South (22.1 %), the Northwest (19.8 %), and the Midwest (11.9 %) which was very

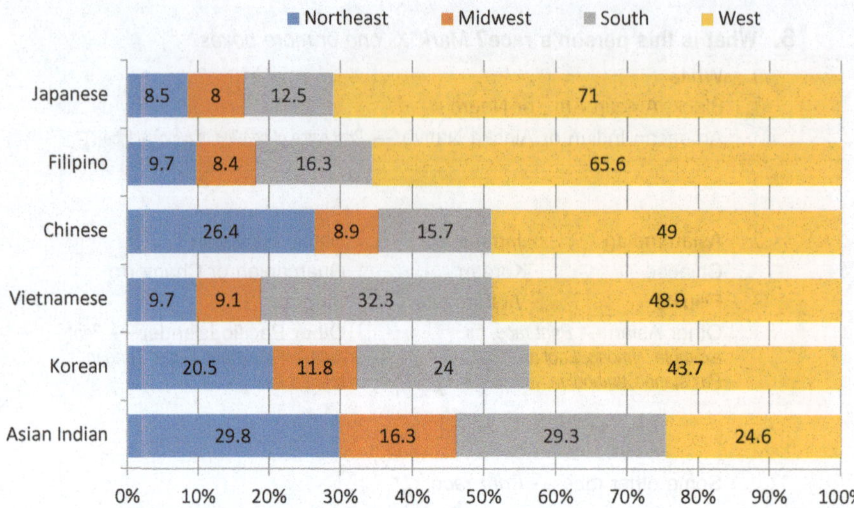

Fig. 2 Percent distribution of geographic location* of detailed Asian subgroups: 2010 US Census [1]. *The Northeast census region includes Connecticut, Maine, Massachusetts, New Hampshire, New Jersey, New York, Pennsylvania, Rhode Island, and Vermont. The Midwest census region includes Illinois, Indiana, Iowa, Kansas, Michigan, Minnesota, Missouri, Nebraska, North Dakota, Ohio, South Dakota, and Wisconsin. The South census region includes Alabama, Arkansas, Delaware, the District of Columbia, Florida, Georgia, Kentucky, Louisiana, Maryland, Mississippi, North Carolina, Oklahoma, South Carolina, Tennessee, Texas, Virginia, and West Virginia. The West census region includes Alaska, Arizona, California, Colorado, Hawaii, Idaho, Montana, Nevada, New Mexico, Oregon, Utah, Washington, and Wyoming

similar to the distribution in 2000. The states with the greatest numbers of Asians in 2010 were California (5.6 million), New York (1.6 million), Texas (1.1 million), New Jersey (0.8 million), Hawaii (0.8 million), Illinois (0.7 million), Washington (0.6 million), Florida (0.6 million), Virginia (0.5 million), and Pennsylvania (0.4 million) [1]. Although the top five cities with the greatest numbers of Asians included New York, NY; Los Angeles, CA; San Jose, CA; San Francisco, CA; and San Diego, CA, the areas experiencing the highest percentage growth in the number of Asians between 2000 and 2010 were located in the South and Midwest.

There were, however, substantial differences in the geographic distribution of the specific Asian ethnic subgroups in 2010. As shown in Fig. 2, 71.0 % of Japanese and 65.6 % of Filipinos lived in the West, followed by close to half of Chinese and Vietnamese, 43.7 % of Koreans, and about a quarter of Asian Indians. Close to a third of Vietnamese and Asian Indians lived in the South, the highest percentages of any of the Asian ethnic subgroups living in that region. Chinese and Asian Indians were the most likely of any of the groups to live in the Northeast (26.4 % and 29.8 %, respectively). Asian Indians, who were distributed the most evenly across the country, also had the highest percentage of any group living in the Midwest (16.3 %). California had the highest proportion of each of these subgroups living in any state, ranging from 43 % of the Filipinos to 19 % of the Asian Indians.

These results provide insights into where studies of migrant populations may be conducted to include the largest numbers of Asians by specific Asian ethnic subgroup and where the most recently arrived migrant populations are located. In addition, the differences in the proportions of mixed race populations among the Asian ethnic subgroups indicate that there may be different genetic factors to consider when studying the Japanese and Filipino populations, for example, which had the highest proportions of multiple race individuals (35.4 % and 22.4 %, respectively), compared to the Vietnamese who had the lowest (6.4 %).

Comparison of Worldwide Cancer Rates

Information on cancer incidence rates in other countries is necessary to compare differences in cancer incidence rates between countries of origin and the USA. The history of comparison of worldwide cancer rates began with Segi [2] and colleagues who produced a series of reports comparing cancer mortality in 24 countries in the 1950s, showing that the distinctive geographical and racial/ethnic variation in cancer occurrence may provide clues to the etiology of cancer. Recognizing the importance of accurate and timely cancer registration, the International Agency for Research on Cancer (IARC) and the International Association of Cancer Registries (IACR) were established. Since 1966, detailed information of cancer recorded by regional or national registries around the world was published in the series "Cancer Incidence in Five Continents" (CI5), which was updated typically every 5 years [3–5]. The CI5 series provides the major sources of information to compute the country-specific cancer incidence rates which are provided in the online, freely accessible database, GLOBOCAN. As cancer rates may vary considerably within a country, GLOBOCAN national rates (incidence, mortality, and prevalence) are estimated using data from the individual contributing registries, taking into account regional and urban/rural patterns. GLOBOCAN 2012 is the fifth and most recent version that presents cancer incidence and mortality in 184 countries [6].

Given that age itself is one of the strongest risk factors for developing cancer and unadjusted or crude incidence rates are highly dependent on the underlying age distribution of the population, age-standardized incidence rates (ASR) are used for comparison of cancer incidence rates between populations. Age standardization in GLOBOCAN and CI5 are typically calculated using world standard population proposed by Segi [2], but age truncation into 5- or 10-year age groups may be used in different studies.

Cancer Incidence and Mortality in Asian Americans

The development of national population-based cancer registries, which included large populations of Asian Americans within the USA, has provided the basis for studies of cancer incidence and mortality. Efforts on the national level to collect incidence and mortality data in a systematic way began with the National Cancer Act of 1971 that mandated the collection and analysis of data useful in the prevention, diagnosis, and treatment of cancer. This mandate led to the formation of SEER (Surveillance Epidemiology and End Results), the program that established population-based cancer registries funded by the National Cancer Institute. Regions in the SEER program were selected to represent the diverse racial ethnic composition of the US population. The inclusion of Hawaii and San Francisco at the outset of the program in 1975 and the subsequent addition of Los Angeles County and four counties in the San Jose/Monterey area in 1992 allowed coverage of Asian-American and Pacific Islander (AAPI) population. In 1988, cancer became a reportable condition in California, leading to the establishment of the California Cancer Registry (CCR), and in 1992, the entire state was included in SEER program. Reporting by SEER registries uses a standardized protocol and is centrally monitored, and participation requires meeting quality control standards including promptness, histologic confirmation, and completeness [7].

Data from the CCR have been used to study cancer patterns of the five most populous Asian subgroups in California (Chinese, Japanese, Filipino, Korean, Vietnamese) [8, 9]. Because of small numbers, cancer patterns for Southeast Asian (Vietnamese, Laotian, Hmong, Kampuchean (Cambodian), Thai, Burmese) and the Indian Continent (Asian Indian, Pakistani, Bangladeshi, Nepalese, Sikkimese, Sri Lankan) are often studied as a group [10]. The Los Angeles County Cancer Surveillance Program (CSP), the SEER population-based cancer registry for Los Angeles County, has the longest history of estimating cancer incidence rates for specific Asian ethnic groups. Since 1976, the CSP has reported on cancer incidence rates for four Asian groups (Chinese, Japanese, Filipino, and Koreans), and this was expanded in 1991 to include four additional AAPI groups (Vietnamese, South Asian, Thai/Hmong/Kampuchean (Cambodian)/Laotian, and Hawaiian/Samoan). Thus, since the early studies of Smith and King [11–16] and others who investigated cancer mortality patterns of Chinese and Japanese residing in California, Hawaii, and New York, there are now data resources to study cancer incidence and mortality patterns in multiple Asian-specific populations on a county (Los Angeles), statewide (California), and nationwide (SEER) level.

Methodologic Considerations in Studies of Asian Americans and Cancer

Taken at face value, changes in cancer incidence and mortality rates observed in an Asian ethnic migrant subgroup compared to rates in their home country imply that disease incidence is affected by risk factors which have changed with moving to the new environment, since the migrant population would be expected to have a similar genetic background to those remaining in the home country. However, there are multiple potential sources of bias that should be considered when conducting studies designed to assess the effects of migration and associated changes in lifestyle on cancer risk. These biases may be specific to the type of study design and are summarized below. Previous reviews have also provided an excellent description of major biases in migrant studies and are still relevant today [17, 18].

All traditional epidemiological observational study designs can be used to study the effect of migration status on cancer risk among Asian Americans, including ecologic, cross-sectional, case series, case-control, and cohort studies and variations such as the nested case-control study [19]. Studies which do not obtain direct individual information or which do not allow for distinguishing the timing between risk factor exposure and disease onset may be considered "descriptive studies" which are helpful for identifying disease patterns and for hypothesis generating or for providing suggestions for possible cause and effect relationships that would require further study to confirm. Analytic designs obtain individual information on exposures of interest and outcome measures, as well as potential confounders. Inference about cause and effect is strengthened if exposure history is available and precedes the outcome being studied. In general, the ecological study and case series are considered to be descriptive studies, while case-control and cohort studies are analytic designs. The cross-sectional design obtains individual information; however, the exposure and outcome are assessed at the same point in time. While this may prevent the assessment of cause and effect for many exposures and outcomes, the temporal sequence between these events can be determined in some circumstances (e.g., exposures occurring in childhood compared to outcomes in adulthood). We present below some examples of the use of the various study designs to investigate the effect of migration on cancer risk among Asian Americans and limitations/potential biases associated with the designs.

Ecological Study Design

This study design is often used in migrant-related studies in which individual data on exposures are not collected and comparisons are based on established datasets including cancer registries, census information, and geographic-based measures of exposures. A comparison of cancer rates between countries and subgroups is used to develop hypotheses about risk factors for cancer based on prevalence of different risk factor profiles between the areas of comparison. No individual level information is obtained.

There are important methodological concerns in the comparison of incidence rates that involve the quality of the numerator and denominator data, as well as the matching of definitions of Asian subgroups between the sources of data.

(a) The ascertainment of the cancer cases (numerator) is related to the quality of cancer registration.

Completeness of case ascertainment may be affected by definitions used to identify cases, diagnostic coding schemes used, rates of histologic confirmation of cases, and criteria used by pathologists [18]. These practices may differ between the country of origin and those in the host country. Differences in the proportion of histologically confirmed cases and death certificate-only cases are two important indicators used to assess the quality of cancer registries. A summary of cancer registry quality indicators and procedures has been described [20, 21]. In addition, the incidence of certain cancers (e.g., prostate, colorectum, breast, thyroid, etc.) may be quite dependent on screening practices [4].

(b) The quality of denominator data may differ between the country of origin and the host country.

The assessment of accuracy of denominator data is important to assure that the comparison of rates between the country of origin and the USA is based on true differences in cancer incidence. If, for example, the denominator data for the country of origin was underestimated and the numerator reflecting cancer incidence was complete, the cancer incidence rate in that country would be overestimated. Conversely, should the denominator be overestimated, the rate based on it would be underestimated (again assuming the numerator data were complete). In addition to providing cancer incidence rates for 184 countries, GLOBOCAN 2012 has also provided an assessment of the quality of rates by country and the sources of data used for each one [6].

In the USA, denominator data for Asian ethnic subgroups are produced every 10 years when the Census is conducted. For the 2010 Census, data by the detailed Asian subgroups as well as mixed race subgroups is provided in the 2010 Census Summary File 1 [1]. Population estimates need to be projected during intercensal years for each of the specific Asian ethnic subgroups.

The different registries in the USA (e.g., SEER, CCR, and Los Angeles CSP) have developed their own intercensal population estimates for their respective regions. Also there are differences in the availability of rates for the detailed Asian subgroups. The SEER program provides US population files that can be used to calculate rates using the SEER* Stat program by county, state, and age group for the year 1969–2013, but this is only provided as a summarized total for Asians and not by specific Asian ethnic subgroup (http://seer.cancer.gov/popdata/download.html). In SEER, AAPI rates are often presented for AAPI combined and not by specific (or disaggregated) Asian-American ethnic groups. Small numbers of individual AAPI populations in earlier years of SEER and unstable rates are reasons to present rates for AAPI as a group. The CCR has also developed its own population estimates for denominators to calculate Asian race-specific rates using population estimates for California obtained from the 1990 and 2000 census [9]. The CSP has similarly developed its own population estimates for denominators to calculate Asian race-specific rates using population estimates for LA County obtained from the 1970, 1980, 1990, and 2000 US population censuses.

With the rapidly growing AAPI population in the USA, there are now concerted efforts to examine cancer patterns of the eight most populous Asian ethnic populations (Asian Indian/Pakistani, Chinese, Filipino, Japanese, Kampuchean (Cambodian), Korean, Laotian, Vietnamese) [22, 23]. Miller and colleagues [22] included cancer diagnoses among AAPI populations from 1998–2002 identified in 14 SEER registries covering 68 % of the total US AAPI population and presented incidence and mortality rates by detailed AAPI groups. Gomez and colleagues [23] expanded this analysis by including data for three study periods (1990–1994, 1998–2002, 2004–2008) which allowed assessment of incidence trends over time. In both studies, methodologies were developed to produce a consistent set of denominators using the 1990 and/or 2000 Census population distributions by age, sex, and detailed Asian-American ethnicity of a given geographic area [22, 23].

(c) Matching numerator and denominator definitions of race.

The specific Asian ethnic definitions must be matched between the numerator and denominator data. The coding of race in cancer registries is based on hospital admission forms which may be based on self-report or observation by the admissions staff or from death certificates. Patients are not specifically asked about multiple races. From the CCR, the proportion of Asians in California with multiple races was substantially lower (7.1 %) than those based on the Census data (15.3 %). Thus, the potential bias would be for cancer incidence rates specific to the Asian in combination population to be underestimated. There is also a greater possibility of misclassification of race in the cancer registry records. Swallen and colleagues [24] reported that approximately 20 % of Vietnamese patients with cancer actually were not Vietnamese but were Chinese or other Asians. Similar misclassification may affect other Asian subgroups, but the extent has not been investigated in all Asian subgroups.

(d) Examples of comparisons of cancer rates between subgroups.

In one example, a study compared cancer rates between Asian Americans in the USA with their countries of origin. Matsuno and colleagues conducted a study to examine age-related differences in breast cancer rates between the USA and Japan [25]. Rates were higher among Japanese in Hawaii (72.4/100,000) compared to Japanese in Osaka (21.8/100,000), but the most striking difference was seen in women over age 50 years, where rates continued to increase with age among Japanese in Hawaii, but leveled off after this age among women in Osaka. This pattern of higher rates among postmenopausal women suggests that the increasing rates of postmenopausal, estrogen receptor-positive breast cancer in Western countries are likely due to Western lifestyle, obesity, and use of menopausal hormones. Another possible reason for the higher rates seen in Hawaii may be related to increased screening for breast cancer in Western countries [26].

Another example illustrates comparisons among Asian Americans based on birthplace. Using the CCR, multiple studies have been done to assess rate differences between US born and non-US born for different cancers including lymphoid malignancies [27], papillary thyroid [28], liver [29], non-small cell lung [30], breast [31], and colorectal cancer [32]. Limitations of these studies include the assumptions made to categorize patients according to nativity and potential misclassification, attribution of ecological characteristics to individuals, and possible mismatches between how immigrant status is categorized between numerator and denominator data, as well as by detailed age-specific Asian ethnic subgroups.

It should be noted that cancer rates estimated for specific Asian ethnic groups in the USA represent a composite of rates of first-generation migrants and US-born descendants. Although information on birthplace is available in registry data, this information is incomplete. In addition, obtaining denominators for US born and foreign born of a specific Asian ethnic subgroup is a challenge. Thus, cancer rates reported for a specific Asian-American ethnic population are sensitive to the proportion of US born vs. foreign born. Even among the foreign born, the pattern of migration (e.g., age at migration, reasons for migration) may differ between different Asian ethnic subgroups.

Differences in rates between US-born Asians and non-US-born Asian Americans may be informative about the importance of timing of exposure. If rates for the non-US born remain relatively unchanged (compared to their country of origin) while rates for the US born approach rates for the host country (i.e., the US), then the factors of etiologic importance may be operating early in life. In contrast, if rates have already changed in the non-US born (becoming more similar to the US rate), this may suggest that factors operating in adult life are important. These same methodologies can also be used to compare and contrast changes in cancer rates by birthplace across different Asian ethnic groups.

(e) Summary of issues to consider for ecologic comparison of incidence rates.

Formation of appropriate comparisons between population groups requires a research infrastructure to provide reliable incidence and mortality data and to turn these data into reliable summary statistics by which populations can be compared. At a minimum, reliable ecologic comparisons require that (1) methods of reporting incident and fatal cancers are based on uniform standards, (2) information about racial/ethnic group membership must be available from death records or incidence reports, (3) the size of the populations contributing deaths or incident cases to the specific counts of interest must be clearly defined, and (4) the age structure of the populations also be known.

In addition to issues related to accurate and comparable calculations of incidence rates, there are important selection factors that may affect assumptions about the effect of migration on cancer risk factors. Migrants leaving their home country are usually a selected group who are migrating for various reasons including job opportunities, education, socioeconomic, religious, political, or other reasons. Thus, they may not have the same health status or risk of cancer as nonmigrants in their home country. Such differences would affect comparisons of migrants with rates in the country of origin but could also affect comparisons within the host country if the migrants differ from the US born in terms of access to screening and medical care.

Finally, as indicated earlier, 15.3 % of Asian Americans listed more than one race in the 2010 US Census, and the highest proportions listing another race were among Japanese (35.4 %) and Filipinos (22.4 %). The most commonly mentioned second race was white. This population mixing occurring between migrant populations and the US population will have important consequences for the validity of the assumption that the migrant and nonmigrant groups are genetically similar. While this still may be true for recent migrants, those that have been in the US for longer periods of time may have less genetic homogeneity with the population in their country of origin. Thus, differences between their cancer rates and those from their country of origin may not be due solely to environmental factors.

Cross-Sectional Study

The cross-sectional study design usually involves a survey which obtains personal information, but in which information on the outcome as well as possible risk factors is obtained at one point in time. For some exposures, it is not possible to determine the sequence of events between the occurrence of the exposure and outcome; thus, identifying a causal relationship between a risk factor and the disease is not possible. However, for some exposures, such as those occurring in childhood, in comparison to an outcome that occurred in adulthood, the temporal sequence can be inferred. This type of study has been routinely used to determine risk factor profiles including smoking [33], alcohol use [34], body mass index [35], as well as factors that are associated with the use of screening programs. As an example, to better understand the lower cancer screening rates among Asian Americans compared to non-Hispanic whites, data from the 2001 California Health Interview Survey was used to determine if this disparity was related to nativity, years in the USA, English language ability, and access to care [36, 37]. Although there are several large cross-sectional surveys in the USA that can provide data on screening and other behaviors related to cancer risk (e.g., diet, physical activity, alcohol consumption, etc.), information on AAPI was added only in recent years [38]. These surveys include the National Health Interview Survey (NHIS), the Behavior Risk Factor Surveillance System (BRFSS), and the National Health and Nutrition Examination Survey (NHANES). Websites for these studies provide additional information about the variables included and how to access data (http://www.cdc.gov/nchs/nhanes.htm; http://www.cdc.gov/brfss/about/about_brfss.htm; http://www.cdc.gov/nchs/nhis.htm). The importance of the recent inclusion of AAPI in these national surveys cannot be overemphasized since these data allow comparison of a range of self-perceived health status, prevalence of selected chronic conditions, and distribution of a number of important biomarkers (in NHANES), as well as the use of health services among AAPI and minority groups in the USA [39, 40].

Case-Only Study

A case-only study consists of review of characteristics of a series of cases, with no comparison to non-diseased persons, and is not linked to population denominators to calculate incidence rates. However, due to the heterogeneous nature of cancer cases, i.e., cancers of a particular anatomic site may have different histological subtypes, the study of cancer cases alone may provide insights into disease risk factors.

Certain subtypes may be more related to diet and environmental exposures than other subtypes. The comparison of the distribution of cancer subtypes between migrants and US-born Asians may provide insights into factors associated with migration that may predict the subtype of cancer that occurs. In a study of cancers of the uterus, US-born Asian women were more likely to be diagnosed with type I cancers, which are mainly low-grade endometrioid adenocarcinomas, and are thought to be associated with unopposed estrogen stimulation, whereas type II cancers are linked to genetic predisposition [41]. These findings suggest that adoption of the Western lifestyle among US-born Asians may be an explanation.

In another study, a comparison of breast cancer subtypes (estrogen/progesterone/epidermal growth factor receptor 2 (ER/PR/HER2)) pointed to differences in subtype distribution by specific Asian ethnic populations, including higher odds of HER2-positive breast cancer subtypes among Korean and other Asian subgroups compared to non-Hispanic White women [42]. Migrant studies may help determine if these differences are due to genetic and/or environmental factors.

Case-Control Study Design

Analytic epidemiologic studies such as case-control studies are necessary to follow-up clues that are suggested by descriptive studies. The case-control study involves a comparison of cases (i.e., those who have the disease of interest) with controls (i.e., those individuals selected to be comparable to the cases but who do not have the disease in question). The goal is to retrospectively assess the differences in exposures of putative risk factors of interest between each of the two groups of individuals, in order to determine if a relationship exists between a risk factor and the disease. This study design has several advantages and disadvantages [43]. In comparison to most cohort studies, it can be conducted relatively quickly, involves fewer subjects, and is less expensive. It can be appropriate to study rare outcomes with longer latency such as cancer, and multiple risk factors or exposures can be studied in association to the outcome of interest. However, drawbacks include finding the appropriate control group, difficulty in validating exposure histories that are based on self-report, and inability to measure all potential confounding variables. Rates of disease in the exposed and unexposed groups cannot be determined. Perhaps of most concern is the possibility of recall bias, where cases may tend to report exposures in more detail than do controls, or they may selectively recall exposures that they think may be related to their disease. When both cases and controls are equally likely to under or overestimate their exposure history, the effect is for the resulting odds ratio to be biased toward the null, and thus the study would be less likely to detect an effect due to the exposure, especially when it is small.

To date, most of the case-control studies of cancer among Asian Americans have been conducted in California or Hawaii where there are existing population-based registries to allow the identification of suitable cases. Identifying suitable control subjects of the same Asian ethnic population remains a challenge in these studies.

The number of cases of a specific Asian ethnic group may be limited in a single geographic area in the USA, and thus recruitment from multiple geographic areas may be necessary.

Despite these challenges, most of the analytic studies on cancer in Asian Americans have been case-control studies, including Japanese, Chinese, or Filipinos but few other Asian ethnic groups. For example, in a series of case-control studies of breast, colorectal, endometrial, gastric, and lung cancers in Hawaii, risk factor prevalence and risk associations between Japanese Americans were compared to other race-ethnic groups in Hawaii [44–48]. To better understand the role of diet and physical activity in the etiology of colorectal cancer, a case-control study was conducted among Chinese in North America and Chinese in China. Sedentary lifestyle, high body mass index, and a high-fat Western diet were major risk factors of colorectal cancer in Chinese Americans, and there were noted differences in risk factor prevalence between Chinese in North America and those in China [49]. A study of prostate cancer among Chinese and Japanese Americans, a low-risk group, allowed the comparison of risk factor prevalence and risk association in Asian Americans with Whites and African Americans who are at intermediate and high risk of prostate cancer, respectively [50]. In a study of breast cancer among Chinese, Japanese, and Filipino women in Hawaii, San Francisco, and Los Angeles County that examined risk factor associations in relation to birth place and history of migration [51], age of menarche, nulliparity, and delay in childbirth, and low soy intake were significant breast cancer risk factors, and the higher prevalence of the at-risk lifestyle factors among Asians in the US compared to their counterparts in Asia is likely contributions to the rising incidence of breast cancer in Asian-American women [52, 53]. A study of breast cancer among Chinese, Japanese, and Filipinos in Los Angeles County allowed the comparison of risk factors separately in the three Asian ethnic groups [54, 55]. Lifetime regular alcohol intake was significantly higher in US-born women, most of whom were Japanese Americans, than in non-US-born Asian-American women, and breast cancer risk was found to increase with increasing alcohol intake among US-born Asian-American women. Since this is a modifiable risk factor, these findings may help prevent the development of breast cancer in this population.

Cohort Study

The cohort study is the ideal type of analytic study in which a population (selected prior to disease onset) is surveyed to determine exposure status and then is followed over time to identify members who develop the disease of interest. Multiple outcomes can be assessed, and incidence rates for disease in exposed and unexposed groups can be determined. In some cohorts, specific exposed and unexposed populations are selected for follow-up, while, in others, all members of specific population may be surveyed for multiple exposures and then followed over time. The prospective cohort involves following a large number of individuals over many years to monitor exposures and development of a sufficient number of outcomes for study. It can be very expensive and withdrawals and loss to follow-up may occur. If loss to follow-up is due to factors associated with outcomes, it can result in selection bias. For example, if immigrant populations returned home when ill, their outcome status may not be recorded, while nonmigrant (or longer-term migrant) populations may no longer leave the USA if they became ill and thus would have more adverse outcomes recorded as a result.

Very few cohort studies of cancer in Asian Americans have been conducted. To our knowledge, the study of Japanese men in Hawaii was the first such study. As part of the Honolulu Heart Study, 8006 men of Japanese ancestry were enrolled in a cohort study [56]. From 1971 to 1975, 6860 of the men were examined again, and blood samples were obtained for measurement of serum cholesterol and other biomarkers. Associations of various lifestyle factors and biomarkers and risk of stomach, lung, colorectal, prostate, and other cancers have been published from this seminal work [57]. A more recent cohort, the Multiethnic Cohort (MEC) study, has been designed to assess ethnic differences in risk factors that may be related to cancer and other disease endpoints [58]. Japanese Americans are one of five race-ethnic groups (African American, Latino, Hawaiians, non-Hispanic whites) included in the MEC. This cohort has allowed the investigation of lifestyle factors, genetic susceptibility, and risk of multiple cancers in Japanese Americans compared to other racial/ethnic groups. Results from this cohort are highlighted in many of the subsequent chapters.

Summary

Asian Americans represent an informative group to study lifestyle and environmental factors related to cancer risk because of their large-scale migration from countries of higher or lower cancer rates (depending on the cancer site) to the USA over time. By 2010, there were over 17 million Asian Americans, and their numbers grew by 46 % between 2000 and 2010 compared to a 9.7 % increase in the US population as a whole. This chapter has provided an overview of issues to consider when using different study designs to assess the role that migration may play in affecting cancer risk. For example, when comparing incidence rates between migrants and their country of origin (or between subgroups within the USA), the quality of numerator and denominator data and the matching of definitions of Asian ethnicity between data sources are highly important. Birthplace is a critical variable in the assessment of the role that timing of exposures may play in cancer risk. Ecological study designs are limited in that they do not obtain individual exposure history, but they are relatively quick and inexpensive studies to conduct and provide important clues regarding cancers that are most affected by change in lifestyle and environment. Analytic studies including case-control and cohort designs are needed to further investigate clues suggested by ecologic and descriptive studies. Many insights have been gained regarding cancer etiology from case-control and cohort studies of Asian populations. While limitations exist in studies involving migrants, such as concerns that Asian Americans may not be genetically identical to their counterparts in the countries of origin due to the increasing numbers of Asians reporting more than one race in the US Census, the use of migrants in observational studies has provided many insights into cancer risk, and these findings are summarized in the following chapters for specific subgroups.

Financial Disclosure None
Authors' declaration of personal interest: None
Declaration of funding interests: None

References

1. Hoeffel E et al (2012) The Asian Population: 2010, E.a.S.A. In: U.S. Department of Commerce, U. S. Census Bureau (ed). U.S. Census Bureau, Washington, DC
2. Segi M (ed) (1960) Cancer mortality for selected sites in 24 countries (1950–57). D.o.P. Health, Tohoku University of Medicine, Sendai
3. Bray F et al (2015) Cancer incidence in five continents: inclusion criteria, highlights from volume X and the global status of cancer registration. Int J Cancer 137(9):2060–2071
4. Parkin DM et al (2010) Fifty years of cancer incidence: CI5 I-IX. Int J Cancer 127(12):2918–2927
5. Shin H-R et al (2010) Cancer in Asia - incidence rates based on data in cancer incidence in five continents IX (1998-2002). Asian Pac J Cancer Prev 11(Suppl 2):11–16
6. Ferlay J et al (2015) Cancer incidence and mortality worldwide: sources, methods and major patterns in GLOBOCAN 2012. Int J Cancer 136(5):E359–E386
7. Hankey BF, Ries LA, Edwards BK (1999) The surveillance, epidemiology, and end results program: a national resource. Cancer Epidemiol Biomark Prev 8(12):1117–1121
8. Kwong SL et al (2005) Asian subgroups and cancer incidence and mortality rates in California. Cancer 104(12 Suppl):2975–2981
9. McCracken M et al (2007) Cancer incidence, mortality, and associated risk factors among Asian Americans of Chinese, Filipino, Vietnamese, Korean, and Japanese ethnicities. CA Cancer J Clin 57(4):190–205
10. Parise C, Caggiano V (2014) Disparities in the risk of the ER/PR/HER2 breast cancer subtypes among Asian Americans in California. Cancer Epidemiol 38(5):556–562
11. Smith RL (1956) Recorded and expected mortality among the Chinese of Hawaii and the United States with special reference to cancer. J Natl Cancer Inst 17(5):667–676
12. Smith RL (1956) Recorded and expected mortality among the Japanese of the United States and Hawaii, with special reference to cancer. J Natl Cancer Inst 17(4):459–473
13. Haenszel W (1961) Cancer mortality among the foreign-born in the United States. J Natl Cancer Inst 26:37–132
14. Haenszel W, Kurihara M (1968) Studies of Japanese migrants. I. Mortality from cancer and other diseases among Japanese in the United States. J Natl Cancer Inst 40(1):43–68
15. King H, Locke FB (1980) Cancer mortality among Chinese in the United States. J Natl Cancer Inst 65(5):1141–1148
16. Locke FB, King H (1980) Cancer mortality risk among Japanese in the United States. J Natl Cancer Inst 65(5):1149–1156
17. Parkin DM, Khlat M (1996) Studies of cancer in migrants: rationale and methodology. Eur J Cancer 32A(5):761–771
18. Kolonel LN, Wilkens LR (2006) Migrant studies. In: Schottenfeld D, Fraumeni JF Jr (eds) Cancer epidemiology and prevention, 3rd edn. Oxford University Press, New York, pp 189–201

19. DiPietro N (2010) Methods in epidemiology: observational study designs. Pharmacotherapy 30:973–984
20. Bray F, Parkin DM (2009) Evaluation of data quality in the cancer registry: principles and methods. Part I: comparability, validity and timeliness. Eur J Cancer 45(5):747–755
21. Parkin DM, Bray F (2009) Evaluation of data quality in the cancer registry: principles and methods Part II. Completeness. Eur J Cancer 45(5):756–764
22. Miller BA et al (2008) Cancer incidence and mortality patterns among specific Asian and Pacific Islander populations in the U.S. Cancer Causes Control 19(3):227–256 [Erratum appears in Cancer Causes Control. 2008;19(3):257-8]
23. Gomez SL et al (2013) Cancer incidence trends among Asian American populations in the United States, 1990-2008. J Natl Cancer Inst 105(15):1096–1110
24. Swallen KC et al (1998) Accuracy of racial classification of Vietnamese patients in a population-based cancer registry. Ethnic Dis 8(2):218–227
25. Matsuno RK et al (2007) Early- and late-onset breast cancer types among women in the United States and Japan. Cancer Epidemiol Biomark Prev 16(7):1437–1442
26. Bleyer A, Welch HG (2013) Effect of screening mammography on breast cancer incidence. N Engl J Med 368(7):679
27. Clarke CA et al (2011) Lymphoid malignancies in U.S. Asians: incidence rate differences by birthplace and acculturation. Cancer Epidemiol Biomark Prev 20(6):1064–1077
28. Horn-Ross PL et al (2011) Papillary thyroid cancer incidence rates vary significantly by birthplace in Asian American women. Cancer Causes Control 22(3):479–485
29. Chang ET et al (2010) Disparities in liver cancer incidence by nativity, acculturation, and socioeconomic status in California Hispanics and Asians. Cancer Epidemiol Biomark Prev 19(12):3106–3118
30. Raz DJ et al (2008) Epidemiology of non-small cell lung cancer in Asian Americans: incidence patterns among six subgroups by nativity. J Thorac Oncol 3(12):1391–1397
31. Gomez SL et al (2010) Hidden breast cancer disparities in Asian women: disaggregating incidence rates by ethnicity and migrant status. Am J Public Health 100(Suppl 1):S125–S131
32. Ladabaum U et al (2014) Colorectal cancer incidence in Asian populations in California: effect of nativity and neighborhood-level factors. Am J Gastroenterol 109(4):579–588
33. Caraballo RS et al (2008) Adult tobacco use among racial and ethnic groups living in the United States, 2002-2005. Prev Chronic Dis 5(3):A78
34. Cook WK, Mulia N, Karriker-Jaffe K (2012) Ethnic drinking cultures and alcohol use among Asian American adults: findings from a national survey. Alcohol Alcoholism 47(3):340–348
35. Lauderdale DS, Rathouz PJ (2000) Body mass index in a US national sample of Asian Americans: effects of nativity, years since immigration and socioeconomic status. Int J Obes Relat Metab Disord 24(9):1188–1194 [Erratum appears in Int J Obes Relat Metab Disord. 2002 Nov;26(11):1521]
36. Kandula NR et al (2006) Low rates of colorectal, cervical, and breast cancer screening in Asian Americans compared with non-Hispanic whites: cultural influences or access to care? Cancer 107(1):184–192
37. Lee S et al (2014) Acculturation and cancer screening among Asian Americans: role of health insurance and having a regular physician. J Community Health 39(2):201–212
38. Giles WH et al (2004) Racial and ethnic approaches to community health (REACH 2010): an overview. Ethnic Dis 14(3 Suppl 1):S5–S8
39. Zhou Y, Boudreau DM, Freedman AN (2014) Trends in the use of aspirin and nonsteroidal anti-inflammatory drugs in the general U.S. population. Pharmacoepidemiol Drug Saf 23(1):43–50
40. Huang B et al (2013) Chronic conditions, behavioral health, and use of health services among Asian American men: the first nationally representative sample. Am J Mens Health 7(1):66–76
41. Simons E et al (2015) Foreign- vs US-born Asians and the association of type I uterine cancer. Am J Obstet Gynecol 212(1):43.e1-6

42. Telli ML et al (2011) Asian ethnicity and breast cancer subtypes: a study from the California Cancer Registry. Breast Cancer Res Treat 127(2):471–478
43. Song JW, Chung KC (2010) Observational studies: cohort and case-control studies. Plast Reconstr Surg 126(6):2234–2242
44. Nomura AM et al (1985) Breast cancer in Caucasian and Japanese women in Hawaii. J Natl Cancer Inst Monogr 69:191–196
45. Hirohata T et al (1987) An epidemiologic study on the association between diet and breast cancer. J Natl Cancer Inst 78(4):595–600
46. Goodman MT et al (2008) Prevalence, acquisition, and clearance of cervical human papillomavirus infection among women with normal cytology: Hawaii Human Papillomavirus Cohort Study. Cancer Res 68(21):8813–8824
47. Goodman MT et al (1997) Association of soy and fiber consumption with the risk of endometrial cancer. Am J Epidemiol 146(4):294–306
48. Galanis DJ et al (1998) Intakes of selected foods and beverages and the incidence of gastric cancer among the Japanese residents of Hawaii: a prospective study. Int J Epidemiol 27(2):173–180
49. Whittemore AS et al (1990) Diet, physical activity, and colorectal cancer among Chinese in North America and China. J Natl Cancer Inst 82(11):915–926
50. Whittemore AS et al (1995) Prostate cancer in relation to diet, physical activity, and body size in blacks, whites, and Asians in the United States and Canada. J Natl Cancer Inst 87(9):652–661
51. Ziegler RG et al (1993) Migration patterns and breast cancer risk in Asian-American women. J Natl Cancer Inst 85(22):1819–1827
52. Wu AH et al (1996) Menstrual and reproductive factors and risk of breast cancer in Asian-Americans. Br J Cancer 73(5):680–686
53. Wu AH et al (1996) Tofu and risk of breast cancer in Asian-Americans. Cancer Epidemiol Biomark Prev 5(11):901–906
54. Wu AH et al (2012) Alcohol and breast cancer risk among Asian-American women in Los Angeles County. Breast Cancer Res 14(6):R151
55. Wu AH, McKean-Cowdin R, Tseng C-C (2011) Birth weight and other prenatal factors and risk of breast cancer in Asian-Americans. Breast Cancer Res Treat 130(3):917–925
56. Nomura A et al (1990) A prospective study of stomach cancer and its relation to diet, cigarettes, and alcohol consumption. Cancer Res 50(3):627–631
57. Nomura A et al (1991) Helicobacter pylori infection and gastric carcinoma among Japanese Americans in Hawaii. N Engl J Med 325(16):1132–1136
58. Kolonel LN et al (2000) A multiethnic cohort in Hawaii and Los Angeles: baseline characteristics. Am J Epidemiol 151(4):346–357

Cancer Incidence and Mortality Patterns Among Chinese Americans

Lihua Liu, Dennis Deapen, and Anna H. Wu

Abstract Chinese is the largest Asian ethnic group in the USA with four million individuals accounting for 23.1 % of the total Asian Americans and 1.3 % of the total US population. Given its large population size and the long history of migration to many countries throughout the world, Chinese immigrants are a valuable resource for epidemiologic investigations of cancer and other diseases to identify environmental and lifestyle risk factors and to understand the interactions between genetics and environment in disease etiology. Using data from population-based cancer registries, this chapter examines the sex-specific cancer incidence and mortality rates of common cancers among Chinese Americans and their relative risks as compared to whites or non-Hispanic (NH) whites. Comparisons of incidence trends and age-specific patterns by cancer type between Chinese Americans and Chinese in China are also provided. For most of the cancers examined, Chinese Americans have lower incidence and mortality rates than the NH whites, but they have substantially higher risk for nasopharyngeal, liver, and stomach cancers and slightly higher risk of gallbladder cancer. Except for lung and colorectal cancer, Chinese Americans display intermediate-risk level between the US whites and Chinese in China. The cancer experience of Chinese Americans highlights the significance of environmental and lifestyle factors in cancer development.

Keywords Chinese American • Cancer • Immigrant • Incidence • Mortality • Trend • Rate ratio

L. Liu, Ph.D. (✉) • D. Deapen, Dr.P.H.
Los Angeles Cancer Surveillance Program, Department of Preventive Medicine, Keck School of Medicine of USC, University of Southern California, Los Angeles, CA 90089, USA
e-mail: lihualiu@usc.edu

A.H. Wu, Ph.D.
Department of Preventive Medicine, Keck School of Medicine of USC, University of Southern California, Los Angeles, CA, USA

A.H. Wu, D.O. Stram (eds.), *Cancer Epidemiology Among Asian Americans*, DOI 10.1007/978-3-319-41118-7_2

History of Chinese Migration to the USA

Chinese immigration to the USA dates back to the 1820s, according to the official US government records [1]. The first wave of a significant number of Chinese immigrants to the USA arrived in California during the 1850s to join the Gold Rush [2]. More came when the Central Pacific Railroad recruited large number of laborers throughout the 1860s until the railroad's completion in 1869. The number of Chinese seeking permanent legal resident status rose from 32 in the 1840s to 133,139 in the 1870s [1]. The early Chinese immigrants were mostly young uneducated men from the Guangdong province in southern China [3]. Demographic data on Chinese in the USA have been collected since the 1860 US population census.

The Chinese Exclusion Act of 1882, as a result of increasing anti-Chinese racial tension coupled with economic depression that started in 1873, effectively ended the immigration of Chinese laborers. The number of Chinese in the USA gradually decreased as many of the immigrants returned home or left for more hospitable places. However, the repeal of the Chinese Exclusion Act of 1943 granted naturalization rights to foreign-born Chinese and established an immigration quota for China. The Immigration and Nationality Act of 1965 abolished racial discrimination in immigration law, beginning a period of renewed Chinese immigration to the USA. The economic reform and Open Door Policy adopted by the Chinese government in the late 1970s resulted in record numbers of young well-educated Chinese students coming to the USA seeking higher education. As the Chinese economy grew, increasing numbers of Chinese emigrate to the USA through business, investment, family reunification, and a variety of venues, besides education. In addition to mainland China, Chinese immigrants may also originate from Taiwan, Hong Kong, Macau, and other regions of the world.

According to the 2010 census, there were 3.5 million Chinese of single race and 0.5 million of multirace living in the USA [4]. Chinese is the largest detailed Asian American group, accounting for 23.1 % of the total Asian Americans and 1.3 % of the total US population. After Spanish, Chinese was the most widely spoken non-English language in the country, with 2.9 million people speaking it at home in 2011 [5]. The number of Chinese speakers in the USA has more than quadrupled since 1980. Among the nation's Chinese speakers, only 44 % reported speaking English "very well." The Chinese-speaking population was found heavily concentrated in the New York, Los Angeles, and San Francisco metro areas [5]. The number of Chinese speakers includes those speaking any of the many Chinese dialects, such as Mandarin and Cantonese.

In comparison to other Asian Americans and the white population, Chinese Americans generally have lower unemployment rate (4.4 % unemployment rate, as compared to 5.2 % for all Asians and 6.5 % for whites), higher median earnings (median weekly earnings in 2013 of $1093, as compared to $987 for Asian Americans and Pacific Islanders (AAPIs) and $865 for whites), higher levels of education (56.8 % of age 25 and older are college graduate, as compared to 53.4 % of all Asians and 31.9 % of whites), but also higher poverty rate (15.2 % during 2000–2012, as compared to 13.0 % for AAPIs and 13.6 % for whites) [6].

History of Studying Cancer Among Chinese Americans

With its large population size and the long history of migration to many countries throughout the world, Chinese immigrants have been recognized as a valuable resource for epidemiologic investigations of cancer and other diseases to identify environmental and behavioral risk factors and to understand the interactions between genetics and environment in disease etiology.

The first systematic national study of cancer occurrence among Chinese Americans was published by Smith and colleagues in 1956 using the cancer mortality data of 1949–1952 [7]. It documented the different cancer risk profiles of Chinese in the USA as compared to the US whites, confirming findings from the few analyses of clinical and autopsy materials reported prior to that time [8]. Studies of cancer patterns among Chinese Americans in the 1950s and 1960s relied on cancer mortality data that were collected consistently through vital statistics with birthplace information of the deceased [7–9]. Those early mortality-based studies were limited by the relatively small number of Chinese deaths in the older age groups and showed the typical male dominance and origin of the early Chinese migrants from southern China [10].

In contrast to cancer mortality data that capture deaths caused by a specific cancer, cancer incidence data record new cases of cancer diagnosis in a given year. Incidence data provide information that is not captured in mortality data. The National Cancer Institute (NCI) conducted three National Cancer Surveys at three points in time, 1937–1939, 1947–1948, and 1969–1971, providing estimates of cancer incidence rates and establishing the field of modern cancer epidemiology [11]. However, cancer incidence data were not systematically collected in the USA until 1973 by the Surveillance, Epidemiology, and End Results (SEER) program that was established by the NCI, as a result of the National Cancer Act of 1971 [12]. Information specific to cancer incidence among Chinese Americans was not systematically available in a meaningful volume until the 1970s through the population-based SEER registries.

The SEER program and its registries have consistently contributed data to the international cancer statistical reports, such as Cancer Incidence in Five Continents (CI5) series that provide internationally comparable cancer incidence information among countries and populations of the world [13]. Although the SEER registries collect detailed racial/ethnic information on cancer patients, the lack of official annual population estimates with corresponding racial/ethnic classification limited the examination of cancer risk specifically among Chinese and other disaggregated Asian American ethnic groups in the SEER program as a whole. However, SEER registries in San Francisco and Los Angeles have had long tradition in monitoring cancer incidence among the large Chinese American communities in their catchment areas.

The SEER registry in Los Angeles, the Los Angeles Cancer Surveillance Program (LACSP), is a population-based cancer registry established in 1972 at the University of Southern California and joined the SEER in 1992. The LACSP is located in the most populous and racially/ethnically diverse county in the country, the Los Angeles County, California. According to the 2010 population census, nearly 0.4 million Chinese lived in the catchment area of LACSP consisting of 12 % of the national total of Chinese Americans. LACSP is the only US registry that has continuously contributed to CI5 cancer incidence data of Chinese and other Asian Americans in Los Angeles, making the comparison of cancer incidence trends between Asians living in the USA and elsewhere possible.

As a result of the growing Asian American population, the increasing interest in and awareness of the heterogeneous cancer burdens among Asian subgroups; SEER has made significant strides in developing necessary population estimates and reporting cancer incidence and mortality statistics among the fast-growing AAPI populations [14–16].

Data Sources and Methods

For this chapter, we utilized a variety of data sources to present a contemporary overview of cancer risk patterns among Chinese Americans. These data sources include recently published information based on SEER registry data, special data files from SEER program, international cancer data in the CI5 series published by the International Association of Cancer Registries (IACR), and up-to-date Chinese-specific cancer information from the LACSP.

Previously Published SEER Data

Using SEER data of 14 registries from 1998 to 2002, Miller et al. (2008) reported the age-adjusted (2000 US standard population) overall and cancer site-specific incidence and mortality rates among specific AAPI populations in the USA in comparison with those of NH whites [14]. We extracted the Chinese-specific case counts and age-adjusted rates by sex and cancer site, along with those of NH whites, and compiled for incidence (Table 1) and mortality (Table 2). The cancer sites in each table are sorted and ranked by the rates from high to low. We also calculated the rate

Table 1 Site-specific cancer incidence counts and age-adjusted (2000 US standard) rates and rate ratios by sex among Chinese Americans and NH Whites, SEER registries, 1998–2002

	Chinese American		NH White		Incidence
	Cases	Rate	Cases	Rate	Rate ratio
Men					
All sites	9,175	348.8	649,731	587.0	0.6
Prostate	2,209	84.8	189,678	170.0	0.5
Colorectal	1,400	54.0	71,656	65.6	0.8
Lung	1,340	53.0	98,625	89.2	0.6
Liver	666	24.0	7,445	6.7	3.6

Table 1 (continued)

	Chinese American		NH White		Incidence
	Cases	Rate	Cases	Rate	Rate ratio
Stomach	461	18.3	10,797	9.9	1.8
Bladder	389	15.7	46,682	43.0	0.4
Non-Hodgkin's Lymphoma	401	14.8	27,294	24.6	0.6
Pancreas	243	9.8	14,220	13.0	0.8
Nasopharynx	277	8.9	717	0.6	14.8
Leukemia	231	8.7	18,718	17.3	0.5
Kidney	192	7.2	19,671	17.5	0.4
Oral	166	6.2	18,462	16.2	0.4
Esophagus	124	4.5	9,079	8.1	0.6
Brain and nervous system	123	4.3	9,893	8.9	0.5
Thyroid	96	3.2	4,996	4.3	0.7
Larynx	78	3.0	8,101	7.1	0.4
Myeloma	74	2.7	7,264	6.6	0.4
Testis	57	1.7	7,816	7.0	0.2
Hodgkin's Lymphoma	40	1.3	3,833	3.5	0.4
Melanoma	35	1.2	32,981	29.3	0.0
Gallbladder	24	0.9	768	0.7	1.3
Women					
All sites	8,817	270.4	617,158	448.5	0.6
Breast	2,652	77.6	195,231	145.2	0.5
Colorectal	1,257	40.2	70,298	47.6	0.8
Lung	923	29.7	83,387	59.0	0.5
Corpus uteri	406	12	35,224	26.0	0.5
Stomach	344	11.1	6,430	4.3	2.6
Thyroid	358	10.0	14,103	11.8	0.8
Ovary	335	10.0	20,736	15.3	0.7
Non-Hodgkin's Lymphoma	316	10.0	24,177	17.2	0.6
Liver	258	8.2	3,689	2.6	3.2
Pancreas	209	6.8	14,520	9.8	0.7
Leukemia	188	5.9	13,800	10.0	0.6
Cervix uteri	193	5.6	9,930	8.1	0.7
Bladder	133	4.4	15,480	10.6	0.4
Kidney	126	4.0	11,787	8.5	0.5
Oral	119	3.6	8,996	6.5	0.6
Nasopharynx	125	3.5	315	0.2	17.5
Brain and nervous system	90	2.7	7,911	6.2	0.4
Myeloma	76	2.5	5,986	4.1	0.6
Gallbladder	41	1.3	1,754	1.2	1.1
Esophagus	32	1.0	3,067	2.1	0.5
Melanoma	32	1.0	24,455	19.3	0.1
Hodgkin's Lymphoma	22	0.7	3,348	2.9	0.2

Source of data: Miller AB et al., Cancer Causes Control 2008; 19:227–256. Appendix 1.

Table 2 Site-specific cancer mortality counts and age-adjusted (2000 US standard) rates and rate ratios by sex among Chinese Americans and NH Whites, SEER registries, 1998–2002

	Chinese American		NH White		Mortality
	Deaths	Rate	Deaths	Rate	Rate ratio
Men					
All sites	5,807	167.8	349,031	241.3	0.7
Lung	1,603	47.0	106,623	72.2	0.7
Liver	761	20.3	9,091	6.1	3.3
Colorectal	657	19.5	35,261	24.6	0.8
Stomach	404	11.7	8,395	5.8	2.0
Prostate	292	10.4	37,137	27.7	0.4
Pancreas	291	8.5	18,399	12.6	0.7
Leukemia	216	6.1	15,119	10.6	0.6
Non-Hodgkin's Lymphoma	205	6.0	15,368	10.6	0.6
Nasopharynx	192	4.5	383	0.3	15.0
Esophagus	134	3.8	11,536	7.7	0.5
Bladder	109	3.6	11,682	8.4	0.4
Kidney	102	2.9	9,135	6.2	0.5
Brain and nervous system	94	2.5	9,477	6.3	0.4
Oral	65	1.8	5,605	3.7	0.5
Myeloma	58	1.7	6,454	4.5	0.4
Larynx	33	0.9	3,316	2.2	0.4
Gallbladder	24	0.7	683	0.5	1.4
Melanoma	21	0.6	6,998	4.7	0.1
Women					
All sites	4,537	107.7	341,117	171.7	0.6
Lung	984	23.8	87,084	44.5	0.5
Colorectal	524	12.8	36,430	17.3	0.7
Breast	564	12.3	53,534	27.8	0.4
Liver	308	7.4	5,546	2.7	2.7
Stomach	305	7.3	5,930	2.8	2.6
Pancreas	273	6.7	19,471	9.5	0.7
Ovary	229	5.2	18,962	9.8	0.5
Non-Hodgkin's Lymphoma	172	4.1	14,024	6.8	0.6
Leukemia	132	3.1	12,132	6.0	0.5
Cervix uteri	93	2.2	4,206	2.4	0.9
Corpus uteri	89	2.1	8,368	4.2	0.5
Brain and nervous system	81	1.8	7,602	4.2	0.4
Kidney	63	1.6	5,611	2.8	0.6
Nasopharynx	65	1.4	245	0.1	14.0
Myeloma	49	1.2	5,948	2.9	0.4
Esophagus	45	1.1	3,766	1.8	0.6
Bladder	38	1.0	5,228	2.4	0.4
Oral	34	0.8	3,142	1.6	0.5
Gallbladder	28	0.7	1,675	0.8	0.9
Thyroid	20	0.5	917	0.5	1.0

Source of data: Miller AB et al., Cancer Causes Control 2008; 19:227–256. Appendix 2.

ratio in each table of the Chinese rate in relation to that of the NH whites by cancer site. In Fig. 1, we combined the rate ratios from Tables 1 and 2 by sex to illustrate the differences or similarities in relative cancer risk between Chinese and NH whites by cancer site using both incidence and mortality data.

Updated SEER Data

Using SEER data of 13 registries from 1990 to 2008, Gomez et al. (2013) published the trends in age-adjusted (2000 US standard population) cancer incidence rates for disaggregated Asian American subgroups, including Chinese and NH whites [15]. While they provided more recent data than Miller et al., it only included the top five cancer sites in each Asian-American subgroup. Taking advantage of the availability of the same database that produced the Gomez et al. report [17], for this chapter, we calculated the age-adjusted (2000 US standard population) cancer incidence rates for Chinese Americans during the period of 2004–2008 for the same cancer sites included in the Miller et al. 2008 article by sex, along with those of NH whites for comparison purposes. The results are shown in Table 3. The rate ratios showing the relative risk of Chinese Americans in relation to NH whites are also provided in Table 3. Because the Miller et al. 2008 study and Gomez et al. 2013 study included different time periods and slightly different SEER registries, the incidence rates generated by the two databases are not directly comparable. Nonetheless, in Fig. 2, we compared the incidence-based rate ratios from these two papers to examine any changes in cancer risk patterns over time from 1998–2002 to 2004–2008.

To provide more recent cancer trends, we used recently released data from SEER to update the cancer incidence rates published in the CI5 series for white population in SEER nine registries, and data from LACSP for Chinese Americans in Los Angeles County. We used the same 1960 world standard population, as used in CI5, and extended the age-adjusted incidence rates to 2012 by sex, year, and cancer site, in order to be compared with the trends data from China as published in CI5.

International Cancer Data

To provide a comparison of cancer risk between Chinese Americans and Chinese in China, we utilized the data published in the CI5. The CI5 series of monographs are results of long-standing collaboration between the International Agency for Research on Cancer (IARC) and the IACR. The CI5 is published every 5 years and is a valuable resource for cancer incidence around the world. The CI5 databases provide access to detailed information on the incidence of cancer as recorded and reported by cancer registries (regional or national) worldwide. The most recent CI5 Volume X covers the time period of 2003–2007, containing average age-specific and age-adjusted (1960 world standard population) site-specific cancer incidence rates by sex for each reporting registry/population [18]. CI5 also offers online

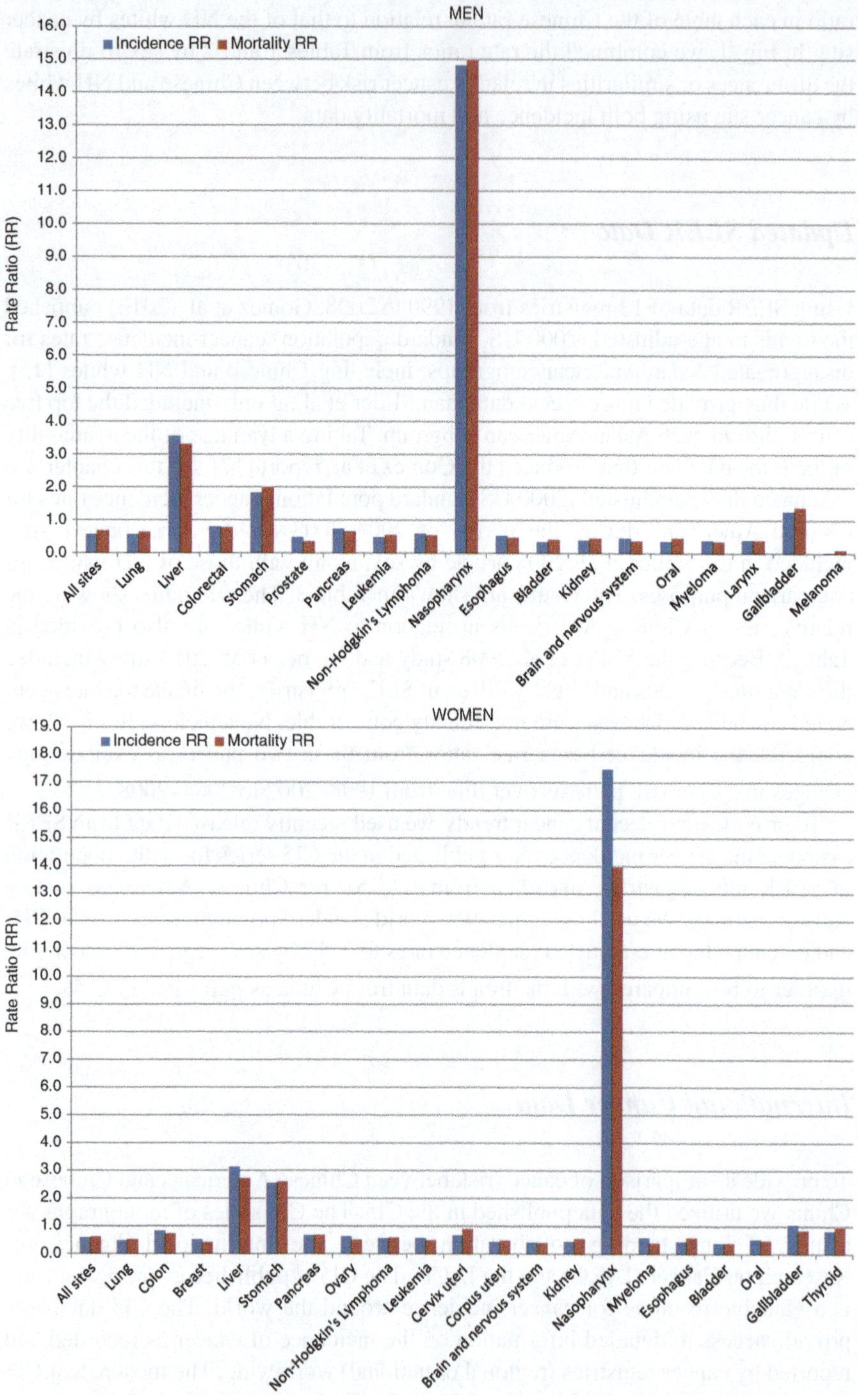

Fig. 1 Comparison of incidence-based rate ratios and mortality-based rate ratios between Chinese Americans and NH whites by cancer site and sex, 1998–2002 (as shown in Tables 1 and 2)

Table 3 Site-specific cancer incidence counts and age-adjusted (2000 US standard) rates and rate ratios by sex among Chinese Americans and NH Whites, SEER registries, 2004–2008

	Chinese American		NH White		Incidence
	Cases	Rate	Cases	Rate	Rate ratio
Men					
All sites	10,705	320.9	572,704	560.2	0.6
Prostate	2,488	74.9	162,504	154.7	0.5
Lung and bronchus	1,678	52.0	74,729	74.0	0.7
Colon and rectum	1,410	42.1	54,752	54.0	0.8
Liver	845	24.1	8,301	7.7	3.1
Stomach	524	16.3	8,832	8.7	1.9
Urinary bladder	506	16.0	43,592	43.8	0.4
Non-Hodgkin Lymphoma	505	14.9	26,059	25.8	0.6
Oral cavity and pharynx	497	13.6	18,112	17.0	0.8
Pancreas	301	9.3	14,086	13.8	0.7
Kidney and renal pelvis	290	8.5	20,888	20.1	0.4
Leukemia	267	7.9	17,055	17.3	0.5
Nasopharynx	282	7.4	590	0.6	12.3
Esophagus	144	4.5	8,722	8.4	0.5
Brain and other nervous system	132	3.7	8,990	9.0	0.4
Thyroid	138	3.6	6,676	6.5	0.6
Myeloma	99	3.1	7,035	6.9	0.4
Larynx	58	1.8	6,050	5.8	0.3
Testis	71	1.7	6,834	7.5	0.2
Melanoma of the skin	43	1.2	37,884	37.1	0.0
Gallbladder	36	1.2	696	0.7	1.7
Hodgkin Lymphoma	34	1.0	3,446	3.6	0.3
Women					
All Sites	11,103	263.4	538,349	440.0	0.6
Breast	3,477	78.8	162,591	135.3	0.6
Colon and rectum	1,447	35.7	53,352	40.6	0.9
Lung and bronchus	1,207	29.9	72,103	56.6	0.5
Corpus uteri	621	14.3	32,452	26.3	0.5
Thyroid	549	12.2	18,712	18.2	0.7
Non-Hodgkin Lymphoma	387	9.4	21,939	17.5	0.5
Stomach	366	9.1	5,058	3.8	2.4
Ovary	352	8.0	17,035	13.9	0.6
Liver	311	7.8	2,898	2.3	3.4
Pancreas	289	7.3	14,013	10.5	0.7
Oral cavity and pharynx	245	5.7	8,119	6.6	0.9
Leukemia	214	5.3	12,586	10.3	0.5
Kidney and renal pelvis	200	4.9	12,288	10.0	0.5
Cervix uteri	209	4.6	6,968	6.8	0.7
Urinary bladder	169	4.3	13,895	10.5	0.4

(continued)

Table 3 (continued)

	Chinese American		NH White		Incidence
	Cases	Rate	Cases	Rate	Rate ratio
Nasopharynx	127	2.8	289	0.2	14.0
Brain and other nervous system	104	2.5	7,006	6.3	0.4
Myeloma	77	1.9	5,249	4.0	0.5
Gallbladder	49	1.2	1,515	1.1	1.1
Esophagus	48	1.2	2,576	2.0	0.6
Melanoma of the skin	43	1.0	27,020	24.3	0.0
Hodgkin Lymphoma	34	0.8	2,996	3.1	0.3

Source of data: Surveillance, Epidemiology, and End Results (SEER) Program (www.seer.cancer.gov) SEER*Stat Database: Incidence—SEER 11, plus Greater CA and NJ, Nov 2010 Sub (1990–2008) detailed API plus White Non-Hispanic—projected from populations, National Cancer Institute, DCCPS, Surveillance Research Program, Cancer Statistics Branch, released June 2011 (updated 10/28/2011), based on the November 2010 submission

analysis tools, CI5plus, for time trends up to 2007 and age-specific curves by time period for selected cancer registries/populations [19]. The LACSP is the only US registry that has consistently reported Chinese American cancer information to CI5 and thus included in the CI5plus. Among the three Chinese cancer registries included in CI5plus, we chose as a comparison the data from China's Shanghai registry for its long history of participation in CI5, large population size, representativeness of urban China, and high-quality data.

We downloaded from CI5plus the China-Shanghai registry annual age-adjusted (1960 world standard population) incidence rates by sex and cancer site for 1988–2007, in order to be compared with current data for whites from SEER (nine registries) and Chinese Americans from LACSP (Figs. 3 and 4). Figures 3 and 4 contain the comparisons of age-specific incidence rates by sex and cancer site for 2003–2007 between Chinese in Los Angeles and Chinese in Shanghai with reference to US whites, as downloaded from the CI5plus online analysis tool.

Cancer Incidence and Mortality Patterns Among Chinese Americans

Overview

Chinese Americans, as compared to NH whites, have lower risk in both cancer incidence (Tables 1 and 3) and mortality (Table 2) for all cancers combined and for many specific cancer sites, regardless of sex. However, their risk for cancers of the nasopharynx, liver, and stomach is noticeably much higher than the NH whites. The relative risk patterns by cancer site between Chinese Americans and NH whites are quite similar in either incidence or mortality data (Fig. 1).

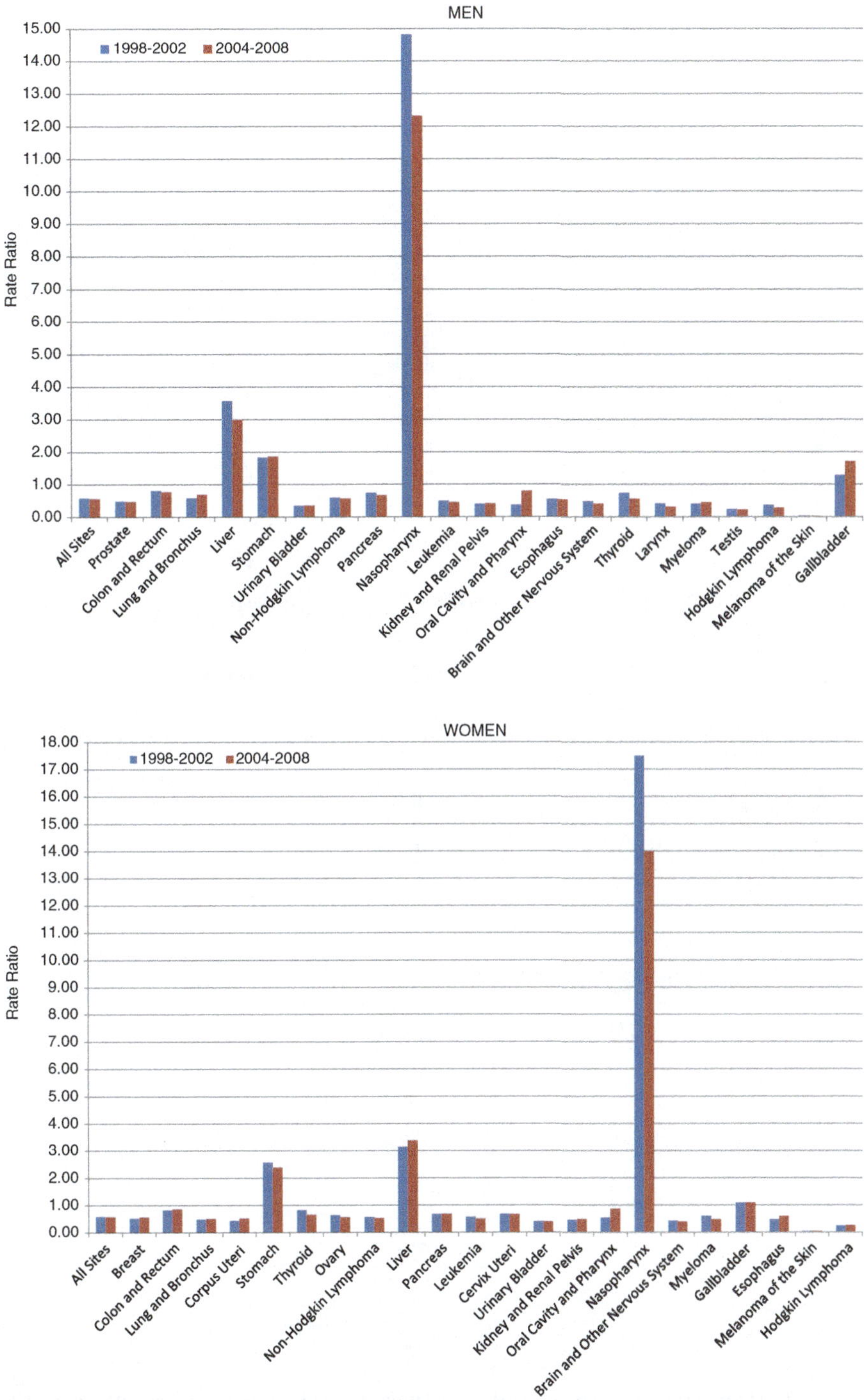

Fig. 2 Comparison of incidence-based rate ratios between Chinese Americans and NH whites by cancer site and sex over time, 1998–2002 vs. 2004–2008 (as shown in Tables 1 and 3)

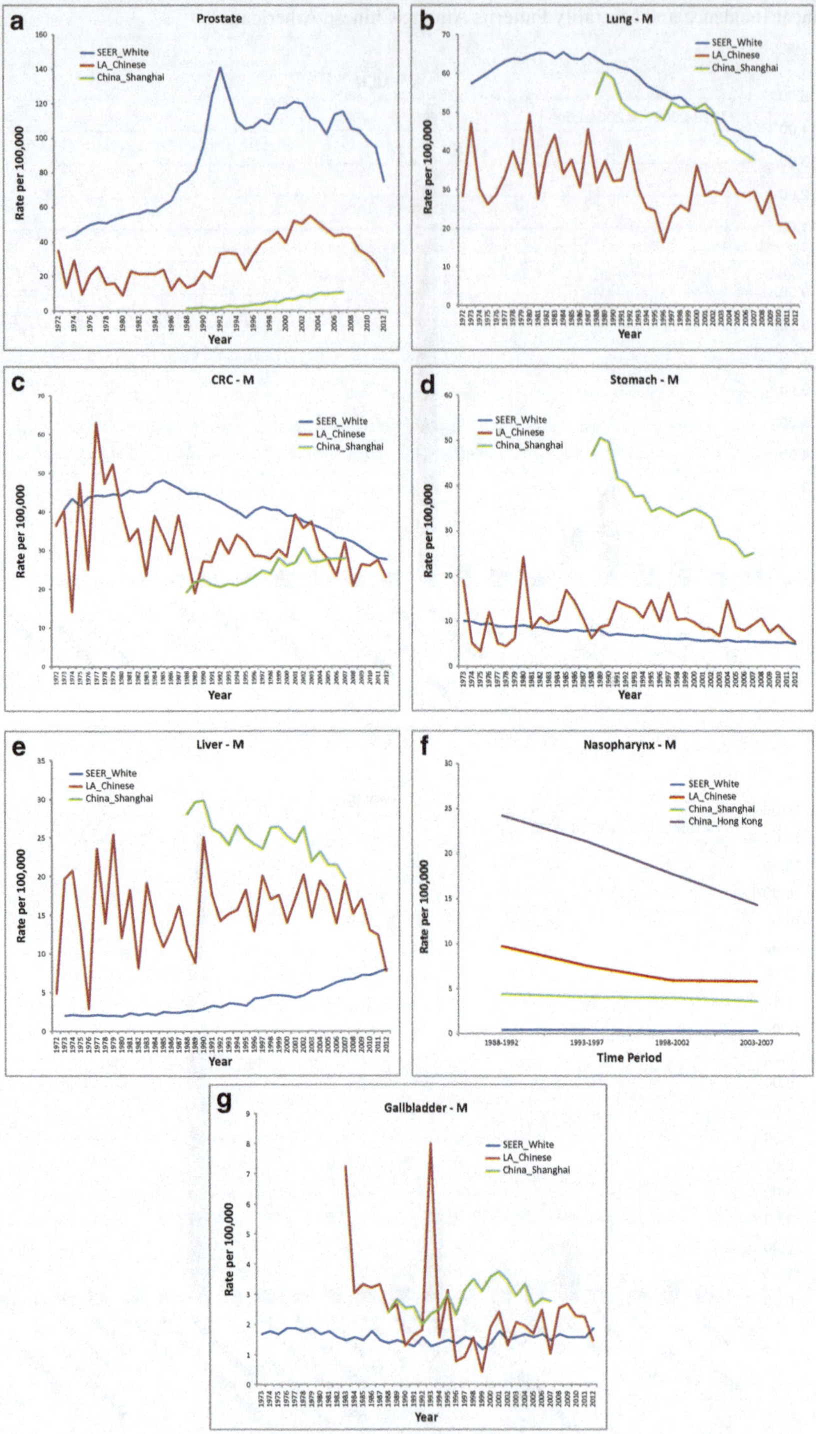

Fig. 3 Time trends of age-adjusted (world population) incidence rates by cancer site among US whites, Chinese in Los Angeles, and Chinese in China-Shanghai, men

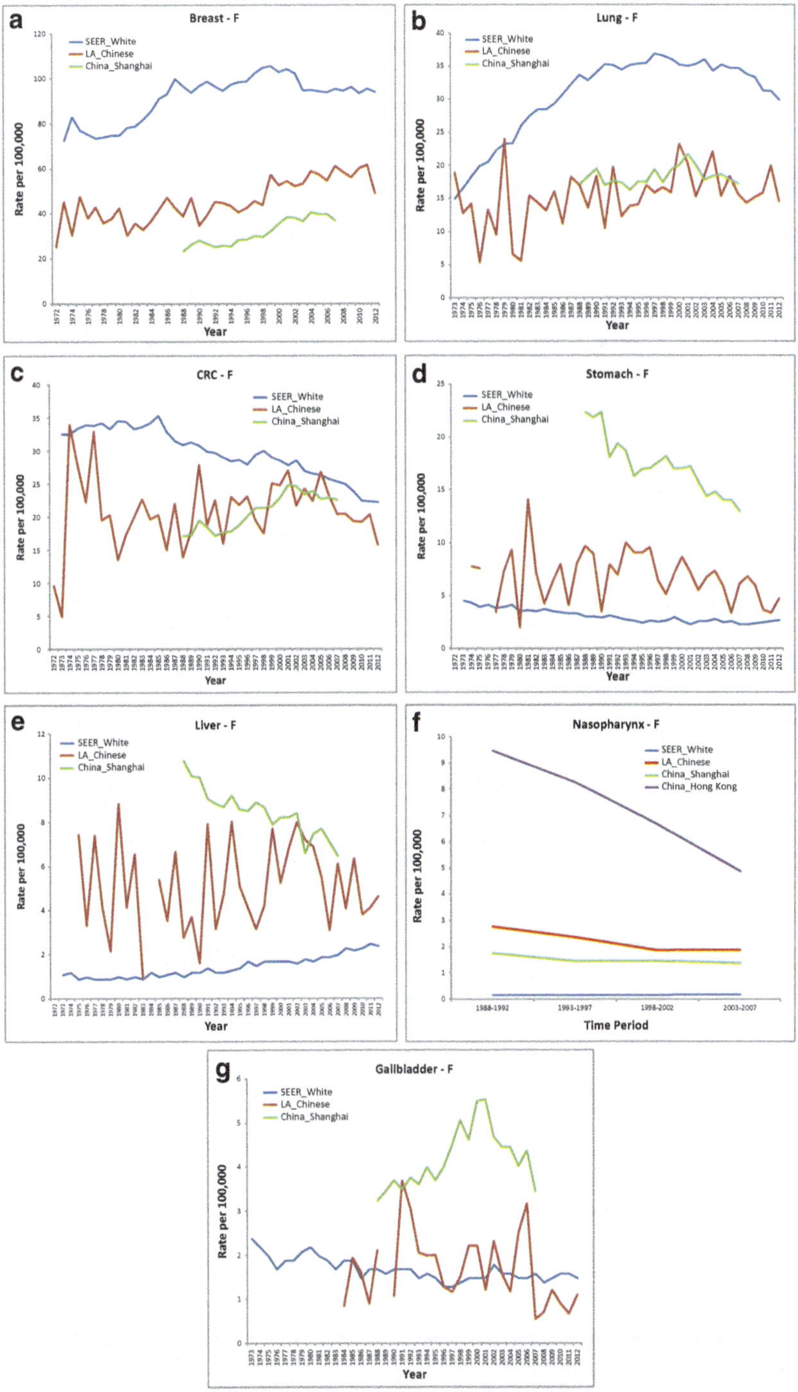

Fig. 4 Time trends of age-adjusted (world population) incidence rates by cancer site among US whites, Chinese in Los Angeles, and Chinese in China-Shanghai, women

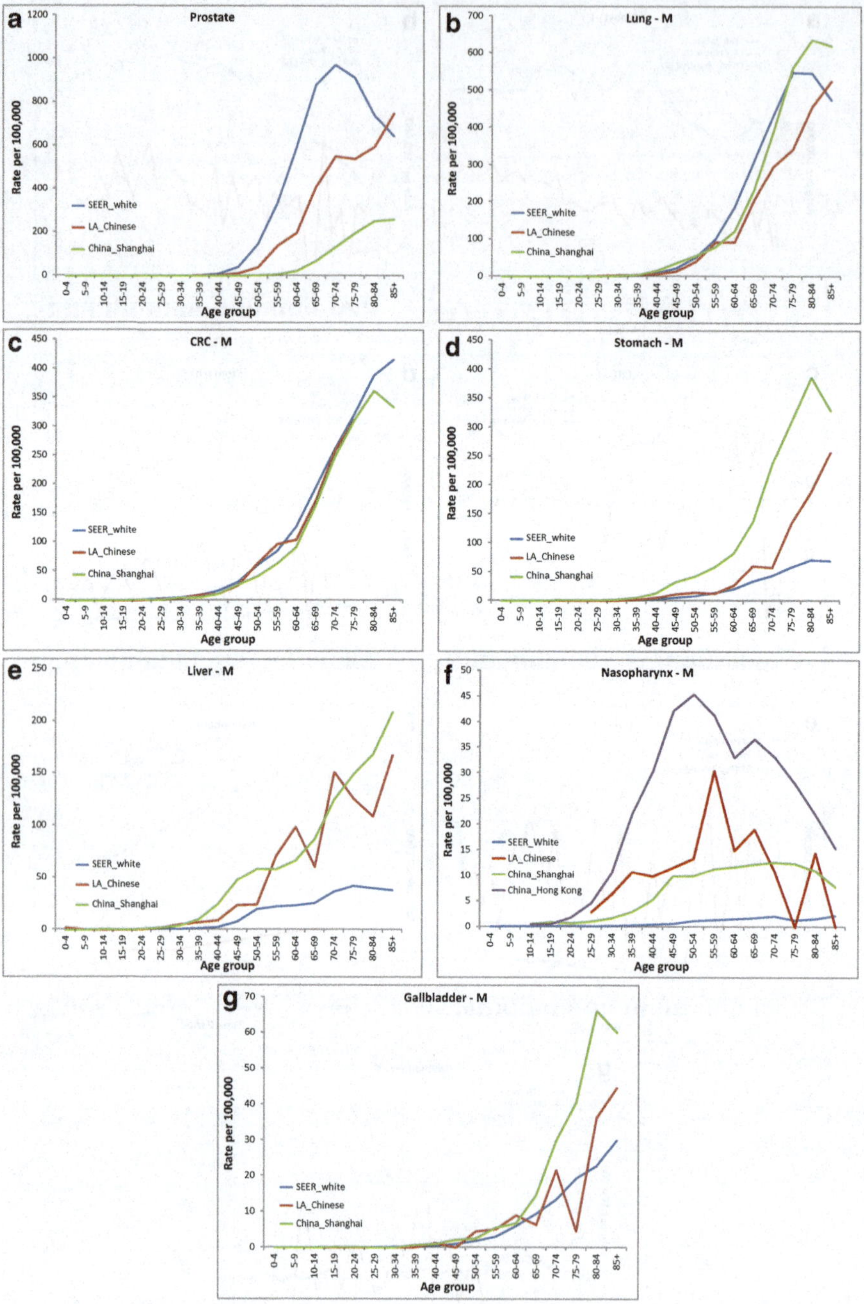

Fig. 5 Age-specific incidence rates by cancer site among US whites, Chinese in Los Angeles, and Chinese in China-Shanghai, men, 2003–2007

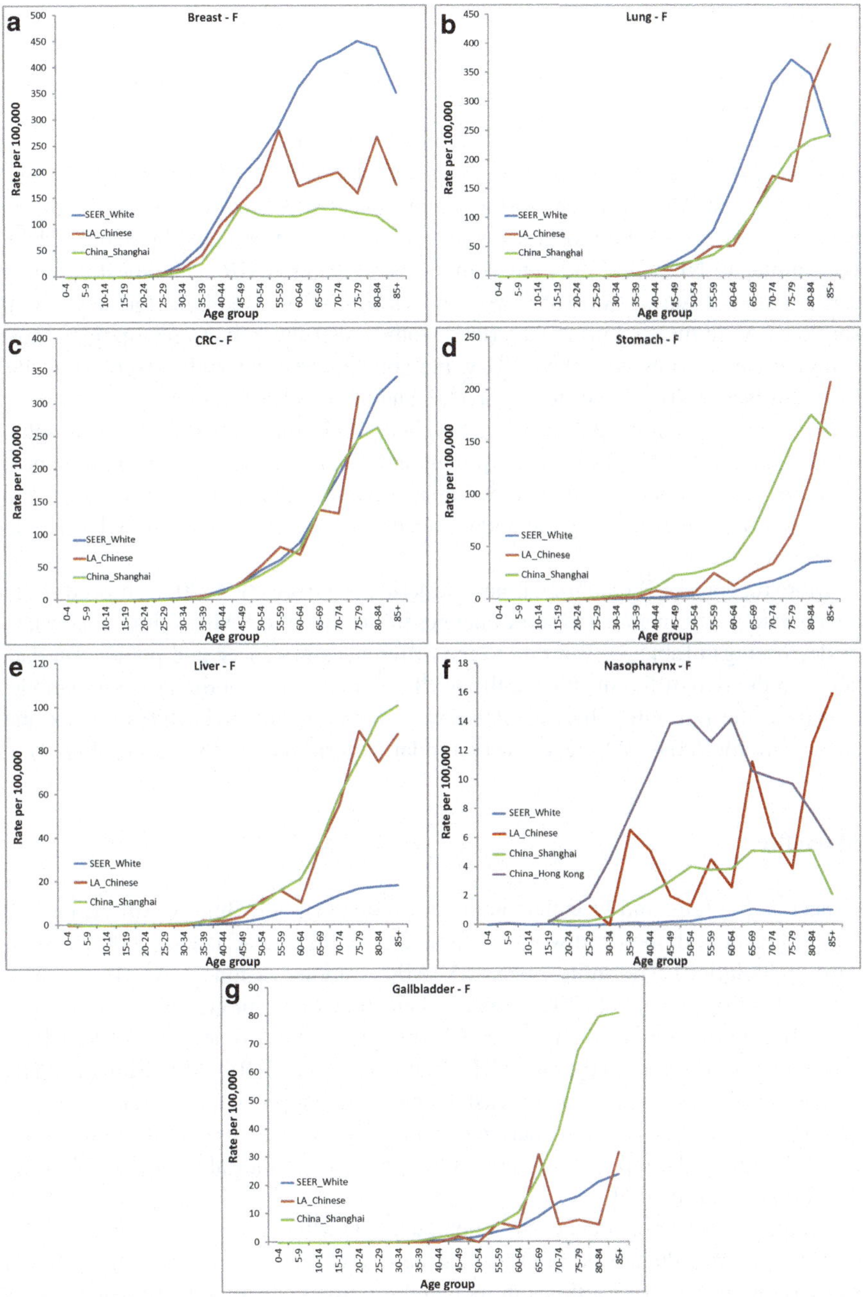

Fig. 6 Age-specific incidence rates by cancer site among US whites, Chinese in Los Angeles, and Chinese in China-Shanghai, women, 2003–2007

Incidence

According to the data published by Miller et al. (2008) for 1998–2002 (Table 1) using SEER registry data [14], the age-adjusted (2000 US standard population) incidence rate (AAIR) among Chinese Americans for all sites combined was 348.8/100,000 in men and 270.4/100,000 in women, about 40 % lower than the AAIR of NH white men or women. The top three most common cancer sites among Chinese-American men were cancers of the prostate, colon and rectum, and lung and bronchus, which was similar to NH white men but with 20–50 % lower AAIRs. The most common cancer among Chinese-American women was breast, followed by colon and rectum and lung. As in men, Chinese-American women also share the same top three most common cancer sites with their NH white counterparts, but with lower risk (50 % lower for breast, 20 % lower for colorectal, and 50 % lower for lung).

In contrast, Chinese Americans had higher AAIRs than NH whites for nasopharyngeal cancer (NPC) (14.8 times in men and 17.5 times in women), liver cancer (3.6 times in men and 3.2 times in women), stomach cancer (1.8 times in men and 2.6 times in women), and gallbladder cancer (1.3 times in men and 1.1 times in women) (Table 1).

More recent SEER data for Chinese Americans during 2004–2008 showed slight decrease in AAIR overall and some changes in site-specific AAIRs (either increasing or decreasing) (Table 3). But due to the differences in cancer and population data between the two different studies, the AAIR estimates are not directly comparable. However, the rate ratios between Chinese Americans and NH whites by sex and cancer site for 2004–2008 reveal very similar patterns as for 1998–2002 (Fig. 2).

Mortality

Cancer of the lung and bronchus is the deadliest for both Chinese Americans and NH whites in both men and women (Table 2), but the age-adjusted (2000 US standard population) mortality rate (AAMR) among Chinese-American men (47.0/100,000) is about 30 % lower than the rate among NH white men (72.2/100,000), while the AAMR for Chinese-American women (23.8/100,000) is about 50 % lower than that of the NH white women (44.5/100,000). Similar to NH whites, colorectal, prostate, and breast are among the top five most common causes of cancer deaths in Chinese-Americans. Unlike NH whites, liver and stomach cancer rank among the top five cancers with higher cancer mortality among Chinese-Americans regardless of sex.

Similar to cancer incidence, as compared to NH whites, Chinese Americans have higher mortality due to nasopharyngeal cancer (15.0 times in men and 14.0 in women), liver cancer (3.3 times in men and 2.7 times in women), stomach cancer (2.0 times in men and 2.6 times in women), and gallbladder cancer (1.4 times in men and 0.9 times in women). For the remaining cancer sites, as well as for all cancer sites combined, Chinese Americans have markedly lower AAMR than NH whites.

The sex-site-specific rate ratios in Chinese Americans relative to NH whites based on incidence closely resemble those based on mortality (Fig. 1).

Incidence Trends and Age Patterns

In the following, we examine the age-adjusted (1960 world standard population) incidence trends and age-specific incidence patterns for the top three most common cancers in Chinese Americans, as well as cancers that show higher risk among Chinese Americans than US whites.

Breast Cancer

Breast cancer is the most commonly diagnosed cancer among Chinese-American women (Table 3). Incidence rate among Chinese in LA has been rising since the 1980s (Fig. 4a); current rates are 60 % of that of the US white women. Rates in Chinese-American women are intermediate across age groups as compared to women in Shanghai and US white women. The differences in rates are particularly pronounced in postmenopausal years. Unlike US whites, breast cancer incidence among Chinese Americans plateaued after menopause, similar to the pattern in Shanghai (Fig. 6a).

Increasing breast cancer risk among Chinese-American women has been reported previously [14, 15, 20, 21]. Acculturation and adoption of Western lifestyles among immigrant Chinese and in many developing countries including China are likely to explain the rising incidence [22–25]. Specifically, the fall in number of births, low physical activity level, and obesity were results of urbanization and westernization that are directly linked with the increase in breast cancer risk in China in recent decades [25–27]. The much higher incidence rates for postmenopausal than premenopausal breast cancer among Chinese in LA as compared to Chinese in Shanghai point to the stronger impact of environmental changes associated with immigration and acculturation on postmenopausal disease and support the suggestion that postmenopausal breast cancer risk is modifiable [28–30].

Prostate Cancer

Prostate cancer is the most common cancer diagnosed in Chinese-American men (Table 3). The incidence trend for Chinese men in LA rose throughout the 1990s and peaked around 2003 before the subsequent downward trend started around 2012 returning to the incidence level observed in the 1980s (Fig. 3a). These changes are clearly associated with the FDA approval of the PSA testing in 1986 and subsequent widespread PSA screening for prostate cancer [32]. However, there was about a 10-year delay in the rise and peaking of the incidence rate among Chinese men in LA as compared to the rates of white men which rose sharply since 1986 and peaked around 2002. Chinese men in Shanghai experienced a steady increasing trend in prostate cancer incidence starting in late 1990. The rise in prostate cancer risk occurred at slightly different ages; rates markedly increased around ages 45–49 among Chinese men in LA, compared to ages 40–45 for white men and ages 55–59 for Chinese men in Shanghai (Fig. 5a). While prostate cancer incidence was highest and peaked at ages 70–74 and then declined in US white men, rates among Chinese men in LA continue to increase with increasing age and surpassed the risk in white men at ages 85+.

The higher prostate cancer risk among Chinese men in LA as compared to Chinese men in Shanghai may be explained, in part, by more widespread PSA screening in the USA [31–33]. Although Western diet (i.e., high calcium, processed meat, milk, and dairy products) has been linked with increased prostate cancer risk [34], while consumption of green tea and soy foods has been associated with decreased prostate cancer risk [35, 36], the evidence for a role of dietary factors in explaining east-west differences in incidence is weak. The consistently lower incidence rate in Chinese American men as compared to white men likely underlines the genetic and etiologic differences between the two populations [37–41].

Lung Cancer

Lung cancer is the second most common cancer among Chinese-American men and third most common cancer among Chinese-American women (Table 3). Lung cancer incidence is lower among Chinese men in LA compared to US white men and Chinese men in Shanghai; all share a similar declining trend in incidence rate (Fig. 3b). Lung cancer risk was lower in Chinese men in LA than US white men across all ages, particularly after age 60 (Fig. 5b). Chinese women in LA and those in Shanghai have comparable rates, which are about half of that of US white women. Rates in all three groups are beginning to decrease (Fig. 4b). The age-specific lung cancer incidence rates are also similar between Chinese women in LA and their counterparts in Shanghai, which are lower than those of US white women, until around 80 years of age (Fig. 6b).

Prevalence of current smokers is low among Chinese Americans with 16.1 % in men and 4.9 % in women, compared to 40.0 % and 26.6 % in US white men and women [42]. Acculturation appeared to have opposite effects on smoking behaviors in immigrant Asian men and women. Smoking rate tends to decrease with acculturation among men but increase with acculturation among women [43], which may partly explain the lower lung cancer risk among Chinese men in LA than Chinese men in Shanghai and the comparable risk level among women between the two locations. Lung cancer incidence in Chinese women appeared to be unusually high given that most were never smokers [44–47]. Besides active smoking, other risk factors, including secondhand smoking, environmental pollution, cooking methods, diet, previous lung diseases, and reproductive and genetic factors, have been implicated [48–57]. The complex risk patterns and disparate trends of lung cancer among subpopulation groups warrant continued surveillance and research among diverse populations [58, 59].

Colorectal Cancer (CRC)

Cancer of the colon and rectum ranks third in Chinese-American men and second among Chinese-American women (Table 3). Compared to NH whites, the risk of developing CRC is about 20 % lower in Chinese-American men and 10 % lower in Chinese-American women (Table 3). With the steady decline in CRC risk among US whites since the 1980s, the risk difference between Chinese Americans and their white counterparts is narrowing in recent years (Figs. 3c and 4c). Chinese in LA and Shanghai and US whites displayed very similar age-specific risk patterns (Figs. 5c and 6c).

Risk of CRC is strongly associated with familial and lifestyle factors [60–64]. Economic development and adoption of Western lifestyle have resulted in the rising incidence of CRC and other cancers in China [65, 66]. Screening has been credited as having considerable impact on the steady reduction in CRC incidence and mortality in the USA since the late 1980s [67]. Differences in access to CRC screening have contributed to the risk disparities among different population groups stratified by racial and socioeconomic characteristics [68–70]. Chinese-Americans are known to underutilize CRC screening [71–73]. Research has shown that education programs specifically designed to address cultural characteristics can significantly improve CRC screening among Chinese-Americans [74].

Stomach Cancer

Stomach cancer is one of the cancers that Chinese-Americans are at higher risk than NH whites; this is particularly striking after age 70 (Figs. 5d and 6d). Chinese-American men and women are 1.9–2.4 times more likely than NH whites to be diagnosed with stomach cancer (Table 3). Stomach cancer incidence rates for Chinese men in LA are about two-thirds lower than rates of Shanghai Chinese men in recent years (Fig. 3d); these differences are observed across all age groups. Risk patterns in women are similar to those in men. Rates in US whites as well as Chinese in LA are declining steadily (Fig. 4d).

The effect of migration on stomach cancer risk reduction among Japanese Americans has been well documented [75–77]. The much lower stomach cancer risk among Chinese in LA than in Shanghai can largely be explained by the lower prevalence of stomach cancer risk factors in the USA, such as *Helicobacter pylori* (*H. pylori*) infection, tobacco consumption, and certain dietary patterns, as well as better food preservation [78–85].

Liver Cancer

Compared to NH whites, liver cancer incidence is 3.1 times higher in Chinese-American men and 3.4 times higher in Chinese-American women (Table 3). In both sexes, the age-adjusted liver cancer risk for Chinese in LA is intermediate between those of Chinese in Shanghai and US whites. In contrast to the clear steady declining incidence among Shanghai Chinese, risk trends appear to be on the rise among US whites and stabilizing among Chinese in LA (Figs. 3e and 4e). Chinese in LA and in Shanghai display almost identical age-specific liver cancer incidence rates that are much higher than those of US whites across all ages, especially in older age groups (Figs. 5e and 6e).

Chronic infection with hepatitis B virus (HBV) causes more than half of liver cancer cases worldwide [86, 87]. While HBV is rare (1 %) in NH whites, 11.5–21.4 % of Chinese Americans carry the virus [88–90]. HBV carriers have much higher risk of developing liver cancer than noncarriers. HBV vaccination has proven to be very effective in reducing liver cancer risk and contributed to the sustained decline in liver cancer incidence around the world, especially in high-risk regions including China [91]. However, studies have shown that knowledge of the relationship between HBV and liver cancer and participation in HBV screening are both low among Chinese-Americans. Over 50 % of Chinese Americans never had HBV test, and about one-third had been vaccinated [92–94]. There are other risk factors of liver cancer including alcohol-related liver diseases, smoking, obesity, diabetes, and infection with hepatitis C virus (HCV) [95–97]. Unlike HBV, currently, there is no vaccination available for HCV. The increase in liver cancer incidence rates among US whites is likely related to the increasing HCV infection in the population [88, 98].

Nasopharyngeal Cancer (NPC)

NPC is a rare cancer worldwide. It ranks as 12th and 16th as the most common cancer among Chinese-American men and women, respectively. However, the incidence rates of NPC among Chinese Americans are 12.3 times higher than NH white men and 14.0 times higher than NH white women (Table 3). Chinese men and women in LA have higher incidence of NPC than both US whites and Chinese in Shanghai, but their risk is lower than that of Chinese in Hong Kong. These risk differentials likely reflect the striking high-risk patterns of NPC in China, particularly in southern coastal China. Incidence of NPC in LA Chinese declined throughout the 1990s and appeared to have now stabilized (Figs. 3f and 4f). The age-specific NPC incidence pattern in Chinese men in LA differs from that of US white men and Chinese men in Shanghai, but resembles that of Chinese men in Hong Kong; incidence peaks between ages 50 and 60. Interestingly, NPC risk appears to continue to increase with age among Chinese women in LA (Figs. 5f and 6f).

Nasopharyngeal cancer is a prevalent disease in southern China, particularly among the Cantonese living in Hong Kong and Guangdong province. Southern Chinese who migrated to low-risk regions still retain a much higher incidence rate compared to local populations [99–102]. But the risk seems to decrease with longer duration of residence and with succeeding generations [103–105]. Such decline in risk may also be attributable to a mixture of Chinese immigrants originating from high- as well as low-risk areas in China [100]. The incidence rates of NPC in China and other high-risk regions have been declining in the past decades, which seem to be associated with rapid economic development in the regions [106–109]. Well-established risk factors for NPC include Epstein-Barr virus (EBV), consumption of salt-preserved fish (particularly during weaning) and vegetables, family history of NPC, tobacco and alcohol consumption, and certain genotypes [99–102]. Despite the strong indication that both environmental factors and genetic traits contribute to the development of this cancer, understanding of its complex etiology is incomplete. Current strategies to reduce the risk of NPC include reducing the consumption of salt-preserved fish and other preserved foods, smoking cessation, reduction of alcohol use, and increase intake of fresh fruits and vegetables.

Gallbladder Cancer

Although generally considered a rare disease, gallbladder cancer has widely varied risk patterns around the world. The incidence rates are low in the USA and most Western and Mediterranean European countries, but high in Asia and Latin America [13]. It is one of the four cancers that Chinese-Americans are at higher risk in incidence than NH whites, more so in men (30 % higher) than in women (10 % higher) (Table 1 and Fig. 1). Regardless of sex, Chinese in LA have much lower incidence rates than Chinese in Shanghai, similar to the NH whites (Figs. 3g and 4g). While incidence in China showed a notable decline in the beginning of the 2000s, it remained relatively stable in the USA. Higher gallbladder cancer risk among Chinese in Shanghai than US whites is consistent across age in both men and women. Between ages 50 and 65, gallbladder cancer risk among Chinese men in LA is comparable to that of Chinese men in Shanghai, higher than that of US white men. The risk reduction for Chinese in LA, as compared to Chinese in Shanghai, seems to occur after age 70 in both sexes (Figs. 5g and 6g).

The risk factors of gallbladder cancer include gallstone, chronic gallbladder inflammation, gallbladder polyps, tobacco use, obesity, and diabetes [110–113]. A family history of gallstone and other gallbladder diseases increases the risk of developing gallbladder cancer [114, 115]. Environmental exposures to heavy metals and radon [116, 117] and a diet high in fried and oily foods have also been implicated in gallbladder cancer incidence [118–120]. The progression of gallbladder cancer is frequently rapid and silent, resulting in late diagnosis and dismal prognosis. Studying the risk variation in different populations, especially immigrants from high-risk regions, will aid identification of genetic and environmental risk factors, early detection, and development of primary prevention strategies to conquer this fatal disease.

Summary

Chinese-Americans demonstrate distinctive cancer risk patterns that are different from the white or NH white population. Although for most of the cancers examined Chinese-Americans have lower incidence and mortality rates than the NH whites, their risk for nasopharyngeal cancer, liver cancer, and stomach cancer is substantially higher, in addition to their slightly higher risk of gallbladder cancer. Except lung and colorectal cancer, Chinese Americans display intermediate-risk level between the US whites and Chinese in China, highlighting the significance of environmental and lifestyle factors in cancer development. Among Chinese-American men, liver cancer incidence seems to be stabilizing. Among women, risk is climbing for breast cancer, lung cancer, and even possibly liver cancer. Continued effort to monitor the cancer trends and develop effective cancer control programs in this special population is both necessary and important. The unique age-specific risk patterns by cancer type among Chinese Americans may offer clues for generating etiologic hypothesis. Focused research on specific racial/ethnic populations with migration history is likely to offer new understanding and opportunities in the fight against cancer.

Financial Disclosure The authors declare no financial benefits in writing this chapter. Work by Liu and Deapen was supported by the National Cancer Institute, National Institutes of Health, Department of Health and Human Services, under Contract No. HHSN261201000035C, and by grant number U58DP003862-10 from the Centers for Disease Control and Prevention. The ideas and opinions expressed herein are those of the authors, and no endorsement by the funding agencies or the federal government is intended or should be inferred.

References

1. United States Department of Homeland Security (2013) Yearbook of immigration statistics: 2012. U.S. Department of Homeland Security, Office of Immigration Statistics, Washington. http://www.dhs.gov/sites/default/files/publications/ois_yb_2012.pdf. Accessed 25 June 2015
2. Kwong P, Miscevic D (2005) Chinese America. The New Press, New York, p 44. ISBN 1-56584-962-0
3. Iris Chang (2003) The Chinese in America. Penguin Books, New York, pp 34–35. ISBN 0-670-03123-2
4. Hoeffel EM, Rastogi S, Kim MO, Shahid H (2012) The Asian population: 2010. 2010 census briefs. U.S. Census Bureau, Suitland, http://www.census.gov/prod/cen2010/briefs/c2010br-11.pdf. Accessed 25 June 2015
5. Ryan C (2013) Language use in the United States: 2011. American community survey reports. U.S. Census Bureau, Suitland, http://www.census.gov/prod/2013pubs/acs-22.pdf. Accessed 25 June 2015
6. United States Department of Labor (2014). The economic status of Asian Americans and Pacific Islanders in the Wake of the Great Recession. http://www.dol.gov/_sec/media/reports/20140828-AAPI.pdf. Accessed 25 June 2015
7. Smith LR (1956) Recorded and expected mortality among the Chinese of Hawaii and the United States with special reference to cancer. J Natl Cancer Inst 17(5):667–676
8. King H, Haenszel W (1973) Cancer mortality among foreign- and native-born Chinese in the United States. J Chronic Dis 26:623–646
9. Fraumeni JF, Mason TJ (1974) Cancer mortality among Chinese Americans, 1950-69. J Natl Cancer Inst 52(3):659–665
10. King H, Li JY, Locke FB, Pollack ES, Tu JT (1985) Patterns of site-specific displacement in cancer mortality among migrants: the Chinese in the United States. Am J Public Health 75(3):237–242

11. Lilienfeld DE (2008) Harold Fred Dorn and the First National Cancer Survey (1937–1939): the founding of modern cancer epidemiology. Am J Public Health 98:2150–2158. doi:10.2105/AJPH.2007.117440
12. Howlader N et al (eds) (2013). SEER Cancer Statistics Review, 1975-2010. National Cancer Institute, Bethesda. http://seer.cancer.gov/csr/1975_2010/, based on November 2012 SEER data submission, posted to the SEER web site, April 2013
13. International Agency for Research on Cancer. CI5Plus. http://ci5.iarc.fr/CI5plus/Default.aspx. Accessed 25 June 2015
14. Miller BA, Chu KC, Hankey BF, Ries LA (2008) Cancer incidence and mortality patterns among specific Asian and Pacific Islander populations in the U.S. Cancer Causes Control 19(3):227–256
15. Gomez SL, Noone AM, Lichtensztajn DY, Scoppa S, Gibson JT, Liu L, Morris C, Kwong S, Fish K, Wilkens L, Goodman M, Deapen D, Miller BA (2013) Cancer incidence trends among Asian American populations in the United States, 1990-2008. J Natl Cancer Inst 105(15):1096–1110
16. Liu L, Noone AM, Gomez SL, Scoppa S, Gibson JT, Lichtensztajn D, Fish K, Goodman M, Wilkens L, Morris C, Kwong S, Deapen D, Miller BA (2013) Cancer Incidence Trends among Native Hawaiians and Other Pacific Islanders in the U.S., 1990-2008. J Natl Cancer Inst 105(15):1086–1095
17. Surveillance, Epidemiology, and End Results (SEER) Program (www.seer.cancer.gov) SEER*Stat Database: Incidence —SEER 11, plus Greater CA and NJ, Nov 2010 Sub (1990–2008) detailed API plus White Non-Hispanic—pops projected from populations, National Cancer Institute, DCCPS, Surveillance Research Program, Cancer Statistics Branch, released June 2011 (updated 10/28/2011), based on the November 2010 submission
18. International Agency for Research on Cancer. CI5: Cancer in five continents. http://ci5.iarc.fr/Default.aspx. Accessed 31 May 2015
19. International Agency for Research on Cancer. CI5plus: Cancer in Five Continents Time Trends. http://ci5.iarc.fr/CI5plus/Pages/online.aspx. Accessed 31 May 2015
20. Deapen D, Liu L, Perkins C, Bernstein L, Ross RK (2002) Rapidly rising breast cancer incidence rates among Asian-American women. Int J Cancer 99:747–750
21. Liu L, Zhang J, Wu AH, Pike MC, Deapen D (2012) Invasive breast cancer incidence trends by detailed race/ethnicity and age. Int J Cancer 130(2):395–404
22. Ferlay J, Shin HR, Bray F, Forman D, Mathers C, Parkin DM (2010) Cancer incidence and mortality worldwide: IARC Cancer Base No.10. GLOBOCAN 2008. International Agency for Research on Cancer, Lyon
23. Fan L, Strasser-Weippl K, Li JJ, St Louis J, Finkelstein DM, Yu KD, Chen WQ, Shao ZM, Goss PE (2014) Breast cancer in China. Lancet Oncol 15(7):e279–e289. doi:10.1016/S1470-2045(13)70567-9
24. Fan L, Zheng Y, Yu KD et al (2009) Breast cancer in a transitional society over 18 years: trends and present status in Shanghai, China. Breast Cancer Res Treat 117:409–416
25. Linos E, Spanos D, Rosner BA et al (2008) Effects of reproductive and demographic changes on breast cancer incidence in China: a modeling analysis. J Natl Cancer Inst 100:1352–1360
26. Zhang Q, Liu LY, Wang F, Mu K, Yu ZG (2012) The changes in female physical and childbearing characteristics in China and potential association with risk of breast cancer. BMC Public Health 12:368. doi:10.1186/1471-2458-12-368
27. Turati F, La Vecchia C (2012) Risk factors for breast cancer in China: similarities and differences with western populations. Arch Med Sci 8:179–182
28. Bertucci F, Birnbaum D (2008) Reasons for breast cancer heterogeneity. J Biol 7(2):6. doi:10.1186/jbiol67
29. Rose DP, Vona-Davis L (2010) Interaction between menopausal status and obesity in affecting breast cancer risk. Maturitas 66(1):33–38
30. Hemminki K, Försti A, Sundquist J, Mousavi S (2011) Preventable breast cancer is postmenopausal. Breast Cancer Res Treat 125:163–167

31. De Angelis D, Rittenhouse HG, Mikolajczyk SD, Shamel LB, Semjonow A (2007) Twenty years of PSA: from prostate antigen to tumor marker. Rev Urol 9(3):113–123
32. Sirovich BE, Schwartz LM, Woloshin S (2003) Screening men for prostate and colorectal cancer in the United States: does practice reflect the evidence? JAMA 289:1414–1420
33. Zhang L, Wu S, Guo LR, Zhao XJ (2009) Diagnostic strategies and the incidence of prostate cancer: reasons for the low reported incidence of prostate cancer in China. Asian J Androl 11(1):9–13
34. World Cancer Research Fund / American Institute for Cancer Research (2007) Food, nutrition, physical activity, and the prevention of cancer: a global perspective. AICR, Washington, pp 305–309, http://www.aicr.org/assets/docs/pdf/reports/Second_Expert_Report.pdf. Accessed 31 May 2015
35. Zheng J, Yang B, Huang T, Yu Y, Yang J, Li D (2011) Green tea and black tea consumption and prostate cancer risk: an exploratory meta-analysis of observational studies. Nutr Cancer 63(5):663–672. doi:10.1080/01635581.2011.570895
36. Yan L, Spitznagel EL (2009) Soy consumption and prostate cancer risk in men: a revisit of a meta-analysis. Am J Clin Nutr 89(4):1155–1163. doi:10.3945/ajcn.2008.27029
37. Sim HG, Cheng CWS (2005) Changing demography of prostate cancer in Asia. Eur J Cancer 41(6):834–845
38. Ito K (2014) Prostate cancer in Asian men. Nat Rev Urol 11:197–212
39. McCracken M, Olsen M, Chen MS Jr, Jemal A, Thun M et al (2007) Cancer incidence, mortality, and associated risk factors among Asian Americans of Chinese, Filipino, Vietnamese, Korean, and Japanese ethnicities. CA Cancer J Clin 57:190–205
40. Kamangar F, Dores GM, Anderson WF (2006) Patterns of cancer incidence, mortality, and prevalence across five continents: defining priorities to reduce cancer disparities in different geographic regions of the world. J Clin Oncol 24:2137–2150
41. Ye DW, Li CL (2007) Epidemiological trends of prostate cancer: retrospect and prospect. China Clin Oncol 17:177–180
42. Caraballo RS, Yee SL, Gfroerer J, Mirza SA (2008) Adult tobacco use among racial and ethnic groups living in the United States, 2002-2005. Prev Chronic Dis 5:A78
43. Choi S, Rankin S, Stewart A, Oka R (2008) Effects of acculturation on smoking behavior in Asian Americans: a meta-analysis. J Cardiovasc Nurs 23:67–73
44. Epplein M, Schwartz SM, Potter JD, Weiss NS (2005) Smoking-adjusted lung cancer incidence among Asian-Americans (United States). Cancer Causes Control 16:1085–1090
45. Le Marchand L, Wilkens LR, Kolonel LN (1992) Ethnic differences in the lung cancer risk associated with smoking. Cancer Epidemiol Biomarkers Prev 1:103–107
46. Torok S, Hegedus B, Laszlo V, Hoda MA, Ghanim B, Berger W et al (2011) Lung cancer in never smokers. Future Oncol 7:1195–1211
47. Zhou W, Christiani DC (2011) East meets West: ethnic differences in epidemiology and clinical behaviors of lung cancer between East Asians and Caucasians. Chin J Cancer 30:287–292
48. Osann KE (1991) Lung cancer in women: the importance of smoking, family history of cancer, and medical history of respiratory disease. Cancer Res 51:4893–4897
49. Samet JM, Avila-Tang E, Boffetta P, Hannan LM, Olivo-Marston S, Thun MJ et al (2009) Lung cancer in never smokers: clinical epidemiology and environmental risk factors. Clin Cancer Res 15:5626–5645
50. Seow A, Poh WT, Teh M, Eng P, Wang YT, Tan WC et al (2000) Fumes from meat cooking and lung cancer risk in Chinese women. Cancer Epidemiol Biomarkers Prev 9:1215–1221
51. Subramanian J, Govindan R (2007) Lung cancer in never smokers: a review. J Clin Oncol 25:561–570
52. Vineis P, Hoek G, Krzyzanowski M, Vigna-Taglianti F, Veglia F, Airoldi L et al (2007) Lung cancers attributable to environmental tobacco smoke and air pollution in non-smokers in different European countries: a prospective study. Environ Health 6:7. doi:10.1186/1476-069X-6-7
53. Xu ZY, Blot WJ, Xiao HP, Wu A, Feng YP, Stone BJ et al (1989) Smoking, air pollution, and the high rates of lung cancer in Shenyang, China. J Natl Cancer Inst 81:1800–1806

54. Lim WY, Chen Y, Chuah KL, Eng P, Leong SS, Lim E et al (2012) Female reproductive factors, gene polymorphisms in the estrogen metabolism pathway, and risk of lung cancer in Chinese women. Am J Epidemiol 175:492–503
55. Zhao B, Seow A, Lee EJ, Poh WT, Teh M, Eng P et al (2001) Dietary isothiocyanates, glutathione Stransferase-M1, -T1 polymorphisms and lung cancer risk among Chinese women in Singapore. Cancer Epidemiol Biomarkers Prev 10:1063–1067
56. Lim WY, Chuah KL, Eng P, Leong SS, Lim E, Lim TK et al (2011) Meat consumption and risk of lung cancer among never-smoking women. Nutr Cancer 63:850–859
57. Lim WY, Chen Y, Ali SM, Chuah KL, Eng P, Leong SS et al (2011) Polymorphisms in inflammatory pathway genes, host factors and lung cancer risk in Chinese female never-smokers. Carcinogenesis 32:522–529
58. Gomez SL, Yang J, Lin SW, McCusker M, Sandler A, Cheng I, Wakelee HA, Patel MI, Clarke CA (2015) Incidence trends of lung cancer by immigration status among Chinese Americans. Cancer Epidemiol Biomarkers Prev 24(8):1157–1164. doi:10.1158/1055-9965
59. Cheng I, Le GM, Noone AM, Gali K, Patel M, Haile RW et al (2014) Lung cancer incidence trends by histology type among Asian American, Native Hawaiian, and Pacific Islander populations in the United States, 1990-2010. Cancer Epidemiol Biomarkers Prev 23:2250–2265
60. Johns LE, Houlston RS (2001) A systematic review and meta analysis of familial colorectal cancer risk. Am J Gastroenterol 96:2992–3003
61. Butterworth AS, Higgins JP, Pharoah P (2006) Relative and absolute risk of colorectal cancer for individuals with a family history: a meta-analysis. Eur J Cancer 42:216–227
62. Lynch HT, de la Chapelle A (2003) Hereditary colorectal cancer. N Engl J Med 348:919–932
63. Larsson SC, Wolk A (2007) Obesity and colon and rectal cancer risk: a meta-analysis of prospective studies. Am J Clin Nutr 86:556–565
64. Wang Y, Jacobs EJ, Patel AV et al (2008) A prospective study of waist circumference and body mass index in relation to colorectal cancer incidence. Cancer Causes Control 19:783–792
65. Chen W, Zheng R, Zeng H, Zhang S, He J (2015) Annual report on status of cancer in China, 2011. Chin J Cancer Res. doi:10.3978/j.issn.1000-9604.2015.01.06
66. Sung JJ, Lau JY, Goh KL, Leung WK (2005) Increasing incidence of colorectal cancer in Asia: implications for screening. Lancet Oncol 6:871–876
67. Zauber AG, Lansdorp-Vogelaar I, Knudsen AB, Wilschut J, van Ballegooijen M, Kuntz KM (2008) Evaluating test strategies for colorectal cancer screening: a decision analysis for the U.S. Preventive Services Task Force. Ann Intern Med 149:659–669
68. Zapka J (2008) Innovative provider—and health system-directed approaches to improving colorectal cancer screening delivery. Med Care 46(9 suppl 1):S62–S67
69. Wu X, Cokkinides V, Chen VW et al (2006) Associations of subsite-specific colorectal cancer incidence rates and stage of disease at diagnosis with county-level poverty, by race and sex. Cancer 107(5 suppl):1121–1117
70. Edwards BK et al (2010) Annual report to the nation on the status of cancer, 1975–2006, featuring colorectal cancer trends and impact of interventions (risk factors, screening, and treatment) to reduce future rates. Cancer 116:544–573
71. Felix-Aaron K, Moy E, Kang M, Patel M, Chesley FD, Clancy C (2005) Variation in quality of men's health care by race/ethnicity and social class. Med Care 43(3 Suppl):I72–I81
72. Sun WY, Basch CE, Wolf RL, Li XJ (2004) Factors associated with colorectal cancer screening among Chinese-Americans. Prev Med 39:323–329
73. Tang TS, Solomon LJ, McCracken LM (2001) Barriers to fecal occult blood testing and sigmoidoscopy among older Chinese-American women. Cancer Pract 9:277–282
74. Tu SP, Taylor V, Yasui Y, Chun A, Yip MP, Acorda E, Li L, Bastani R (2006) Promoting culturally appropriate colorectal cancer screening through a health educator: a randomized controlled trial. Cancer 107(5):959–966
75. Haenszel W, Kurihara M (1968) Studies of Japanese migrants. I mortality from cancer and other diseases among Japanese in the United States. Natl Cancer Inst 40(1):43–68

76. Kolonel LN, Hinds MW, Hankin JH (1980) Cancer patterns among migrant and native-born Japanese in Hawaii in relation to smoking, drinking, and dietary habits. In: Gelboin HV (ed) Genetics and environmental factors in experimental and human cancer. University Park Press, Baltimore, pp 327–340
77. Maskarinec G, Noh JJ (2004) The effect of migration on cancer incidence among Japanese in Hawaii. Ethn Dis 14:431–439
78. Peleteiro B, La Vecchia C, Lunet N (2012) The role of Helicobacter pylori infection in the web of gastric cancer causation. Eur J Cancer Prev 21(2):118–125
79. Bertuccio P, Chatenoud L, Levi F, Praud D, Ferlay J, Negri E, Malvezzi M, La Vecchia C (2009) Recent patterns in gastric cancer: a global overview. Int J Cancer 125:666–673
80. Yamaguchi N, Kakizoe T (2001) Synergistic interaction between Helicobacter pylori gastritis and diet in gastric cancer. Lancet Oncol 2(2):88–94
81. Lee SA, Kang D, Shim KN, Choe JW, Hong WS, Choi H (2003) Effect of diet and Helicobacter pylori infection to the risk of early gastric cancer. J Epidemiol 13(3):162–168
82. Ladeiras-Lopes R, Pereira AK, Nogueira A, Pinheiro-Torres T, Pinto I, Santos-Pereira R, Lunet N (2008) Smoking and gastric cancer: systematic review and meta-analysis of cohort studies. Cancer Causes Control 19:689–701
83. Shikata K, Doi Y, Yonemoto K, Arima H, Ninomiya T, Kubo M, Tanizaki Y, Matsumoto T, Iida M, Kiyohara Y (2008) Population-based prospective study of the combined influence of cigarette smoking and Helicobacter pylori infection on gastric cancer incidence: the Hisayama Study. Am J Epidemiol 168:1409–1415
84. Bertuccio P, Rosato V, Andreano A, Ferraroni M, Decarli A, Edefonti V, La Vecchia C (2013) Dietary patterns and gastric cancer risk: a systematic review and meta-analysis. Ann Oncol 24:1450–1458
85. Park B, Shin A, Park SK, Ko KP, Ma SH, Lee EH, Gwack J, Jung EJ, Cho LY, Yang JJ, Yoo KY (2011) Ecological study for refrigerator use, salt, vegetable, and fruit intakes, and gastric cancer. Cancer Causes Control 22(11):1497–1502. doi:10.1007/s10552-011-9823-7
86. Parkin DM (2006) The global health burden of infection-associated cancers in the year 2002. Int J Cancer 118(12):3030–3044
87. El-Serag HB (2012) Epidemiology of viral hepatitis and hepatocellular carcinoma. Gastroenterology 142(6):1264–1273
88. IOM (Institute of Medicine) (2010) Hepatitis and liver cancer: a National Strategy for Prevention and Control of Hepatitis B and C. The National Academies Press, Washington, http://www.cdc.gov/hepatitis/PDFs/IOM-HepatitisAndLiverCancerReport.pdf. Accessed 31 May 2015
89. Centers for Disease Control and Prevention (2006) Screening for chronic hepatitis B among Asian/Pacific Islander populations—New York City, 2005. MMWR Morb Mortal Wkly Rep 55(18):505–509
90. Chao S, Lee PV, Prapong W, Su J, So S (2004) High prevalence of chronic hepatitis B (HBV) infection in adult Chinese Americans living in California. Hepatology 40(Suppl 1):717A
91. Gao S, Yang WS, Bray F, Va P, Zhang W, Gao J et al (2012) Declining rates of hepatocellular carcinoma in urban Shanghai: incidence trends in 1976–2005. Eur J Epidemiol 27(1):39–46
92. Strong C, Lee S, Tanaka M, Juon HS (2012) Ethnic differences in prevalence and barriers of HBV screening and vaccination among Asian Americans. J Community Health 37:1071–1080
93. Taylor VM, Tu SP, Woodall E et al (2006) Hepatitis B knowledge and practices among Chinese immigrants to the United States. Asian Pac J Cancer Prev 7(2):313–317
94. Thompson MJ, Taylor VM, Jackson JC, Yasui Y, Kuniyuki A, Tu SP, Hislop TG (2002) Hepatitis B knowledge and practices among Chinese American women in Seattle, Washington. J Cancer Educ 17:222–226
95. Shih WL, Chang HC, Liaw YF, Lin SM, Lee SD, Chen PJ et al (2012) Influences of tobacco and alcohol use on hepatocellular carcinoma survival. Int J Cancer 131(11):2612–2621
96. Ezzati M, Riboli E (2013) Behavioral and dietary risk factors for noncommunicable diseases. N Engl J Med 369(10):954–964

97. Chuang SC, La Vecchia C, Boffetta P (2009) Liver cancer: descriptive epidemiology and risk factors other than HBV and HCV infection. Cancer Lett 286(1):9–14
98. Zhang Y, Ren JS, Shi JF, Li N, Wang YT, Qu C, Zhang Y, Dai M (2015) International trends in primary liver cancer incidence from 1973 to 2007. BMC Cancer 15:94. doi:10.1186/s12885-015-1113-4
99. Tsao SW, Yip YL, Tsang CM, Pang PS, Lau VM, Zhang G, Lo KW (2014) Etiological factors of nasopharyngeal carcinoma. Oral Oncol 50(5):330–338. doi:10.1016/j.oraloncology.2014.02.006
100. Chang ET, Adami HO (2006) The enigmatic epidemiology of nasopharyngeal carcinoma. Cancer Epidemiol Biomarkers Prev 15(10):1765–1777
101. Lo KW, To KF, Huang DP (2004) Focus on nasopharyngeal carcinoma. Cancer Cell 5(5):423–428
102. Yu MC, Yuan JM (2002) Epidemiology of nasopharyngeal carcinoma. Semin Cancer Biol 12(6):421–429
103. Warnakulasuriya KA, Johnson NW, Linklater KM, Bell J (1999) Cancer of mouth, pharynx and nasopharynx in Asian and Chinese immigrants resident in Thames regions. Oral Oncol 35:471–475
104. McCredie M, Williams S, Coates M (1999) Cancer mortality in East and Southeast Asian migrants to New South Wales, Australia, 1975-1995. Br J Cancer 79:1277–1282
105. Buell P (1974) The effect of migration on the risk of nasopharyngeal cancer among Chinese. Cancer Res 34:1189–1191
106. Jia WH, Huang QH, Liao J, Ye W, Shugart YY, Liu Q et al (2006) Trends in incidence and mortality of nasopharyngeal carcinoma over a 20-25 year period (1978/1983-2002) in Sihui and Cangwu counties in southern China. BMC Cancer 6:178
107. Cao SM, Simons MJ, Qian CN (2011) The prevalence and prevention of nasopharyngeal carcinoma in China. Chin J Cancer 30:114–119
108. Hsu C, Shen YC, Cheng CC, Hong RL, Chang CJ, Cheng AL (2006) Difference in the incidence trend of nasopharyngeal and oropharyngeal carcinomas in Taiwan: implication from age-period-cohort analysis. Cancer Epidemiol Biomarkers Prev 15(5):856–861
109. Singapore Cancer Registry (2010) Trends in cancer incidence in Singapore 1968–2007. Singapore Cancer Registry Report No. 7. https://www.nrdo.gov.sg/docs/librariesprovider3/Publications-Cancer/inc_report_v8.pdf?sfvrsn=0. Accessed 2 Feb 2016
110. Misra S, Chaturvedi A, Misra NC, Sharma ID (2003) Carcinoma of the gallbladder. Lancet Oncol 4:167–176
111. Pandey M (2003) Risk factors for gallbladder cancer: a reappraisal. Eur J Cancer Prev 12:15–24
112. Hundal R, Shaffer EA (2014) Gallbladder cancer: epidemiology and outcome. Clin Epidemiol 6:99–109. doi:10.2147/CLEP.S37357
113. Lai CH, Lau WY (2008) Gallbladder cancer—a comprehensive review. Surgeon 6:101–110
114. Dutta U, Nagi B, Garg PK, Sinha SK, Singh K, Tandon RK (2005) Patients with gallstones develop gallbladder cancer at an earlier age. Eur J Cancer Prev 14(4):381–385
115. Hsing AW, Bai Y, Andreotti G et al (2007) Family history of gallstones and the risk of biliary tract cancer and gallstones: a population-based study. Int J Cancer 121:832–838
116. Pandey M (2006) Environmental pollutants in gallbladder carcinogenesis. J Surg Oncol 93(8):640–643
117. Darby SC, Whitley E, Howe GR, Hutchings SJ, Kusiak RA, Lubin JH et al (1995) Radon and cancers other than lung cancer in underground miners: a collaborative analysis of 11 studies. J Natl Cancer Inst 87(5):378–384
118. Rai A, Mohapatra SC, Shukla HS (2004) A review of association of dietary factors in gallbladder cancer. Indian J Cancer 41:147–151
119. Jain K, Sreenivas V, Velpandian T, Kapil U, Garg PK (2012) Risk factors for gallbladder cancer: a case-control study. Int J Cancer 132(7):1660–1666
120. Kato K, Akai S, Tominaya KS, Kato J (1989) A case control study of biliary tract cancer in Niigata Prefecture, Japan. Jpn J Cancer Res 80:932–938

Cancer Incidence and Mortality Among Filipinos in the USA and the Philippines: Patterns and Trends

Scarlett Lin Gomez, Meg A. McKinley, Caroline A. Thompson, Rita Leung, Iona Cheng, Anne-Michelle Noone, Latha Palaniappan, Mark Cullen, Christina A. Clarke, Theresa H.M. Keegan, and Sally L. Glaser

Abstract Background Filipino Americans are the second largest Asian-American ethnic group, comprising 3.4 million persons in 2010. This population has grown rapidly, nearly doubling in size from 2000 to 2010. With their varied migration patterns over time, sociodemographic diversity in the USA, and growing presence,

S.L. Gomez (✉) • C.A. Clarke • S.L. Glaser
Cancer Prevention Institute of California, 2201 Walnut Avenue, Suite 300, Fremont, CA 94538, USA

Stanford Cancer Institute, Stanford, CA, USA
e-mail: scarlett@cpic.org

M.A. McKinley • R. Leung
Cancer Prevention Institute of California, 2201 Walnut Avenue, Suite 300, Fremont, CA 94538, USA

C.A. Thompson
Graduate School of Public Health, San Diego State University, San Diego, CA, USA

Palo Alto Medical Foundation Research Institute, Palo Alto, CA, USA

I. Cheng
Cancer Prevention Institute of California, 2201 Walnut Avenue, Suite 300, Fremont, CA 94538, USA

A.-M. Noone
Division of Cancer Control and Population Sciences, National Cancer Institute, Bethesda, MD, USA

L. Palaniappan
Palo Alto Medical Foundation Research Institute, Palo Alto, CA, USA

School of Medicine, Stanford University, Stanford, CA, USA

M. Cullen
School of Medicine, Stanford University, Stanford, CA, USA

T.H. Keegan
Stanford Cancer Institute, Stanford, CA, USA

Division of Hematology and Oncology, Department of Internal Medicine, University of California Davis School of Medicine, Sacramento, CA, USA

A.H. Wu, D.O. Stram (eds.), *Cancer Epidemiology Among Asian Americans*,
DOI 10.1007/978-3-319-41118-7_3

this group is a significant Asian-American population in which to evaluate cancer incidence and mortality patterns.

Methods Two decades (1990–2010) of incidence data from the NCI Surveillance, Epidemiology, and End Results (SEER) registry and population estimate data from the 1990, 2000, and 2010 US Census are used to calculate incidence rates and trends. Incidence rates from available registries in the Philippines, obtained from the Cancer Incidence in Five Continents database, are presented. US cancer mortality rates from 36 states (from 2003 to 2011) are also presented. All rates and 95 % confidence intervals (CI) are calculated as cases or deaths per 100,000 persons. Annual rates are presented as trends, determined using joinpoint regression models to identify distinct changes in trends.

Results Overall, cancer rates are higher for males than females in both the USA and the Philippines. Among US Filipino males, the five most common cancer sites are (1) prostate, (2) lung and bronchus, (3) colon and rectum, (4) non-Hodgkin lymphomas (NHL), and (5) liver, while these sites among males in the Philippines are (1) lung and bronchus, (2) prostate, (3) colon and rectum, (4) liver, and (5) stomach. Among US Filipina females, the three most common sites are (1) breast, (2) colon and rectum, and (3) lung and bronchus, with thyroid and corpus uterus changing as the fourth and fifth most common sites across the time period; in contrast, these sites among females in the Philippines are (1) breast, (2) cervix uteri, (3) colon and rectum, (4) lung and bronchus, and (5) ovary in 1993–1997 and (1) breast, (2) colon and rectum, (3) lung and bronchus, (4) cervix uteri, and (5) corpus uteri in 2003–2007. With regard to cancer mortality, lung, colorectal, prostate, liver, and pancreatic cancers were the five sites contributing most to cancer-related deaths among Filipino males in the USA and Philippines, while lung, breast, colorectal, pancreatic, and ovarian cancers were the five most common sites of cancer-related deaths for females in both populations. Incidence of breast, lung, thyroid, kidney, and bladder cancers is increasing among US Filipinas, and incidence of kidney cancer is increasing among US Filipino males.

Conclusions The incidence and mortality patterns and trends presented for Filipinos in this chapter provide data to support targeted areas for cancer prevention, such as obesity for reducing the risks of uterine, colorectal, and breast cancers, and smoking prevention and cessation for lung, kidney, oral cavity and pharyngeal, bladder, and pancreatic cancers. For those sites that demonstrate changing trends or dramatic differences between Filipinos in the USA and in the Philippines, further targeted studies can leverage these incidence patterns to elucidate environmental and modifiable risk factors.

Keywords Cancer • Philippines • Filipino • Incidence • Mortality • Race • Asian Pacific Islander • SEER • Cancer Incidence in Five Continents

Introduction

Filipino Americans are the second largest Asian-American ethnic group, comprising 3.4 million persons in 2010, and exceeded in numbers only by Chinese Americans at 4.0 million [1]. In recent years, the Filipino American population has grown rapidly, nearly doubling between 2000 and 2010 and now representing nearly 20 % of the total Asian-American population. Among Filipinos in the USA, 43 % live in California (where they are the largest Asian-American ethnic group), 10 % live in Hawaii, and 4 % live each in Illinois, Texas, and Washington State. In the 2010 Census, Filipinos had the second highest proportion (25 %), after Japanese, self-reporting as multiple race: 19 % identified with another non-Asian race, 4 % with multiple Asian groups and another non-Asian race, and 3 % with multiple Asian race groups.

The sociodemographic characteristics of the contemporary Filipino American population reflect their historical migration patterns to the USA. During the American colonial period (approximately between 1899 and 1946), when Filipinos were US nationals, the first Filipino migrants arrived in the mainland USA primarily as laborers. The 1934 Philippine Independence Act then restricted immigration to 50 Filipinos per year. However, with the 1964 Immigration Act, which abolished national-origins quotas and allowed 170,000 immigrants per year from Asia [2], came a second large wave of Asian immigration. Filipino immigrants in this wave were more likely to be women, to come from cities than the countryside, and arrived in the USA to settle permanently. Between 1966 and 1970, 65 % of nearly 40,000 Filipinos admitted to the USA under the occupational category were professional or technical workers, emigrating to escape the regime of Ferdinand Marcos and to seek better employment opportunities. Among these immigrant professionals, the majority were physicians and nurses; however, for physicians, the costs to obtain a US medical license were prohibitive, and many Filipino doctors were underemployed in the USA as nurses, nurses' aides, or laboratory assistants, for which licensure was less involved [2].

According to data from the 2010 Census and 2007–2009 American Community Survey, 53 % of Filipino Americans in this time period were foreign-born. Although 57 % spoke a language other than English at home, 82 % also reported speaking English very well, reflecting the widespread use of English in the Philippines [3]. Because Filipino Americans comprised a large number of skilled laborers after 1964, they are relatively well-educated, with a bachelor's or graduate/professional degree obtained by 46 % (compared with 29 % of the non-Hispanic White population and 49 % of the Asian combined population). However, at $25,799, Filipinos' per capita household income was lower than that of non-Hispanic Whites and all Asians combined ($29,418 and $28,342, respectively). 5 % of Filipino American households lived in poverty (relative to 8 % of non-Hispanic Whites and 8 % of Asians combined), and 11 % lacked health insurance (relative to 13 % of non-Hispanic Whites and 14 % of Asians combined).

With their varied migration patterns over time, contemporary diversity in the USA, and growing presence, Filipino Americans represent a significant Asian-American population in which to evaluate cancer incidence and mortality patterns. The vast heterogeneity among Asian-American ethnic groups translates into substantial variability in cancer incidence and mortality patterns [4–6]. Therefore, examining cancer patterns for distinct ethnic populations is necessary for identifying disparities and effectively targeting future research, health policies, and intervention efforts [7]. To provide a broad overview of cancer occurrence among US Filipinos, this chapter presents incidence and mortality rates and trends over approximately 20 years, for the ten most common cancer sites in each gender/outcome group. These statistics are based on data from the National Cancer Institute's Surveillance, Epidemiology, and End Results (SEER) program, the National Center for Health Statistics (NCHS), and the US Census. For comparison, we present incidence rates from the International Agency for Research on Cancer (IARC) for two regions in the Philippines.

Methods

US Cancer Incidence Data

Cancer incidence data for all invasive cancers newly diagnosed during the 21-year period 1990–2010 were obtained from 13 US SEER cancer registries (Table 1) [8]. Catchment areas for these population-based registries cover nearly two-thirds of the Filipino American population [9]. SEER data on race and Hispanic ethnicity are generally based on patients' medical records; for this analysis, Filipinos were included regardless of Hispanic ethnicity. Based on an algorithm developed by the North American Association for Central Cancer Registries, information on birthplace and surname was used to assign race/ethnicity when a specific race designation was lacking [10].

US Mortality Data

Mortality rates are based on the underlying causes of death in Filipino decedents from 36 US states over the period 2003–2011, as reported in detail in [11]. Death counts were obtained from the NCHS; the 36 states were chosen based on adoption of the 2003 death certificate standard, which captures detailed coded Asian race categories [12]. Death certificates are completed by medical examiners and may be subject to misclassification of race/ethnicity [13, 14].

US Population Data

Detailed population data for Filipino Americans are available from the 1990, 2000, and 2010 US censuses. Intercensal estimates were developed from linear interpolation between censuses [15]. Due to Hawaii's mixed Asian-American population, the SEER Hawaii registry developed state population estimates derived from sample

Table 1 Annual counts and distribution of Filipino populations by Surveillance, Epidemiology, End Results (SEER) registry and Census year

Census Year		N	%
	1990	1,040,610	–
	2000	1,420,523	–
	2010	1,793,997	–
1990			
	California	768,495	73.85%
	Connecticut	5,319	0.51%
	Atlanta (Metropolitan)	2,184	0.21%
	Hawaii	152,957	14.70%
	Iowa	1,574	0.15%
	Detroit (Metropolitan)	9,689	0.93%
	New Jersey	54,591	5.25%
	New Mexico	2,154	0.21%
	Utah	1,958	0.19%
	Seattle (Puget Sound)	41,689	4.01%
2000			
	California	1,017,248	71.61%
	Connecticut	8,938	0.63%
	Atlanta (Metropolitan)	5,681	0.40%
	Hawaii	200,386	14.11%
	Iowa	2,959	0.21%
	Detroit (Metropolitan)	13,743	0.97%
	New Jersey	91,022	6.41%
	New Mexico	3,895	0.27%
	Utah	4,310	0.30%
	Seattle (Puget Sound)	72,341	5.09%
2010			
	California	1,341,360	74.77%
	Connecticut	14,291	0.80%
	Atlanta (Metropolitan)	8,963	0.50%
	Hawaii	169,694	9.46%
	Iowa	4,851	0.27%
	Detroit (Metropolitan)	17,444	0.97%
	New Jersey	119,314	6.65%
	New Mexico	6,784	0.38%
	Utah	8,241	0.46%
	Seattle (Puget Sound)	103,055	5.74%

survey data collected by the Hawaii Department of Health [16]. Population data for mortality rates were calculated from the 2000 and 2010 Censuses, with interpolated population estimates for years between surveys, and the interpolated value for 2007 as the interval average [17].

Population counts of Filipinos by SEER region for the three censal years (1990, 2000, and 2010) are shown in Table 1.

Cancer Incidence and Population Data in the Philippines

Cancer incidence data for the Philippines were available from the Cancer Incidence in Five Continents (CI5) database, a collaboration between the International Agency for Research on Cancer (IARC) and the International Association of Cancer Registries (IACR) [18, 19]. This database provides detailed information on cancer incidence recorded by registries worldwide for 5-year time periods; indices of data quality are available by cancer site and registry (http://ci5.iarc.fr/CI5I-X/Pages/Quality_sel.aspx). For the Philippines, data are included in CI5 from two registries: (1) Manila, including the highly urbanized city of Manila, and several local cities and municipalities (population approximately 29 million) and (2) Rizal province, representing 14 municipalities (population approximately 32 million) (Table 2) [18, 19]. As these registries collected data for different time periods, we limited our analyses to the two time periods (1993–1997, 2003–2007) when both registries contributed data. The data, which were available as 5-year aggregated case counts and population totals by registry, sex, cancer site, and age at diagnosis (5-year age group), were converted into a SEER*Stat database for computing incidence rates for comparison to US Filipino rates [20]. Percent change was calculated between the two time periods.

The Manila and Rizal registries provided case counts for 16 or 17 age groups, depending on the time period. Given that there are 18 age groups for cancer case numerator data, we combined cases in age groups for which no population data were available (80–84, 85+, unknown age) [21]. Using the combined oldest age groups, we produced incidence rates for the two Philippine registries age-standardized to the US 2000 Standard Million population.

Table 2 Annual counts and distributions of Filipinos in the Philippines (Manila and Rizal), based on the Cancer Incidence in Five Continents (CI5) database

5-Year Period in CI5		N	%
	1993–1997	51,646,820	–
	2003–2007	61,915,826	–
1993–1997			
	Manila	25,379,745	49.14%
	Rizal	26,267,075	50.86%
2003–2007			
	Manila	29,280,897	47.29%
	Rizal	32,643,929	52.72%

Statistical Analysis

All rates and 95 % confidence intervals (CI) were calculated as cases or deaths per 100,000 persons. Incidence rates were calculated using SEER*Stat software (http://seer.cancer.gov/seerstat/). Mortality rates were computed in R. Rates were suppressed for case counts <10 [22]. Annual rates are shown graphically as trends, determined using joinpoint regression models to identify distinct slopes in the trends. Annual percentage change (APC) statistics (95 % confidence intervals (CI)) are used to characterize the trends' magnitude and direction [23]. A maximum of five joinpoints were allowed based on single year data. Rate estimates and trend lines from the trends based on joinpoint analyses are plotted on a semilogarithmic scale [24, 25].

Results and Discussion of Incidence and Mortality Patterns

Overview of the Most Common Cancer Sites and Trends

Overall cancer rates were higher for males than females in both the USA and the Philippines. Among US Filipino males, the five most common cancer sites were (1) prostate, (2) lung and bronchus, (3) colon and rectum, (4) non-Hodgkin lymphomas (NHL), and (5) liver (Table 3). The relative rank order of these five sites remained unchanged over the 21-year period. Among US Filipino females, the three most common sites were (1) breast, (2) colon and rectum, and (3) lung and bronchus, with thyroid and corpus uterus changing as the fourth and fifth most common sites across the time period (Table 4).

In contrast, the most common cancer sites among Filipino males in the Philippines differ somewhat, with the five most common sites for the two periods (1993–1997 and 2003–2007) being (1) lung and bronchus, (2) prostate, (3) colon and rectum, (4) liver, and (5) stomach (Table 5). Among females in the Philippines, the five most

Table 3 Age-adjusted incidence rates and 95 % confidence intervals (CI) of the top ten cancer sites, by time period, Filipino males, United States

1990–1995			
Rank	Site	Count	Rate (95 % CI)
	All Sites	8,823	399.2 (390.8, 407.7)
1	Prostate	2,757	133.1 (128.1, 138.2)
2	Lung and Bronchus	1,521	68.8 (65.3, 72.3)
3	Colon and Rectum	1,024	46.7 (43.9, 49.7)
4	Non-Hodgkin Lymphoma	427	18.5 (16.8, 20.4)
5	Liver	299	13 (11.6, 14.6)
6	Leukemia	297	11.8 (10.5, 13.3)
7	Urinary Bladder	234	10.9 (9.5, 12.4)
8	Pancreas	225	10.7 (9.4, 12.2)
9	Stomach	236	10.7 (9.4, 12.2)
10	Oral Cavity and Pharynx	251	10.6 (9.3, 12.0)

(continued)

Table 3 (continued)

1996–2000

Rank	Site	Count	Rate (95 % CI)
	All Sites	8,883	392 (383.4, 400.1)
1	Prostate	2,628	121.2 (116.6, 126.0)
2	Lung and Bronchus	1,623	72.3 (68.8, 75.9)
3	Colon and Rectum	1,096	48.1 (45.2, 51.0)
4	Non-Hodgkin Lymphoma	450	19.3 (17.5, 21.2)
5	Liver	340	14.2 (12.7, 15.9)
6	Urinary Bladder	264	12.3 (10.9, 13.9)
7	Stomach	243	10.9 (9.6, 12.4)
8	Oral Cavity and Pharynx	271	10.8 (9.5, 12.2)
9	Leukemia	261	10.6 (9.3, 12.0)
10	Kidney and Renal Pelvis	231	9.7 (8.4, 11.0)

2001–2005

Rank	Site	Count	Rate (95 % CI)
	All Sites	10,219	369.6 (362.3, 377.0)
1	Prostate	3,182	117.7 (113.5, 122.0)
2	Lung and Bronchus	1,795	66.9 (63.8, 70.1)
3	Colon and Rectum	1,312	47 (44.5, 49.7)
4	Non-Hodgkin Lymphoma	513	18.4 (16.8, 20.2)
5	Liver	419	14.6 (13.2, 16.2)
6	Urinary Bladder	299	11.4 (10.1, 12.8)
7	Leukemia	278	9.6 (8.5, 10.8)
8	Oral Cavity and Pharynx	279	9.4 (8.3, 10.6)
9	Kidney and Renal Pelvis	283	9.2 (8.2, 10.4)
10	Pancreas	228	8.7 (7.6, 9.9)

2006–2010

Rank	Site	Count	Rate (95 % CI)
	All Sites	11,576	352.2 (345.6, 358.9)
1	Prostate	3,350	101.9 (98.3, 105.5)
2	Lung and Bronchus	1,879	60.3 (57.5, 63.1)
3	Colon and Rectum	1,488	44.6 (42.3, 47)
4	Non-Hodgkin Lymphoma	587	18.2 (16.7, 19.8)
5	Liver	532	15.7 (14.3, 17.1)
6	Kidney and Renal Pelvis	487	13.7 (12.5, 15.0)
7	Urinary Bladder	330	10.7 (9.6, 12.0)
8	Pancreas	318	10 (8.9, 11.1)
9	Oral Cavity and Pharynx	337	9.5 (8.5, 10.6)
10	Leukemia	308	9.5 (8.4, 10.6)

Table 4 Age-adjusted incidence rates and 95 % confidence intervals (CI) of the top ten cancer sites, by time period, Filipina females, United States

1990–1995

Rank	Site	Count	Rate (95 % CI)
	All Sites	7978	273.8 (267.4, 280.3)
1	Breast	2702	85.7 (82.4, 89.2)
2	Colon and Rectum	728	28.1 (25.9, 30.4)
3	Lung and Bronchus	608	23.1 (21.2, 25.2)
4	Thyroid	532	15.6 (14.2, 17.0)
5	Corpus and Uterus, NOS	456	14.3 (13.0, 15.8)
6	Non-Hodgkin Lymphoma	329	12.6 (11.1, 14.1)
7	Cervix Uteri	401	12.4 (11.1, 13.7)
8	Ovary	346	11 (9.8, 12.3)
9	Leukemia	220	7.8 (6.7, 9.0)
10	Pancreas	166	7.1 (5.9, 8.3)

1996–2000

Rank	Site	Count	Rate (95 % CI)
	All Sites	9091	280.5 (274.6, 286.5)
1	Breast	3371	97.2 (94.0, 100.6)
2	Colon and Rectum	842	27.8 (25.9, 29.9)
3	Lung and Bronchus	703	24.1 (22.3, 26.0)
4	Corpus and Uterus, NOS	590	17.1 (15.7, 18.6)
5	Thyroid	595	16.7 (15.4, 18.2)
6	Non-Hodgkin Lymphoma	359	12.1 (10.8, 13.4)
7	Ovary	352	10.5 (9.4, 11.7)
8	Cervix Uteri	360	10.3 (9.2, 11.4)
9	Pancreas	183	6.6 (5.6, 7.7)
10	Leukemia	186	6 (5.2, 7.0)

2001–2005

Rank	Site	Count	Rate (95 % CI)
	All Sites	11,725	286.1 (280.9, 291.5)
1	Breast	4,142	96.1 (93.2, 99.1)
2	Colon and Rectum	1,147	29.5 (27.8, 31.3)
3	Lung and Bronchus	1,000	26.1 (24.5, 27.9)
4	Corpus and Uterus, NOS	866	19.8 (18.5, 21.2)
5	Thyroid	805	18.5 (17.2, 19.8)
6	Non-Hodgkin Lymphoma	467	12.1 (11, 13.3)
7	Ovary	433	10.4 (9.4, 11.4)
8	Cervix Uteri	358	8.4 (7.6, 9.3)
9	Pancreas	278	7.5 (6.6, 8.4)
10	Leukemia	237	6.1 (5.3, 7.0)

(continued)

Table 4 (continued)

2006–2010

Rank	Site	Count	Rate (95 % CI)
	All Sites	14,852	298.9 (294.0, 303.8)
1	Breast	5,190	100.2 (97.4, 103.0)
2	Colon and Rectum	1,407	29.2 (27.6, 30.7)
3	Lung and Bronchus	1,358	28.6 (27.1, 30.2)
4	Thyroid	1,195	23.8 (22.4, 25.2)
5	Corpus and Uterus, NOS	1,174	22.2 (20.9, 23.5)
6	Non-Hodgkin Lymphoma	598	12.6 (11.5, 13.6)
7	Ovary	506	10 (9.2, 10.9)
8	Pancreas	397	8.7 (7.8, 9.6)
9	Cervix Uteri	355	7 (6.3, 7.8)
10	Leukemia	312	6.7 (6.0, 7.5)

Table 5 Age-adjusted incidence rates and 95 % confidence intervals (CI) of the top ten cancer sites, by 5-year time period (1993–1997 and 2003–2007), males, Philippines (Manila and Rizal)

1993–1997

Rank	Site	Count	Rate (95 % CI)
	All Sites	23,476	314.6 (309.3–319.9)
1	Lung and Bronchus	5,429	77.9 (75.4–80.5)
2	Prostate	1,601	40.0 (37.8–42.3)
3	Colon and Rectum	2,356	33.6 (31.9–35.4)
4	Liver	2,629	32.0 (30.4–33.6)
5	Stomach	994	15.7 (14.5–17.0)
6	Non-Hodgkin Lymphoma	859	9.0 (8.2–9.9)
7	Larynx	626	8.9 (8.1–9.8)
8	Nasopharynx	936	8.6 (7.8–9.3)
9	Bladder	483	8.0 (7.2–9.0)
10	Leukemia	1,281	7.6 (7.0–8.3)

2003–2007

Rank	Site	Count	Rate (95 % CI)
	All Sites	32,398	335.6 (330.8–340.3)
1	Lung and Bronchus	6,347	71.3 (69.2–73.5)
2	Prostate	3,708	63.4 (61.1–65.8)
3	Colon and Rectum	4,175	43.9 (42.2–45.7)
4	Liver	3,269	30.6 (29.3–32.0)
5	Stomach	1,052	12.5 (11.5–13.4)
6	Non-Hodgkin Lymphoma	1,125	9.4 (8.6–10.1)
7	Leukemia	1,763	8.8 (8.2–9.5)
8	Bladder	622	8.0 (7.2–8.8)
9	Larynx	726	7.7 (7.0–8.4)
10	Nasopharynx	1,072	7.2 (6.6–7.8)
10	Skin	648	7.2 (6.5–7.9)

Table 6 Age-adjusted incidence rates and 95 % confidence intervals (CI) of the top ten cancer sites, by time period (1993–1997 and 2003–2007), females, Philippines (Manila and Rizal)

1993–1997			
Rank	Site	Count	Rate (95 % CI)
	All Sites	29,632	268.2 (264.6–271.9)
1	Breast	7,975	66.8 (65.1–68.5)
2	Cervix uteri	3,400	26.6 (25.5–27.6)
3	Colon and Rectum	2,187	25.8 (24.5–27.0)
4	Lung and Bronchus	1,807	21.4 (20.3–22.6)
5	Ovary	2,079	15.6 (14.8–16.4)
6	Corpus and Uterus, NOS	1,331	12.2 (11.5–13.0)
7	Thyroid	1,646	11.7 (11.0–12.4)
8	Liver	928	10.8 (10.0–11.7)
9	Stomach	726	8.6 (7.9–9.4)
10	Leukemia	1,123	6.2 (5.7–6.8)

2003–2007			
Rank	Site	Count	Rate (95 % CI)
	All Sites	44,776	295.1 (291.9–298.3)
1	Breast	13,051	80.4 (78.8–81.9)
2	Colon and Rectum	3,846	32.3 (31.1–33.5)
3	Lung and Bronchus	2,684	22.8 (21.9–23.8)
4	Cervix uteri	3,999	22.4 (21.6–23.2)
5	Corpus and Uterus, NOS	2,655	16.2 (15.5–16.9)
6	Ovary	2,776	16.0 (15.3–16.7)
7	Thyroid	3,056	15.2 (14.6–15.9)
8	Liver	1,369	11.8 (11.1–12.5)
9	Leukemia	1,644	8.0 (7.5–8.5)
10	Stomach	839	7.2 (6.6–7.8)

common sites were (1) breast, (2) cervix uteri, (3) colon and rectum, (4) lung and bronchus, and (5) ovary in 1993–1997 and (1) breast, (2) colon and rectum, (3) lung and bronchus, (4) cervix uteri, and (5) corpus uteri in 2003–2007 (Table 6).

From 1990 through 2010, US Filipino males experienced a decrease (APC=–1.2 %, 95 % CI:–1.5, –0.9) and US Filipinas experienced an increase (APC=0.6, 95 % CI: 0.4, 0.7) in cancer incidence overall (Tables 7 and 8). Among males, the decrease reflected a decline in the most common cancers (e.g., lung and prostate (Table 7, Fig. 1)). However, the incidence of less common cancers, including kidney and liver, increased notably over the 21-year period (Fig. 2), with kidney cancer ranking as the sixth most common cancer among US Filipino males in 2006–2010 (Table 3). In contrast, leukemia dropped from being the sixth most common cancer in the early 1990s to being the tenth most common cancer in the most recent 5-year period for US Filipino males (Table 3). Among US Filipinas, the most common cancers, including breast, lung, thyroid, and corpus and uteri, increased in incidence over the 21-year

Table 7 Annual Percent Change (APC) and 95 % confidence intervals (CI) in cancer incidence rates from 1990 to 2010, Filipino males, USA

Site	Time Period	APC (95 % CI)
All Sites	1990–1993	6.4 (1.5, 11.5)
	1993–2010	−1.2 (−1.5, −0.9)
Prostate	1990–1993	13.6 (0.6, 28.3)
	1993–2010	−2.3 (−3, −1.6)
Lung and Bronchus	1990–1996	3.0 (−0.6, 6.6)
	1996–2010	−1.9 (−2.7, −1.0)
Colon and Rectum	1990–2010	−0.4 (−1.0, 0.2)
Non-Hodgkin Lymphoma	1990–2010	−0.2 (−0.9, 0.6)
Liver	1990–2010	1.1 (0.2, 2.0)
Kidney and Renal Pelvis	1990–2010	3.4 (2.3, 4.5)
Leukemia	1990–2010	−1.4 (−2.3, −0.5)
Oral Cavity and Pharynx	1990–2010	−1.0 (−2.1, 0.2)
Urinary Bladder	1990–2010	−0.1 (−1.1, 0.9)
Pancreas	1990–2010	−0.3 (−1.6, 1.0)

APCs are computed using the SEER Joinpoint program, which identifies changes in trends

Table 8 Annual Percent Change (APC) and 95 % confidence intervals (CI) in cancer incidence rates from 1990 to 2010, Filipina females, USA

Site	Time Period	APC (95 % CI)
All Sites	1990–2010	0.6 (0.4, 0.7)
Breast	1990–2010	0.8 (0.4, 1.1)
Colon and Rectum	1990–2010	0.3 (−0.5, 1.1)
Lung and Bronchus	1990–2010	1.5 (0.9, 2.1)
Thyroid	1990–2004	1.4 (0.4, 2.4)
	2004–2010	6.4 (3.8, 9.1)
Corpus and Uterus, NOS	1990–2010	2.8 (2.2, 3.4)
Non-Hodgkin Lymphoma	1990–2010	0.2 (−0.8, 1.2)
Ovary	1990–2010	−0.6 (−1.7, 0.5)
Cervix Uteri	1990–2010	−3.8 (−5.0, −2.6)
Pancreas	1990–2010	1.5 (0.4, 2.7)
Leukemia	1990–2010	−0.4 (−2.1, 1.2)
Kidney and Renal Pelvis	1990–2010	2.5 (1.0, 4.1)
Urinary Bladder	1990–2010	1.9 (0.1, 3.7)

APCs are computed using the SEER Joinpoint program, which identifies changes in trends.

Fig. 1 Trends in incidence of the five most common cancers in US Filipinos, 1990–2010, males

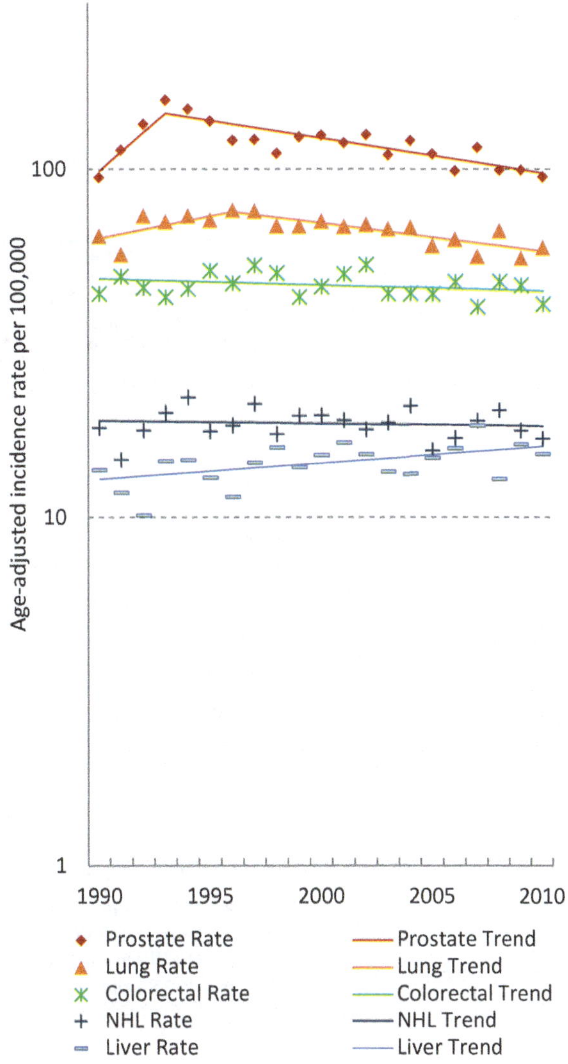

period (Table 8, Fig. 3). For thyroid cancer, the increase was dramatic, averaging 6.4 % (95 % CI: 3.8–9.1) per year from 2004 through 2010. Less common cancers (pancreas, kidney, and bladder) also showed slight increases in incidence over time (Fig. 4). The only notable rate decrease among Filipinas was for cervical cancer, declining 3.8 % per year (95 % CI:–5.0,–2.6). For NHL and colorectal and ovarian cancer, incidence rates were relatively stable (Figs. 3 and 4).

In the Philippines, overall cancer incidence increased between 1993–1997 and 2003–2007. Among males, the greatest increases occurred for prostate cancer and colorectal cancer, while lung and stomach cancer rates declined. Among females,

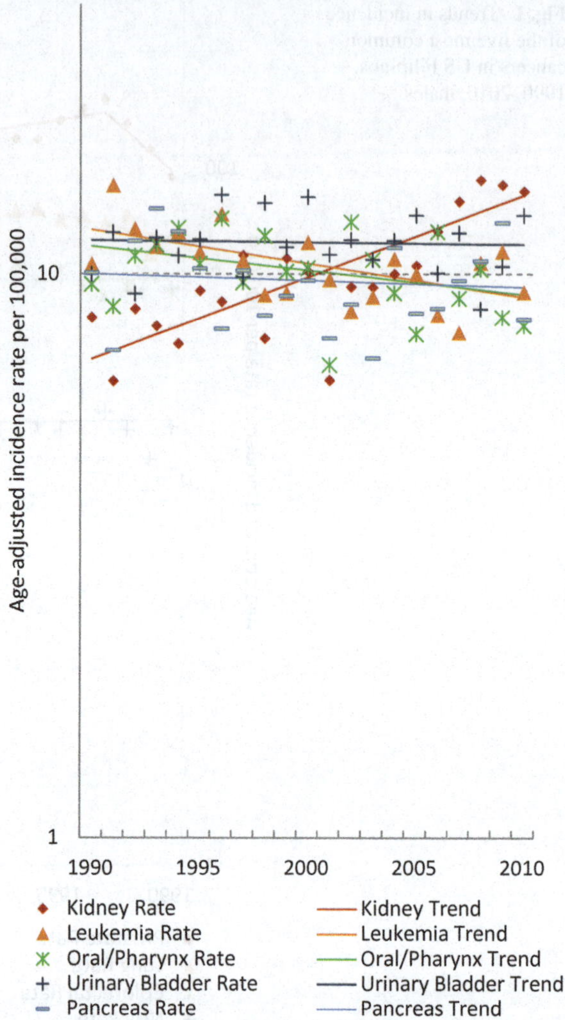

Fig. 2 Trends in incidence of the next five most common cancers in US Filipinos, 1990–2010, males

rates of cancers of the breast, colorectum, and thyroid, and of leukemia increased, while rates of cervical and stomach cancers declined. Incidence rates of NHL and liver cancer were stable in both males and females during this time (Fig. 5).

With regard to cancer mortality among Filipinos in the USA, lung, colorectal, prostate, liver, and pancreatic cancers were the five sites contributing most to cancer-related deaths among males (Table 9), while lung, breast, colorectal, pancreatic, and ovarian cancers were the five most common sites of cancer-related deaths for females (Table 10).

Fig. 3 Trends in incidence of the five most common cancers in US Filipinos, 1990–2010, females

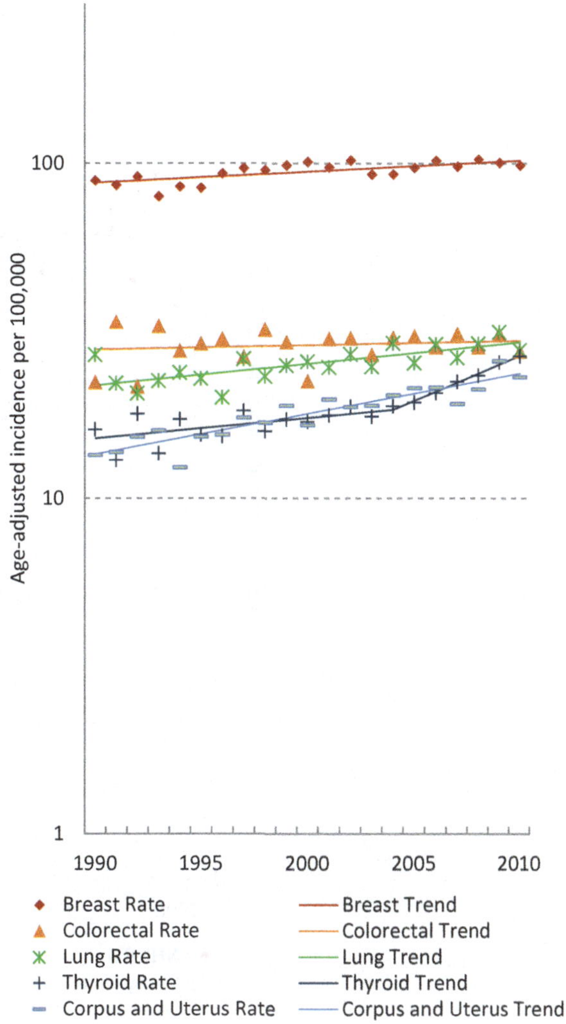

Site-Specific Patterns and Trends

Prostate Cancer

Prostate cancer ranked as the most common cancer site among US Filipino males over the entire 21-year period, despite steady rate declines after 1993 (APC=–2.3 %, 95 % CI:–3.0,–1.6), representing the largest incidence decrease of any cancer site (Fig. 1). In contrast, among males in the Philippines, the rate of prostate cancer increased by 50 % from 1993–1997 (40.0 per 100,000) to 2003–2007 (63.4 per 100,000), while remaining considerably lower than in the

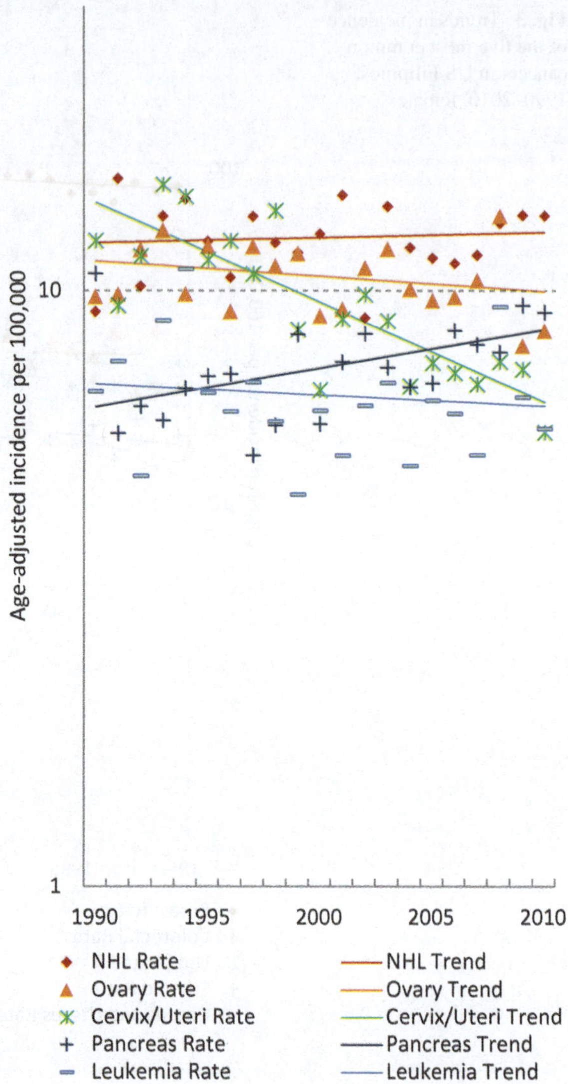

Fig. 4 Trends in incidence of the next five most common cancers in US Filipinos, 1990–2010, females

USA (101.9 per 100,000). Increased PSA screening has been attributed as the cause of much of the incidence differential between the two countries. While very little is known about nongenetic risk factors for prostate cancer, the dramatic differences in incidence between Filipinos in the USA and in the Philippines suggest that environmental factors may be relevant. Given the high burden of this disease and the migrant experience of Filipinos, research in this population may help to elucidate the etiologic role of lifestyle factors such as increased consumption of animal protein and dietary fat and decreased consumption of phytochemicals common in traditional Asian diets [26] (Fig. 6).

Fig. 5 Trends in mortality of the five most common cancer deaths in US Filipinos, 2003–2011, males

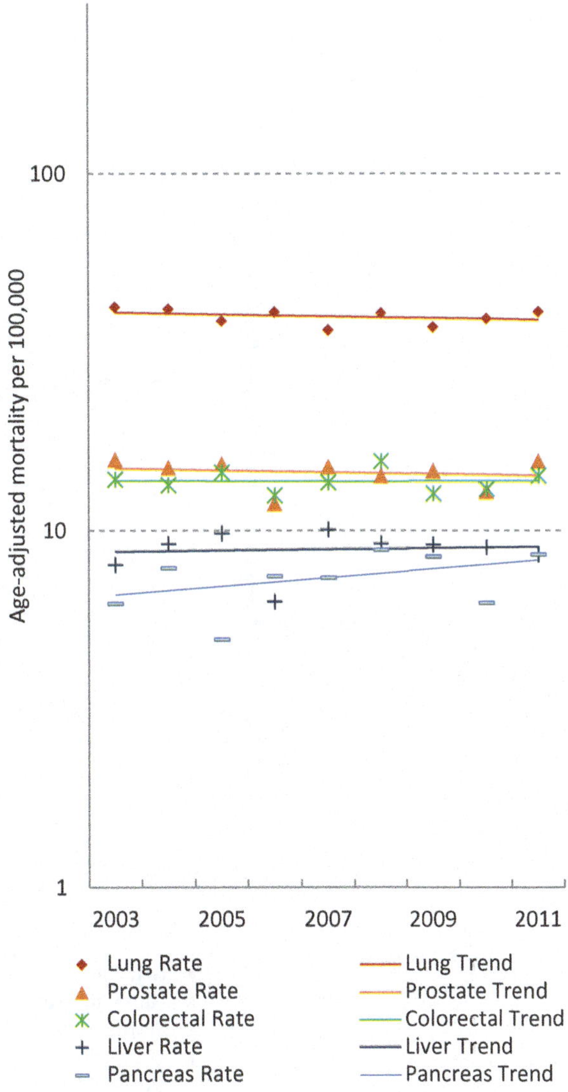

Fig. 6 Trends in mortality of the next five most common cancer deaths in US Filipinos, 2003–2011, males

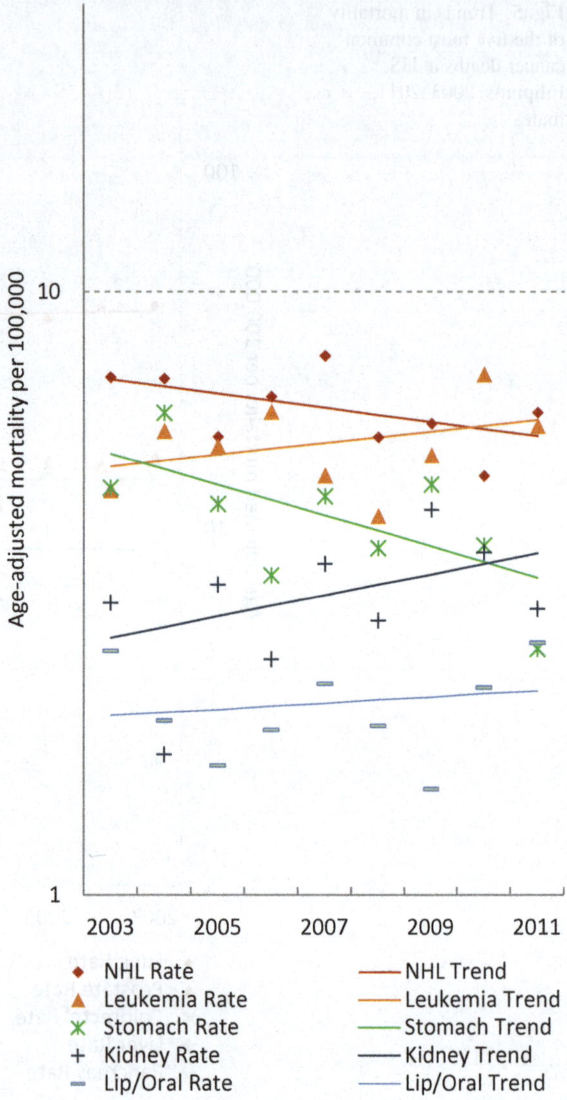

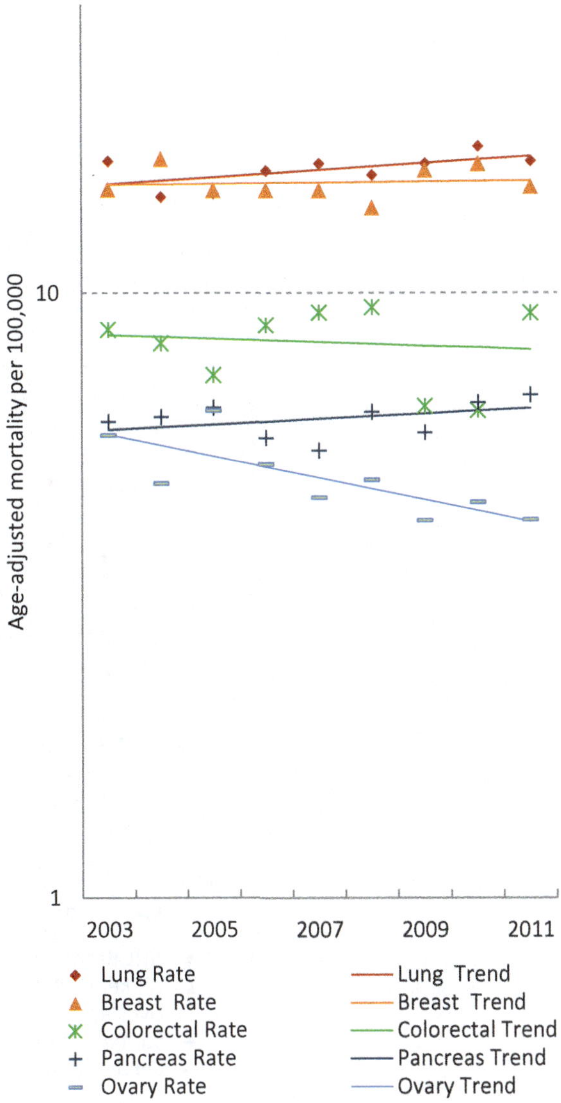

Fig. 7 Trends in mortality of the five most common cancer deaths in US Filipinos, 2003–2011, females

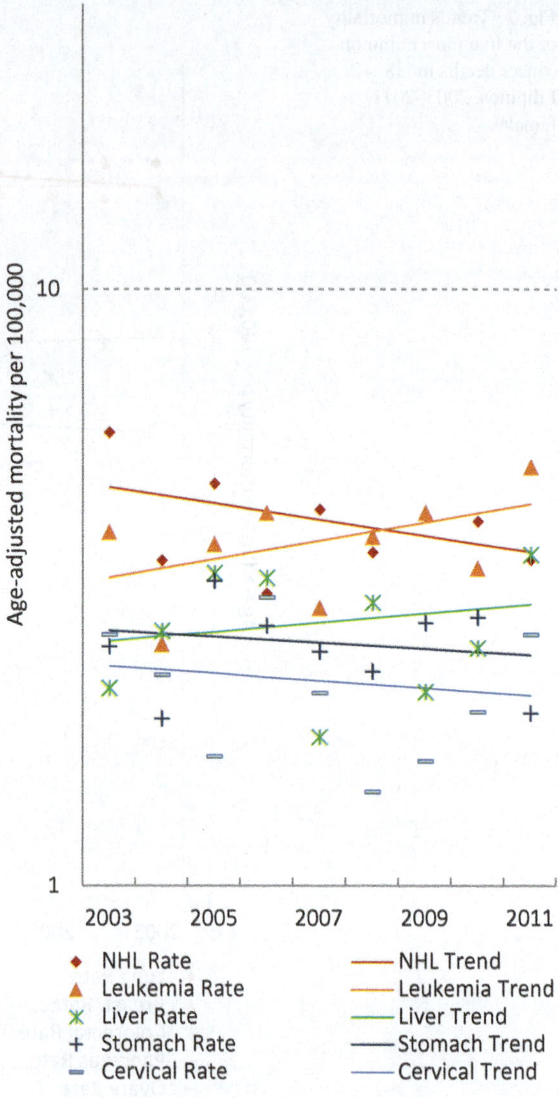

Fig. 8 Trends in mortality of the next five most common cancer deaths in U.S. Filipinos, 2003–2011, females

Breast Cancer

Among Filipina females in the USA and in the Philippines, breast cancer is the most commonly diagnosed cancer, with rates steadily increasing from 1990 to 2010 (APC=0.8 %, 95 % CI: 0.4, 1.1), or by almost 15 % from the 1990–1995 rate to the 2006–2010 rate (Fig. 3). In the Philippines, the rate increased by 20 % from 1993–1997 to 2003–2007 (Tables 4 and 6). The increasing trends in breast cancer incidence contrast with the well-documented declines among US non-Hispanic White women [27–29] but are consistent with reports showing considerable differences in

Table 9 Age-adjusted mortality rates and 95% confidence intervals (CI)for total cancers and top 10 cancer sites in Filipinos, 2003-2011, males, United States

2003–2011			
Rank	Site	Count	Rate (95%CI)
	All Sites	9526	131.6 (128.8, 134.3)
1	Lung and Bronchus	2926	39.9 (38.4, 41.4)
2	Prostate	849	14.6 (13.5, 15.6)
3	Colon and Rectum	1027	13.8 (12.9, 14.7)
4	Liver	721	8.8 (8.2, 9.5)
5	Pancreas	545	7.4 (6.8, 8.1)
6	Non-Hodgkins Lymphoma	444	6.4 (5.8, 7)
7	Leukemia	409	5.6 (5.1, 6.2)
8	Stomach	296	4.2 (3.7, 4.7)
9	Kidney	254	3.1 (2.7, 3.6)
10	Lip/Oral cavity	166	2.1 (1.7, 2.4)

Table 10 Age-adjusted mortality rates and 95% confidence intervals (CI) for total cancers and top 10 cancer sites in Filipinos, 2003-2011, females, United States

2003–2011			
Rank	Site	Count	Rate (95% CI)
	All Sites	10360	87 (85.2, 88.7)
1	Lung and Bronchus	1871	16.1 (15.3, 16.8)
2	Breast	2023	15.2 (14.5, 15.9)
3	Colon and rectum	935	8.2 (7.7, 8.8)
4	Pancreas	692	6.2 (5.7, 6.7)
5	Ovary	621	4.9 (4.5, 5.3)
6	Non-Hodgkin Lymphoma	446	4 (3.6, 4.4)
7	Leukemia	434	3.8 (3.5, 4.2)
8	Liver	303	2.7 (2.4, 3.1)
9	Stomach	292	2.5 (2.2, 2.8)
10	Cervix uteri	287	2.1 (1.9, 2.4)

California rates between US-born and foreign-born Filipinas and dramatic increases in incidence over time among US-born Filipinas [30, 31]. The secular trends seen here for Filipinas in the USA and the Philippines are consistent with the increases seen among women living in other Asian countries [32, 33]. Because mortality rates have not declined (Fig. 7), it is likely that these incidence patterns reflect changes in lifestyle risk factors, including menstrual and reproductive factors, diet, obesity, and physical activity, and, to a lesser extent, increases in mammographic screening. As US Filipinas are diagnosed with proportionally more tumors that are positive for Her2Neu relative to non-Hispanic Whites [34], it would be worthwhile to examine trends in incidence rates by breast cancer subtypes (Fig. 8).

Colorectal Cancer

Among US Filipinos, colorectal cancer incidence was stable in males and females from 1990 through 2010 (Figs. 1 and 3). However, a recent study of cancer incidence for the period 1988–2007 in California reported an increase in colorectal cancer incidence in Filipinas (APC = 1.6 %, 95 % CI: 0.5, 2.6) and stable rates among Filipinos [35]. In recent years (2006–2010), colorectal cancer was the third most commonly diagnosed cancer among US Filipinos (44.6 per 100,000) and second among US Filipinas (29.2 per 100,000) and the second and third most common cause of cancer death among US Filipinos and Filipinas, respectively. In the Philippines, colorectal cancer incidence rates increased considerably since the 1990s for both men and women, such that in 2003–2007, they were comparable to the US rates. In the USA, rates of colon and rectal cancer separately were stable over this time period for both Filipino males and females (data not shown). Some hereditary traits are important risk factors for this disease, including familial polyposis (formation of numerous polyps in the colon), familial nonpolyposis colorectal cancer (HNPCC), history of inflammatory bowel disease, and first-degree family history of colorectal cancer [36]. Additional risk factors include excessive alcohol use, obesity, and smoking [37]. Data from the California Health Interview Survey (CHIS) show increases from 2007 to 2014 in the percentage of adults who are overweight for both Filipino males and females (BMI > 25: 56.2 %–69.5 % among males, 31.5 %–38.7 % among females), although data for Asian-specific BMI cut points are not available. Future research efforts should focus on the prevention (both through lifestyle modifications and screening) and early detection of colorectal cancer in this population, in addition to evaluating the role of specific cultural dietary effects on colorectal cancer incidence in this population.

Lung Cancer

Among US Filipinos, lung cancer was the second most common cancer among males and third among females, but it was the leading cause of cancer death among both genders. In the Philippines, lung cancer is the most common cancer among males (71.3 per 100,000), with rates higher than for US Filipino males (60.3 per 100,000). Among Filipinas, rates are slightly lower in the Philippines (22.8 per 100,000) than in the USA (28.6 per 100,000). The trends of lung cancer in the USA also differ by gender, with a significantly declining trend among males (APC = −1.9 %, 95 % CI: −2.7,−1.0) during 1996–2010 and an increasing trend among females (APC = 1.5 %, 95 % CI: 0.9, 2.1) during 1990–2010 (Tables 7 and 8). Incidence trends varied, however, by tumor histology, reflecting the relative role of tobacco use in lung cancer occurrence in this population [38]. Among US Filipino males, rates of adenocarcinoma were unchanged over time, while rates of other subtypes (including small cell, squamous cell, and unspecified histology) declined significantly over time [38]. In contrast, rates of adenocarcinoma among females increased significantly over time. While all histologic subtypes are strongly associated with tobacco use, adenocarcinoma is less strongly associated with tobacco use, which is consistent with findings from a recent population-based case series that 70 % of Asian-American women diagnosed with lung cancer were lifetime never-smokers (in contrast to 14 % of Asian-American men) [39]. Although tobacco use appears to decrease with acculturation among Asian-American males (not specific to Filipinos), it increases with acculturation among Asian-American females [40]. This pattern with acculturation among women is suggested in the CHIS data, with higher prevalence of current smokers by English language fluency (very well vs. poor/well) among Filipinas (11 % vs. 1 %) [41]. Therefore, smoking prevention, particularly among US Filipinas, is imperative. However, given their low smoking prevalence, and the few known lung cancer risk factors among US never-smoker populations (some risk factors such as tuberculosis and other previous lung diseases, exposure to second-hand smoke, and other indoor and outdoor air pollution have been identified in Asia), additional research into etiologic risk factors may elucidate knowledge and progress against lung cancer among never-smokers.

Cervical Cancer

From 2006 through 2010, cervical cancer was the ninth most common cancer diagnosed in US Filipinas and the fourth most common cancer diagnosed among females in the Philippines. The incidence rate in the Philippines was threefold higher than the USA (22.4 vs. 7.5 per 100,000) during the time period 2003–2007. While cervical cancer was significantly more common in the Philippines, the rate declined by 16 % from 1993–1997 to 2003–2007. A significant decline also occurred from 1990 through 2010 among US Filipinas (APC=–3.8, 95 % CI:–5.0,–2.6) (Table 8, Fig. 4). Cervical cancer was the tenth most common cause of cancer-related death in US Filipinas, but a leading cause of cancer-related death among women in the Philippines [42, 43]. Stage at diagnosis differed considerably between the USA and the Philippines; the majority of cases in the USA are diagnosed at the localized or regional stage, while in the Philippines, the majority are diagnosed at a late stage (stage III) [42]. The most important risk factor is infection with types 16 and 18 of the human papillomavirus (HPV), which are associated with sexual behavior variables. HPV infection is reported to cause approximately 70 % of cervical cancers worldwide [44, 45]. In the Philippines, these high-risk HPV types are commonly found in women with cervical cancer [42]. While HPV prevalence among US Filipinas has not been reported, among women of all races in the USA, the most common high-risk HPV type is 53 (5.8 %), followed by 16 (4.2 %); type 18 is less common (1.8 %) [46]. The variation in prevalence of high-risk HPV types may explain the incidence rate disparity between the two populations. Other risk factors include a history of cigarette smoking and high parity [47, 48]. Differences in rates of screening (Pap smears), treatment options, and survival between the US Filipina population and women in the Philippines have been reported, with 5-year survival significantly lower in the Philippines (68.8 % vs. 42.9 %) [49]. Future research should focus on prevention measures, including the effects of screening guidelines and vaccination against HPV.

Thyroid Cancer

Among US Filipinos, thyroid cancer was the 4th most common cancer among females and the 12th most common among males from 2006 through 2010 (Table 4). Among US Filipinas, rates increased rapidly since 2004 by an annual average of 6.4 % (95 % CI: 3.8, 9.1) (Table 8, Fig. 3). The incidence rates for women (15.2 per 100,000) and for men (5.0 per 100,000) in the Philippines were lower than rates in the USA for Filipino women and men (23.8 and 7.3 per 100,000, respectively) but mirror the increasing trends in the USA in more recent years (14 % increase from the period 1993–1997 to 2003–2007 among women in the Philippines). While screening for thyroid cancer has become extensive in Asian countries such as Korea and Japan and hypothesized to account for some of the large incidence (but not mortality) rate increases over the past decade [50], we are not aware of similar expansion in thyroid cancer screening in the Philippines. Although changes in diagnostic imaging and over-screening may account for some of the increase in the USA, it has been a subject of debate whether better diagnostics and increased screening behavior alone account for the increase [51–53]. Known risk factors for thyroid cancer include exposure to ionizing radiation, a family history of thyroid cancer, and high body mass index; hormonal and reproductive factors, such as age at menarche and reproductive history, have also been implicated [51, 54–57]. Dietary factors such as consumption of fish and shellfish have been suggested to decrease risk, while low iodine increases risk of follicular thyroid cancer [58–60]. However, how diet influences thyroid function and thyroid hormone levels remains incompletely understood.

Corpus and Uteri Cancer

Cancer of the corpus and uteri (among which the vast majority is uterine (endometrial) cancer) is the most commonly diagnosed gynecologic cancer in women [61]. Incidence rates of uterine cancer in US Filipinas had risen 2.8 % per year (95 % CI: 2.2, 3.4) from 1990 to 2010, from 14.3 to 22.2 cases per 100,000, making uterine cancer the fifth most commonly diagnosed cancer. In the Philippines, rates were lower, but uterine cancer incidence also increased over time. Uterine cancer is believed to be caused by exposure to unopposed estrogen, through early age of menarche, nulliparity, late age at first birth, estrogen-only hormone therapy, or high-dose estrogen in oral contraceptive pills are also implicated. Obesity is one of the strongest and most important modifiable risk factors for this cancer, and US Filipinas have the highest body mass index of all Asian-American ethnicities [62, 63], with prevalence of obesity rising sharply in the past 20 years. Recent immigrants have been disproportionately affected due to adoption of high-fat western diet and reduced physical activity. In 2008, the 15-year increase in obesity prevalence was 164 % in long-term Filipino immigrants and 256 % in recent Filipino immigrants, representing the most dramatic increases of any Asian group [64]. Efforts should be taken to prevent weight gain and obesity prevalence among Filipinas in the U.S. and Philippines.

Liver Cancer

Liver cancer was the fifth most commonly diagnosed cancer among US Filipino males (15.7 per 100,000) and the fourth leading cause of cancer death in this group from 1990 through 2010. This cancer is comparatively less common among Filipinas, as the 14th most common cancer and eighth leading cause of cancer deaths. Incidence rates among US Filipino males increased by an average of 1.1 % per year (95 % CI: 0.2, 2.0) since 1990. In the Philippines, the incidence rate during the time period 2003–2007 was almost twice the US rate (30.6 vs. 15.7 cases per 100,000) among males, ranking as the fourth most common cancer. Liver cancer among women in the Philippines was also more common than among Filipinas in the USA (11.8 per vs. 4.6 cases per 100,000; 2003–2007). The most significant risk factor for liver cancer worldwide is infection with hepatitis B virus (HBV); coinfection with hepatitis C virus (HCV) increases risk further [65]. A recent study of hepatitis B surface antigen seroprevalence in the Philippines determined that 16.7 % of randomly sampled adults were seropositive, corresponding to an estimated 7.3 million infected people, which likely explains some proportion of the higher rates in the Philippines as compared to the USA [66]. Additional risk factors, particularly among Filipinos in the USA, include excessive alcohol intake over a long period of time, cirrhosis of the liver (often a result of excessive alcohol intake), and obesity. Immunization against HBV, especially in newborns, reduces the incidence of liver cancer [65, 67]. Successful efforts to provide HBV immunizations and education regarding HBV transmission will impact future liver cancer incidence worldwide.

Kidney and Renal Pelvis Cancer

Kidney and renal pelvis cancer is currently the sixth most commonly diagnosed cancer among US Filipino males and the ninth leading cause of death. In males, the incidence rate in the most recent 5-year period (2006–2010) was 13.7 per 100,000, having increased steadily by an average of 3.4 % per year since 1990 (95 % CI: 2.3, 4.5) (Table 7, Fig. 2). In females, the incidence rate was less than half that for males (4.5 per 100,000) but also rose steadily since 1990 (2.5 % per year; 95 % CI: 1.0, 4.1). From 2003 through 2007, incidence rates for US Filipinos were twice those for males and females in the Philippines (6.2 and 2.8 cases per 100,000, respectively). In addition to increasing age, other established risk factors for kidney and renal pelvis cancer are cigarette smoking, obesity, and hypertension [68]. According to 2011/2012 data from the CHIS, 18.1 % of Filipino men in California are current smokers, while 27.9 % are former smokers [41], with little change since 2007 [69]. For women, smoking prevalence was low but appears to be increasing, up from 4.6 to 7.8 % from 2007 to 2011/2012. CHIS data show increases from 2007 to 2011/2012 in the percentage of adults who are overweight for both Filipino males and females (BMI > 25: 57.7–69.5 % among males, 32.4–42.4 % among females). While it is not clear why kidney cancer incidence rates are higher in Filipinos in the USA than in the Philippines, differences in smoking rates and increase in body weight due to acculturation, in addition to increased screening rates and changes in diagnostic procedures, may be relevant.

Non-Hodgkin Lymphomas (NHL)

NHL was the fourth most common cancer among US Filipino men and the sixth most common cancer among US Filipino women from 2003 through 2007. In the USA, it ranked as the sixth most common cause of cancer death among Filipino men and women. Incidence rates were higher for Filipino males and females in the USA (18.2 and 12.7 per 100,000, respectively) than in the Philippines (9.4 and 7.1 per 100,000, respectively) during 2003–2007. A prior assessment in California found nearly identical incidence rates for foreign-born and US-born Filipinos [70]. NHL incidence trends have been stable since the 1990s. Risk factors for NHL are not well understood, but rates were higher among men than among women, both in the USA and in the Philippines, and it is slightly more common among men older than 65 years of age. Immune system deficiency, such as that occurs with infection with HIV, is associated with an increased risk. Rates of NHL are substantially lower among Filipinos (and all Asian ethnic groups in the USA and Asia) than non-Hispanic Whites [71]. As NHL represents an assortment of subtypes heterogeneous with respect to histologic, clinical, prognostic, and (likely) etiologic characteristics, incidence of distinct NHL subtypes should be assessed among Filipinos. Evidence from a prior analysis of NHL subtype incidence in all Asians combined showed increasing risks of indolent lymphoma subtypes (follicular lymphoma, chronic lymphocytic leukemia/small cell lymphoma) among Asians with US birthplace and neighborhood acculturation indicators, pointing to an important influence of environmental factors that change with immigration and acculturation to a Westernized lifestyle [70].

Ovarian Cancer

In recent years, ovarian cancer was the seventh most common cancer type among US Filipinas and the sixth most common cancer type among women in the Philippines; in the USA, it was the fifth leading cause of cancer death. The incidence rate was lower in the USA (10.0 cases per 100,000) than in the Philippines (16.0 cases per 100,000) from 2003 through 2007, but incidence rates have remained stable in both populations. Risk factors for ovarian cancer include increasing age (55 years and older), nulliparity, and the use of hormone replacement therapy. A family history of ovarian cancer is also a strong risk factor; it is estimated that heredity constitutes 5–10 % of all ovarian cancers [72–77]. Factors that reduce risk include the use of oral contraceptives, surgical tubal ligation, and hysterectomy [76]. Study of the prevalence of these risk factors, specifically the use of oral contraceptives and postmenopausal hormone replacement therapy, as well as certain genetic mutations (e.g., BRCA) among the US Filipina and Philippines populations, should be conducted to better understand the higher incidence of ovarian cancer in the Philippines vs. US Filipinas.

Leukemia

From 1990 to 2010, the incidence of leukemia in US Filipino males declined. In the early 1990s, this cancer ranked as the sixth most commonly diagnosed cancer among Filipino males and in the most recent time period (2006–2010) as the tenth most common cancer, with an incidence rate of 9.5 cases per 100,000. Among US Filipinas, the rate has remained stable or declined slightly; for 2006–2010, it was 6.7 cases per 100,000. Leukemia is ranked as the seventh leading cause of cancer death in both Filipinos and Filipinas in the USA. From 2003 through 2007, the incidence rates for males in the Philippines and in the USA were similar (8.8 vs. 9.2 cases per 100,000, respectively), but among females, the incidence rate in the Philippines was 80 % higher than the US rate (8.0 vs. 6.3 cases per 100,000, respectively). For the period 1973–1986, incidence rates similarly had been reported as higher in the Philippines than in the USA among females, but not males [78]. Smoking and exposure to radiation and certain chemicals, particularly benzene, are risk factors for leukemia [79, 80]. However, risk factors differ by leukemia subtype, so future studies should compare incidence rates of leukemia by subtype in the Philippines and the USA to better understand the geographical differences in incidence among females.

Oral Cavity and Pharyngeal Cancers

Cancers of the oral cavity and pharynx were the ninth most common type of cancer among US Filipino males but, at 15th, was considerably less common among females. From 2006 to 2010, the incidence rate for US Filipino males was twice that for females (9.5 vs. 4.2 per 100,000), and this group of cancers is ranked the tenth leading cause of cancer death among US Filipino males (2.5 per 100,000). From 1990 through 2010, the incidence rate in the USA declined significantly among females (APC=–2.8 %; 95 % CI:–4.0,–1.5) and was stable among males. Only nasopharyngeal cancer incidence rates are reported in the Philippines data, which were slightly lower than the US rates for oral and pharyngeal cancers among males and females (7.2 and 2.9 per 100,000, respectively) [18, 19]. Risk factors for these cancers include diet, cigarette smoking, and chewing tobacco, as well as heavy alcohol use and infection with Epstein-Barr virus and HPV [81, 82]. As described above, smoking prevalence among US Filipino males has remained relatively stable in recent years but increased among females, which may have an effect on future trends of oral and pharyngeal cancer in this group [41].

Bladder Cancer

Bladder cancer was the 7th most common cancer diagnosed in US Filipino males and the 17th most common cancer in US Filipinas from 2006 through 2010. The incidence rate among US Filipino males in the most recent 5-year period was more than three times that among females (10.7 vs. 2.9 per 100,000). For males, annual rates have been stable, while for females, rates increased by an average 1.9 % per year from 1990 through 2010 (95 % CI: 0.1, 3.7). Bladder cancer incidence rates were slightly lower in the Philippines than in the USA for males (8.0 per 100,000) and similar for females (2.8 per 100,000) during 2003–2007. Cigarette smoking, occupational exposures, various medical conditions, and related treatment are major risk factors for this cancer [83, 84]. The increasing incidence rates among US Filipinas may be related to smoking patterns, given evidence of increases in smoking rates among Filipinas [41, 69]. In the USA, approximately 80 % of bladder cancer diagnoses are considered noninvasive or "superficial," meaning many of these cancers may be cured [83]; indeed, mortality is low and the 5-year survival for this cancer in the general population is estimated to be 77 % [85]. Further study into differences in smoking patterns between the USA and Philippines and its impact on bladder cancer (and other smoking-related cancers) warrant study.

Pancreatic Cancer

Pancreatic cancer was the eighth most common cancer in US Filipino males and females from 2006 through 2010, and the fifth and fourth leading cause of cancer death, respectively. Although US Filipino males had a higher incidence rate than Filipinas (10.0 and 8.7 per 100,000), incidence has increased among females since 1990 (1.5 % per year; 95 % CI: 0.4, 2.7) and was stable in males. Incidence of this cancer in the Philippines (7.1 and 6.7 per 100,000) from 2003 to 2007 was slightly lower than in the USA for both males and females (10.0 and 8.7 per 100,000) from 2006 to 2010. Risk factors for pancreatic cancer are not well understood, but they include cigarette smoking, obesity, chronic pancreatitis, diabetes, family history of pancreatitis or pancreatic cancer, and mutations in the BRCA2 gene [86, 87]. This cancer has a poor prognosis in all racial/ethnic groups, with approximately only 7 % of all diagnoses surviving 5 years. Current smoking patterns may affect future incidence of pancreatic cancer, particularly increasing prevalence with acculturation among US Filipino females. It has recently been shown that pancreatic cancer risk dropped quickly after smoking cessation, suggesting that smoking may be a late-stage carcinogen [88].

Summary

The incidence and mortality patterns and trends presented for Filipinos in this chapter provide data to support targeted areas for cancer prevention, such as obesity for reducing the risks of uterine, colorectal, and breast cancers, and smoking prevention and cessation for lung, kidney, oral cavity and pharyngeal, bladder and pancreatic cancers. The continuing increases in rates of breast, lung, thyroid, kidney, and bladder cancers among Filipinas and of kidney cancer among Filipino males are of particular concern and warrant further attention. For those sites that demonstrate changing trends or dramatic differences between Filipinos in the USA and in the Philippines, further targeted studies can leverage these incidence patterns to elucidate environmental and modifiable risk factors.

Financial Disclosure This work was supported by the Stanford Cancer Institute (to S. Glaser), National Institute on Minority Health and Health Disparities (grant number R01 MD007012 to M. Cullen and L. Palaniappan), and the NIH National Center for Advancing Translational Sciences 1-KL2-TR-001444 (to C. Thompson). The collection of cancer incidence data used in this study was supported by the California Department of Health Services as part of the statewide cancer reporting program mandated by California Health and Safety Code Section 103885; the National Cancer Institute's Surveillance, Epidemiology, and End Results Program under contract HHSN261201000140C awarded to the Cancer Prevention Institute of California, contract HHSN261201000035C awarded to the University of Southern California, and contract HHSN261201000034C awarded to the Public Health Institute; and the Centers for Disease Control and Prevention's National Program of Cancer Registries, under agreement #1U58 DP000807-01 awarded to the Public Health Institute.

References

1. U.S. Census Bureau (2012) The Asian population: 2010. 2010 census briefs. U.S. Department of Commerce, Washington, DC
2. Takaki R (1989) Strangers from a different shore: a history of Asian Americans. Penguin, New York
3. Asian & Pacific Islander American Health Forum 1986-2011. Demographic and socioeconomic profiles of Asian Americans, Native Hawaiians, and Pacific Islanders in the United States. http://www.apiahf.org/sites/default/files/Demographic_Socioeconomic_Profiles_AANHPI.pdf2011.
4. Gomez SL, Noone AM, Lichtensztajn DY et al (2013) Cancer incidence trends among Asian American populations in the United States, 1990-2008. J Natl Cancer Inst 105(15):1096–1110
5. Miller BA, Chu KC, Hankey BF, Ries LA (2008) Cancer incidence and mortality patterns among specific Asian and Pacific Islander populations in the U.S. Cancer Causes Control 19(3):227–256
6. McCracken M, Olsen M, Chen MS Jr et al (2007) Cancer incidence, mortality, and associated risk factors among Asian Americans of Chinese, Filipino, Vietnamese, Korean, and Japanese ethnicities. CA Cancer J Clin 57(4):190–205
7. Gomez SL, Glaser SL, Horn-Ross PL et al (2014) Cancer research in Asian American, Native Hawaiian, and Pacific Islander populations: accelerating cancer knowledge by acknowledging and leveraging heterogeneity. Cancer Epidemiol Biomarkers Prev 23(11):2202–2205
8. Surveillance, Epidemiology, and End Results (SEER) Program (www.seer.cancer.gov) SEER*Stat Database: Incidence—SEER 11, plus Greater CA and NJ, Nov 2012 Sub (1990-2010) detailed API plus White non-Hispanic—pops projected from populations (no HTR adjustment). Surveillance Research Program, Cancer Statistics Branch, released May 2013, based on the November 2012 submission
9. Surveillance Epidemiology and End Results web site, http://seer.cancer.gov/registries/data.html. SEER Registries. [Internet]. Accessed December 2010; http://seer.cancer.gov/registries/data.html
10. NAACCR Race and Ethnicity Workgroup (2011) NAACCR Asian Pacific Islander Identification Algorithm [NAPIIA v1.2.1]. North American Association of Central Cancer Registries, Springfield, IL. http://www.naaccr.org/LinkClick.aspx?fileticket=3HnBhlmhkBs%3D&tabid=92&mid=432;August 2011

11. Thompson CA, Gomez SL, Hastings, KG, Kapphahn K, Yu P, Shariff-Marco S, Bhatt AS, Wakelee HA, Patel MI, Cullen MR, Palaniappan LP. The burden of cancer in Asian Americans: a report of national mortality trends by Asian ethnicity. Cancer Epidemiol Biomarkers Prev in press
12. Hoyert DL, Kung HC (1997) Asian or Pacific Islander mortality, selected states, 1992. Mon Vital Stat Rep 46(1 Suppl):1–63
13. Rosenberg HM, Maurer JD, Sorlie PD et al (1999) Quality of death rates by race and Hispanic Origin: a summary of current research, 1999. Series 2: Data Evaluation and Methods Research No. 128. National Center for Health Statistics, Hyattsville
14. Sorlie PD, Rogot E, Johnson NJ (1992) Validity of demographic characteristics on the death certificate. Epidemiology 3(2):181–184
15. U.S. Census Bureau (2001) Appendix H. Characteristic Iterations. Census 2000 Summary File 2 Technical Documentation, U.S. Census Bureau, p H-1. www.census.gov/prod/cen2000/doc/sf2.pdf. Accessed Jan 2011
16. American Cancer Society (2010) Cancer Research Center of Hawai'i, Hawai'i State Department of Health. Hawai'i Cancer Fact & Figures 2010. http://www.uhcancercenter.org/research/research-highlightsreports. Accessed 4 Feb 2013
17. U.S. Census Bureau (2011) Asian alone by selected groups. American Community Survey 1-year estimates
18. Curado MP, Edwards BK, Shin HR et al (2007) Cancer incidence in five continents, vol IX. IARC Scientific, Lyon
19. Parkin DM, Whelan SL, Ferlay J, Raymond L, Young J (eds) (1997). Cancer in five continents, vol. VII. IARC Scientific, Lyon
20. Surveillance Research Program (2014) National Cancer Institute SEER*Stat software (seer.cancer.gov/seerstat) version v 8.1.5. Database name: cancer in five continents—only Asian Countries, Vols. VII, VIII, IX and X
21. Personal communication with Jacques Ferlay (Section of Cancer Surveillance). IARC, Lyon. October 3, 2014.
22. Brillinger DR (1986) The natural variability of vital rates and associated statistics. Biometrics 42:693–734
23. Kim HJ, Fay MP, Feuer EJ, Midthune DN (2000) Permutation tests for joinpoint regression with applications to cancer rates. Stat Med 19:335–351; correction: 2001;2020:2655
24. Devesa SS, Donaldson J, Fears T (1995) Graphical presentation of trends in rates. Am J Epidemiol 141(4):300–304
25. Jatoi I, Anderson WF, Rao SR, Devesa SS (2005) Breast cancer trends among black and white women in the United States. J Clin Oncol 23(31):7836–7841
26. Sim HG, Cheng CW (2005) Changing demography of prostate cancer in Asia. Eur J Cancer 41(6):834–845
27. Clarke CA, Glaser SL (2007) Declines in breast cancer after the WHI: apparent impact of hormone therapy. Cancer Causes Control 18(8):847–852
28. Edwards BK, Ward E, Kohler BA et al (2010) Annual report to the nation on the status of cancer, 1975-2006, featuring colorectal cancer trends and impact of interventions (risk factors, screening, and treatment) to reduce future rates. Cancer 116(3):544–573
29. Kurian AW, Clarke CA, Carlson RW (2009) The decline in breast cancer incidence: real or imaginary? Curr Oncol Rep 11(1):21–28
30. Gomez SL, Quach T, Horn-Ross PL et al (2010) Hidden breast cancer disparities in Asian women: disaggregating incidence rates by ethnicity and migrant status. Am J Public Health 100(Suppl 1):S125–S131
31. Reynolds P, Hurley S, Goldberg D, Quach T, Rull R, Von Behren J (2011) An excess of breast cancer among young California-born Asian women. Ethn Dis 21(2):196–201
32. Shin HR, Joubert C, Boniol M et al (2010) Recent trends and patterns in breast cancer incidence among Eastern and Southeastern Asian women. Cancer Causes Control 21(11): 1777–1785

33. Ziegler RG, Anderson WF, Gail MH (2008) Increasing breast cancer incidence in China: the numbers add up. J Natl Cancer Inst 100(19):1339–1341
34. Telli ML, Chang ET, Kurian AW et al (2011) Asian ethnicity and breast cancer subtypes: a study from the California Cancer Registry. Breast Cancer Res Treat 127(2):471–478
35. Giddings BH, Kwong SL, Parikh-Patel A, Bates JH, Snipes KP (2012) Going against the tide: increasing incidence of colorectal cancer among Koreans, Filipinos, and South Asians in California, 1988-2007. Cancer Causes Control 23(5):691–702
36. Colon Cancer Treatment (PDQ). http://www.cancer.gov/cancertopics/pdq/treatment/colon/ Accessed 13 Jan 2015. U.S. Department of Health and Human Services, National Cancer Institute, Bethesda, MD. http://www.cancer.gov/cancertopics/pdq/treatment/colon/HealthProfessional
37. A snapshot of colorectal cancer, incidence and mortality. http://www.cancer.gov/researchand-funding/snapshots/colorectal Accessed 13 Jan 2015. U.S. Department of Health and Human Services, National Cancer Institute, Bethesda, MD. http://www.cancer.gov/cancertopics/pdq/treatment/colon/HealthProfessional
38. Cheng I, Le GM, Noone AM et al (2014) Lung cancer incidence trends by histology type among Asian American, Native Hawaiian, and Pacific Islander populations in the United States, 1990-2010. Cancer Epidemiol Biomarkers Prev 23(11):2250–2265
39. Gomez SL, Chang ET, Shema SJ et al (2011) Survival following non-small cell lung cancer among Asian/Pacific Islander, Latina, and Non-Hispanic white women who have never smoked. Cancer Epidemiol Biomarkers Prev 20(3):545–554
40. Choi S, Rankin S, Stewart A, Oka R (2008) Effects of acculturation on smoking behavior in Asian Americans: a meta-analysis. J Cardiovasc Nurs 23(1):67–73
41. CHIS 2011–2012 Adult Public Use File. UCLA Center for Health Policy Research, Los Angeles, CA. Accessed 16 Jan 2015. http://healthpolicy.ucla.edu/Pages/home.aspx
42. Domingo EJ, Dy Echo AV (2009) Epidemiology, prevention and treatment of cervical cancer in the Philippines. J Gynecol Oncol 20(1):11–16
43. Laudico A, Medina VM, Mirasol-Lumague MR et al (2010) 2010 Philippine Cancer Facts and Estimates. Manila Cancer Registry, Manila
44. Clifford GM, Smith JS, Plummer M, Munoz N, Franceschi S (2003) Human papillomavirus types in invasive cervical cancer worldwide: a meta-analysis. Br J Cancer 88(1):63–73
45. Bosch FX, Manos MM, Munoz N et al (1995) Prevalence of human papillomavirus in cervical cancer: a worldwide perspective. International biological study on cervical cancer (IBSCC) Study Group. J Natl Cancer Inst 87(11):796–802
46. Hariri S, Unger ER, Sternberg M et al (2011) Prevalence of genital human papillomavirus among females in the United States, the National Health and Nutrition Examination Survey, 2003-2006. J Infect Dis 204(4):566–573
47. Cervical Cancer Prevention (PDQ). http://www.cancer.gov/cancertopics/pdq/prevention/cervical/Patient/page3#_16 Accessed: 16 Jan 2015. U.S. Department of Health and Human Services, National Cancer Institute, Bethesda, MD. http://www.cancer.gov/cancertopics/pdq/prevention/cervical/Patient/page3#_16.
48. Munoz N, Franceschi S, Bosetti C et al (2002) Role of parity and human papillomavirus in cervical cancer: the IARC multicentric case-control study. Lancet 359(9312):1093–1101
49. Redaniel MT, Laudico A, Mirasol-Lumague MR, Gondos A, Brenner H (2011) Cancer survival differences between European countries and an urban population from the Philippines. Eur J Public Health 21(2):221–228
50. Vaccarella S, Dal Maso L, Laversanne M, Bray F, Plummer M, Franceschi S (2015) The impact of diagnostic changes on the rise in thyroid cancer incidence: a population-based study in selected high-resource countries. Thyroid 25(10):1127–1136
51. Horn-Ross PL, Lichtensztajn DY, Clarke CA et al (2014) Continued rapid increase in thyroid cancer incidence in California: trends by patient, tumor, and neighborhood characteristics. Cancer Epidemiol Biomarkers Prev 23(6):1067–1079
52. Ahn HS, Kim HJ, Welch HG (2014) Korea's thyroid-cancer "epidemic"—screening and overdiagnosis. N Engl J Med 371(19):1765–1767
53. Lee JH, Shin SW (2014) Overdiagnosis and screening for thyroid cancer in Korea. Lancet 384(9957):1848

54. Horn-Ross PL, Morris JS, Lee M et al (2001) Iodine and thyroid cancer risk among women in a multiethnic population: the Bay Area Thyroid Cancer Study. Cancer Epidemiol Biomarkers Prev 10(9):979–985
55. Horn-Ross PL, McClure LA, Chang ET et al (2011) Papillary thyroid cancer incidence rates vary significantly by birthplace in Asian American women. Cancer Causes Control 22(3):479–485
56. Davies L, Welch HG (2006) Increasing incidence of thyroid cancer in the United States, 1973-2002. JAMA 295(18):2164–2167
57. Pellegriti G, Frasca F, Regalbuto C, Squatrito S, Vigneri R (2013) Worldwide increasing incidence of thyroid cancer: update on epidemiology and risk factors. J Cancer Epidemiol 2013:965212
58. Dal Maso L, Bosetti C, La Vecchia C, Franceschi S (2009) Risk factors for thyroid cancer: an epidemiological review focused on nutritional factors. Cancer Causes Control 20(1): 75–86
59. Choi WJ, Kim J (2014) Dietary factors and the risk of thyroid cancer: a review. Clin Nutr Res 3(2):75–88
60. Liu ZT, Lin AH (2014) Dietary factors and thyroid cancer risk: a meta-analysis of observational studies. Nutr Cancer 66(7):1165–1178
61. American Cancer Society (2014) Cancer facts & figures 2014. American Cancer Society, Atlanta
62. Gomez SL, Kelsey JL, Glaser SL, Lee MM, Sidney S (2004) Immigration and acculturation in relation to health and health-related risk factors among specific Asian subgroups in a health maintenance organization. Am J Public Health 94(11):1977–1984
63. Klatsky AL, Armstrong MA (1991) Cardiovascular risk factors among Asian Americans living in northern California. Am J Public Health 81(11):1423–1428
64. Singh GK, Siahpush M, Hiatt RA, Timsina LR (2011) Dramatic increases in obesity and overweight prevalence and body mass index among ethnic-immigrant and social class groups in the United States, 1976-2008. J Community Health 36(1):94–110
65. General Information about Adult Primary Liver Cancer.http://www.cancer.gov/cancertopics/pdq/treatment/adult-primary-liver/Patient#Keypoint2 Accessed 26 Nov 2014. U.S. Department of Health and Human Services, National Cancer Institute, Bethesda
66. Wong SN, Ong JP, Labio ME et al (2013) Hepatitis B infection among adults in the Philippines: a national seroprevalence study. World J Hepatol 5(4):214–219
67. Chang MH, Chen TH, Hsu HM et al (2005) Prevention of hepatocellular carcinoma by universal vaccination against hepatitis B virus: the effect and problems. Clin Cancer Res 11(21):7953–7957
68. Chow WH, Dong LM, Devesa SS (2010) Epidemiology and risk factors for kidney cancer. Nat Rev Urol 7(5):245–257
69. CHIS 2007 Adult Public Use File. UCLA Center for Health Policy Research, Los Angeles, CA. Accessed 16 Jan 2015. http://healthpolicy.ucla.edu/Pages/home.aspx
70. Clarke CA, Glaser SL, Gomez SL et al (2011) Lymphoid malignancies in U.S. Asians: incidence rate differences by birthplace and acculturation. Cancer Epidemiol Biomarkers Prev 20(6):1064–1077
71. Carreon JD, Morton LM, Devesa SS et al (2008) Incidence of lymphoid neoplasms by subtype among six Asian ethnic groups in the United States, 1996-2004. Cancer Causes Control 19(10):1171–1181
72. Canchola AJ, Chang ET, Bernstein L et al (2010) Body size and the risk of ovarian cancer by hormone therapy use in the California Teachers Study cohort. Cancer Causes Control 21(12):2241–2248
73. Chang ET, Lee VS, Canchola AJ et al (2007) Diet and risk of ovarian cancer in the California Teachers Study cohort. Am J Epidemiol 165(7):802–813
74. Chang ET, Lee VS, Canchola AJ et al (2008) Dietary patterns and risk of ovarian cancer in the California Teachers Study cohort. Nutr Cancer 60(3):285–291
75. Horn-Ross PL, Whittemore AS, Harris R, Itnyre J (1992) Characteristics relating to ovarian cancer risk: collaborative analysis of 12 U.S. case-control studies. VI. Nonepithelial cancers among adults. Collaborative Ovarian Cancer Group. Epidemiology 3(6):490–495

76. National Cancer Institute. Ovarian Cancer. http://www.cancer.gov/cancertopics/types/ovari-anAccessed 3 Dec 2014. U.S. Department of Health and Human Services, National Cancer Institute, Bethesda, MD
77. Rodriguez C, Patel AV, Calle EE, Jacob EJ, Thun MJ (2001) Estrogen replacement therapy and ovarian cancer mortality in a large prospective study of US women. JAMA 285(11):1460–1465
78. Pang JW, Cook LS, Schwartz SM, Weis NS (2002) Incidence of leukemia in Asian migrants to the United States and their descendants. Cancer Causes Control 13(9):791–795
79. Leukemia & Lymphoma Society (2014) Facts Spring 2014. Leukemia & Lymphoma Society, White Plains. https://www.lls.org/content/nationalcontent/resourcecenter/freeeducationmaterials/generalcancer/pdf/facts.pdf
80. National Cancer Institute (2014) A snapshot of leukemia. Cancer snapshots: disease focused and other snapshots. http://www.cancer.gov/researchandfunding/snapshots/leukemia Accessed 13 Nov 2014
81. National Cancer Institute (2014).Oral cancer prevention. http://www.cancer.gov/cancertopics/pdq/prevention/oral/HealthProfessional. Accessed: 3 Dec 2014. U.S. Department of Health and Human Services, National Cancer Institute, Bethesda, MD
82. National Cancer Institute: PDQ® Oral Cancer Prevention. Bethesda, MD: National Cancer Institute. Date last modified 07/02/2014 http://cancer.gov/cancertopics/pdq/prevention/oral/HealthProfessional. Accessed 13 Nov 2014
83. Bladder Cancer Treatment (PDQ). http://www.cancer.gov/cancertopics/pdq/treatment/bladder. Accessed 3 Dec 2014. U.S. Department of Health and Human Services, National Cancer Institute, Bethesda, MD. http://seer.cancer.gov/statfacts/html/urinb.html.
84. Polednak AP (2009) Trends in incidence rates of tobacco-related cancer, selected areas, SEER Program, United States, 1992-2004. Prev Chronic Dis 6(1):A16
85. SEER Cancer Statistics Factsheets: Bladder. http://seer.cancer.gov/statfacts/html/urinb.html. Accessed 3 Dec 2014. U.S. Department of Health and Human Services, National Cancer Institute, Bethesda, MD. http://seer.cancer.gov/statfacts/html/urinb.html.
86. SEER Cancer Statistics Factsheets: Pancreas Cancer. http://seer.cancer.gov/statfacts/html/pancreas.html. Accessed 29 Jan 2014. U.S. Department of Health and Human Services, National Cancer Institute, Bethesda, MD. http://seer.cancer.gov/statfacts/html/pancreas.html
87. van Asperen CJ, Brohet RM, Meijers-Heijboer EJ et al (2005) Cancer risks in BRCA2 families: estimates for sites other than breast and ovary. J Med Genet 42(9):711–719
88. Lynch SM, Vrieling A, Lubin JH et al (2009) Cigarette smoking and pancreatic cancer: a pooled analysis from the pancreatic cancer cohort consortium. Am J Epidemiol 170(4):403–413

Cancer Screening Among Asian Americans

Annette E. Maxwell, Victoria M. Taylor, and Roshan Bastani

Abstract Cancer screening tests such as mammograms, Pap smears, and colonoscopies can help detect cancer at an early stage, before symptoms appear. Some screening tests such as colonoscopy and Pap smears can also detect precancerous abnormal tissue, which if removed can prevent the occurrence of cancer. Generally, the earlier cancer is detected, the easier it is to treat. Survival and mortality outcomes are also much better for cancer detected at an early versus late stage. However, in addition to benefits, some screening tests carry risks, and finding the cancer early does not always improve the person's health or help the person live longer [1].

This chapter will examine the utilization of cancer screening tests among selected Asian American ethnic groups and describe the research on factors that are associated with screening. We will give examples of interventions to promote cancer screening that have been tested in Asian American populations and summarize both the scientific knowledge and research gaps regarding cancer screening. The chapter will close with recommendations and next steps for research and practice on cancer screening among Asian Americans.

Keywords Chinese Americans • Japanese Americans • Filipino Americans • Southeast Asians • Vietnamese Americans • Korean Americans • Hmong • Breast cancer screening • Cervical cancer screening • Colorectal cancer screening • Hepatitis B virus testing • Correlates of screening • Interventions to promote cancer screening

---

A.E. Maxwell, Dr. P.H. (✉) • R. Bastani, Ph.D.
Jonsson Comprehensive Cancer Center, UCLA Kaiser Permanente Center for Health Equity, Fielding School of Public Health, University of California at Los Angeles, 650 Charles Young Dr, A2-125 CHS, Los Angeles, CA 90095-6900, USA
e-mail: amaxwell@ucla.edu

V.M. Taylor, M.D., M.P.H.
Division of Public Health Sciences, Fred Hutchinson Cancer Research Center, Department of Health Services, University of Washington, Seattle, WA, USA

A.H. Wu, D.O. Stram (eds.), *Cancer Epidemiology Among Asian Americans*,
DOI 10.1007/978-3-319-41118-7_4

Introduction

Cancer screening tests such as mammograms, Pap smears, and colonoscopies can help detect cancer at an early stage, before symptoms appear. Some screenings tests such as colonoscopy and Pap smears can also detect precancerous abnormal tissue, which if removed can prevent the occurrence of cancer. Generally, the earlier cancer is detected, the easier it is to treat. Survival and mortality outcomes are also much better for cancer detected at an early versus late stage. However, some screening tests carry risks, and finding the cancer early does not always improve the person's health or help the person live longer.

Many organizations, including the American Cancer Society, issue cancer screening guidelines, but the guidelines issued by the US Preventive Services Task Force are the most commonly referenced and utilized. The US Preventive Services Task Force, which is an independent, volunteer panel of national experts in prevention and evidence-based medicine, develops recommendations for or against screening tests based on a review of high-quality scientific evidence and by weighing the potential benefits and harms of each screening test. The Task Force also periodically updates its recommendations based on new scientific evidence [2]. Table 1 shows the current recommendations relevant for cancer screening. Only tests that receive a Grade A or B are recommended.

Few studies have examined utilization of cancer screening tests among Asian American populations, and most have focused on utilization of *mammograms* for early detection of breast cancer, *Pap smears* for early detection of cervical cancer, and *fecal occult blood tests and colonoscopies* for the prevention and early detection of colorectal cancer. Compared to other racial/ethnic groups in the USA, Asian Americans have a relatively high risk of infection with hepatitis B virus (HBV), which accounts for 80 % of liver cancer cases in this group. HBV testing can lead to earlier detection and hence potentially reduce the onset of serious sequelae of chronic liver disease. In addition, testing and, if indicated, vaccination can reduce HBV transmission (*see* Chap. 10). Thus, *hepatitis B testing* is recommended for Asian American populations, and studies have been conducted on this topic in a number of Asian American ethnic groups.

There is scant research among Asian Americans on *human papillomavirus (HPV) testing*, on the utilization of *lung cancer screening* and on *BRCA risk assessment* for high-risk Asian American groups. Asian Americans experience high incidence and mortality rates of stomach cancer (see Chap. 11). *Stomach cancer screening* using photofluorography or upper endoscopy is recommended in some Asian countries (e.g., Japan and South Korea). However, we will not discuss screening for stomach cancer in this chapter since there is no screening recommendation in the USA. *Prostate cancer screening* using prostate-specific antigen is no longer recommended by the US Preventive Services Task Force and will also not be discussed.

As described in the previous and subsequent chapters, specific Asian ethnic groups in the USA exhibit varying risk profiles of cancer incidence and mortality due to differences in migration history, lifestyle, and environmental exposures. In addition, there are vast differences among Asian ethnic groups with respect to

Table 1 US Preventive Services Task Force recommendations relevant for cancer screening

Topic	Description (date of most recent recommendation)	Grade
Breast cancer screening	The USPSTF recommends biennial screening mammography for women aged 50–74 years (November 2009)	B
Cervical cancer screening	The USPSTF recommends screening for cervical cancer in women aged 21–65 years with cytology (Pap smear) every 3 years or, for women aged 30–65 years who want to lengthen the screening interval, screening with a combination of cytology and human papillomavirus (HPV) testing every 5 years (March 2012)	A
Colorectal cancer screening	The USPSTF recommends screening for colorectal cancer using fecal occult blood testing (annually), sigmoidoscopy (every 5 years), or colonoscopy (every 10 years) in adults beginning at age 50 years and continuing until age 75 years. The risks and benefits of these screening methods vary (October 2008)	A
Lung cancer screening	The USPSTF recommends annual screening for lung cancer with low-dose computed tomography in adults aged 55–80 years who have a 30 pack-year smoking history and currently smoke or have quit within the past 15 years. Screening should be discontinued once a person has not smoked for 15 years or develops a health problem that substantially limits life expectancy or the ability or willingness to have curative lung surgery (December 2013)	B
Hepatitis B screening: nonpregnant adolescents and adults	The USPSTF recommends screening for hepatitis B virus infection in persons at high risk for infection (May 2014)	B
Hepatitis B screening: pregnant women	The USPSTF strongly recommends screening for hepatitis B virus infection in pregnant women at their first prenatal visit (June 2009)	A
BRCA risk assessment and genetic counseling/testing	The USPSTF recommends that primary care providers screen women who have family members with breast, ovarian, tubal, or peritoneal cancer with one of several screening tools designed to identify a family history that may be associated with an increased risk for potentially harmful mutations in breast cancer susceptibility genes (*BRCA1* or *BRCA2*). Women with positive screening results should receive genetic counseling and, if indicated after counseling, BRCA testing (December 2013)	B
Prostate cancer screening	The USPSTF recommends against prostate-specific antigen (PSA)-based screening for prostate cancer (May 2012)	D

Notes. A: The USPSTF recommends the service. There is high certainty that the net benefit is substantial
B: The USPSTF recommends the service. There is high certainty that the net benefit is moderate or there is moderate certainty that the net benefit is moderate to substantial
D: The USPSTF recommends against the service. There is moderate or high certainty that the service has no net benefit or that the harms outweigh the benefits

socioeconomic status, acculturation, access to care, and other factors that are known to impact cancer screening rates. Therefore, it is important to examine cancer screening in specific Asian ethnic groups, rather than in all Asian ethnic groups combined, to obtain a fine-grained picture of screening uptake as well as factors that may facilitate or impede screening.

Data Sources to Estimate Cancer Screening Rates

There is no national resource that allows for estimation of cancer screening rates among Asians in the USA. Therefore, screening estimates must be compiled from a patchwork of sources of varying breadth and quality. Most information on cancer screening for the general US population is obtained from survey research, and this is the case for information on Asians as well. Among Asian Americans, surveys have generally been conducted by telephone or in face-to-face settings. Some surveys have included randomly selected samples of participants (population-based sample), while others have utilized convenience samples, often recruited with the help of community organizations that serve members of the target population. In both type of surveys, screening is assessed through self-reports, which may suffer from recall bias and social desirability response bias.

Very few *population-based surveys* that assess cancer screening have included sufficient Asian American participants, thereby limiting ability to analyze data and report screening rates for specific Asian American groups [3]. Some surveys such as the California Health Interview Survey have included adequate samples of a few of the largest Asian ethnic groups to be able to obtain subgroup level estimates of screening rates. The California Health Interview Survey is a telephone survey that has been conducted every 2 years since 2001 in English, Spanish, Chinese (Mandarin and Cantonese dialects), Vietnamese, and Korean. The survey oversamples Asian ethnic groups so that each group‘s total sample of adults reaches a target of 500 [4]. Because California is home to about 5.5 million Asian Americans, almost one third of all Asian Americans in the USA [5], and because the California Health Interview Survey is conducted in four Asian languages which allows non-English speakers to participate, its data are frequently used to estimate cancer screening among Asian Americans nationally (e.g., [6–8]). However, even population-based surveys including the California Health Interview Survey have several limitations: Recent immigrants who may have limited English fluency and who do not speak one of the survey languages cannot participate. Surveys usually include only a few questions each on a large number of topics and do not provide much detail on cancer screening and on factors that are associated with screening such as awareness of a screening test or barriers to screening. Since these surveys are designed to assess health issues in the general population, they may only ask questions on health topics that are relevant for the majority of respondents; health issues that are important for Asian Americans but not for all racial/ethnic groups, such as hepatitis B testing and vaccination, may not be assessed in these surveys. Population-based surveys typically do not provide data on smaller Asian American groups such as the Hmong, Thai, Native Hawaiians, and Pacific Islander populations.

Community surveys are often conducted in specific Asian American ethnic groups in various Asian languages, typically with help from Asian American community organizations. While some community surveys recruit participants in a systematic fashion, such as through community directories or by selecting common names from telephone directories [9, 10], others use snowball sampling or recruit individuals at specific locations such as faith-based organizations, Asian grocery stores, and nail salons [11, 12]. Surveys are often conducted face-to-face, taking advantage of existing relationships with community members and allowing interviewers to establish some rapport with respondents. These convenience samples often include individuals with low levels of income and education and recent immigrants who may be less likely to respond if they received a "cold call" from a university or survey firm asking them to participate in a survey. Many of these surveys are conducted in a single Asian American ethnic group, but comparison of screening rates across Asian ethnic groups and across surveys is usually possible because most surveys assess cancer screening using standard questions such as "have you ever had (specific screening test)?" and, if yes, "when did you receive the last (specific screening test) for routine screening?" Comparison of knowledge and beliefs related to specific screening tests across Asian ethnic groups can be more challenging because there is less homogeneity in how questions are phrased and because translations into many different Asian languages can introduce small differences in meaning. Few community-based surveys include more than one Asian American ethnic group [13–15].

Both population-based samples and convenience samples have strengths and limitations. Therefore, we use both as data sources for reporting screening rates and factors that are associated with screening among Asian Americans. More recently, *electronic health records* have been utilized to assess cancer screening and to conduct comparisons among members of various racial/ethnic groups [16]. Electronic health records are usually considered the gold standard for assessing receipt of medical care and don't suffer the limitations of self-report. However, even if obtained from a large health-care organization serving an ethnically diverse patient population, electronic health records only include patients with access to care, and some reports are further limited to "active" patients who have used at least one primary care-related visit during a specific time period, for example, the past 2 years [16]. While these data sources are informative, many patients without health insurance, who often have the lowest cancer screening rates [17], are not included in electronic health records.

Cancer Screening Rates Among Asian Americans

Mammography Screening

Although some organizations such as the American Cancer Society recommend mammography screening for women 40 years and older, the US Preventive Services Task Force currently recommends biennial mammography screening only for women between 50 and 74 years of age. Many reports on mammography screening include women 40 years and older, especially if they are based on studies that were conducted before the US Preventive Services Task Force changed their guidelines from women 40 years and over to women 50–74 years of age. Estimates for screening rates vary among different surveys, but most surveys indicate that Asian American women underutilize mammography screening relative to White and

Table 2 Breast and cervical cancer screening rates among Asian American ethnic groups, California Health Interview Survey 2011–2012 (mammogram in past 2 years) and 2007 (Pap test in past 3 years), % (95 % confidence interval)

Asian American ethnic group	Had a mammogram in the past 2 years (women 40+)	Had a Pap test in the past 3 years (women 18+)
Filipina	78.2 (70.2–86.2)	75.4 (68.7–82.2)
Vietnamese	75.6 (67.8–83.4)	76.2 (66.1–86.3)
Chinese	72.8 (66.9–78.7)	64.9 (58.8–71.0)
Korean	51.8 (42.6–60.9)	71.0 (63.4–78.5)
South Asian	68.8 (57.0–80.6)	73.4 (63.3–83.5)
Japanese	84.1 (77.3–90.9)	75.2 (66.3–84.1)

Source: http://healthpolicy.ucla.edu/publications/Documents/PDF/2014/mammogramsfactsheet_apr2014.pdf and AskCHIS

African American women. For example, in the 2010 National Health Interview Survey, 64 % of Asian American women 50–74 years of age reported receipt of a mammogram in the past 2 years, compared to 73 % of non-Hispanic White and African American women [3].

Based on the data from the 2011–2012 California Health Interview Survey (http://healthpolicy.ucla.edu/publications/Documents/PDF/2014/mammograms-factsheet_apr2014.pdf, accessed 11/12/14), 72 % of Asian American women 40 years and older reported receipt of a recent mammogram in the past 2 years, compared to 83 % of African American, 81 % of White, and 77 % of Latina women. Screening rates among women 40 years and older from different Asian American ethnic groups ranged from 52 % (95 % confidence interval 43–61 %) among Korean American women to 84 % (95 % confidence interval 77–91 %) among Japanese American women (see Table 2), a difference of 32 % points. Screening rates are slightly higher among women 50 years and older, but the screening pattern remains unchanged.

One of the Healthy People 2020 national goals for improving the health of Americans is to increase the proportion of women who receive a mammogram according to the guidelines to 81 % (https://www.healthypeople.gov/2020/topics-objectives/topic/cancer/objectives, accessed 11/20/14). Japanese American women residing in California have already achieved this goal and Filipina-, Vietnamese-, and Chinese Americans residing in California can potentially achieve this goal. However, given the current screening rate, it is unlikely that South Asian- and Korean American women will achieve this goal by 2020.

Cervical Cancer Screening

Asian American women also underutilize cervical cancer screening, but disparities among Asian American ethnic groups are less pronounced than for mammography screening. Based on the 2007 California Health Interview Survey, which assessed receipt of a Pap test but not HPV screening, adherence to screening guidelines ranges from 65 % among Chinese American women to 76 % among Vietnamese women, a difference of 11 % points (see Table 2). Screening rates in all Asian American groups are substantially lower than rates among non-Hispanic Whites (87 %), African Americans (88 %), and Latinas (85 %). The Healthy People 2020 goal is to increase the proportion of women who receive cervical cancer screening according to the guidelines to 93 %. Given the current screening rate, it is unlikely that any Asian American ethnic group will achieve this goal by 2020.

Colorectal Cancer Screening

The American Cancer Society recommends receipt of a guaiac-based fecal occult blood test (FOBT) or fecal immunochemical test (FIT) ever year, *or* flexible sigmoidoscopy every 5 years, *or* colonoscopy every 10 years, *or* double-contrast barium enema every 5 years, *or* CT colonography (virtual colonoscopy) every 5 years for men and women 50 years and over at average risk for developing colorectal cancer. The US Preventive Services Task Force recommends colorectal cancer screening tests only for individuals between age 50 and 75. Between 2001 and 2009, the California Health Interview survey assessed receipt of a stool blood test and sigmoidoscopy or colonoscopy in five cross-sectional surveys. Figure 1 shows the proportion of respondents 50 years of age and older who are adherent to colorectal cancer screening guidelines based on receipt of a fecal occult blood test within the past 12 months or a colonoscopy or sigmoidoscopy within the past 5 years, since not all survey years distinguished between these two procedures. Estimates include colorectal cancer screening for any reason to maintain consistency across survey years and are standardized to the age and gender distribution of the 2001 California population. Analyses were conducted using survey replicate weights for Asian ethnic groups with sufficient sample size [18].

As shown in Fig. 1, there is an upward trend in colorectal cancer screening utilization among all racial/ethnic groups. The proportion of Asian Americans that are up to date with colorectal cancer screening is estimated to be above 60 % in 2009, which is slightly lower than the estimate for Whites and African Americans. The lower panel in Fig. 1 suggests that disparities in colorectal cancer screening widened from 2001 to 2005 and narrowed between 2005 and 2009. In 2009, the last survey year in which colorectal cancer screening was assessed in the California Health Interview Survey, higher screening rates were observed among Japanese-, Chinese-, and Vietnamese Americans and lower screening rates among Korean- and Filipino Americans. There were no statistically significant differences in screening rates between males and females in any of these Asian ethnic groups (AskCHIS).

The Healthy People 2020 goal is to increase the proportion of adults 50–75 years who receive a colorectal cancer screening according to the guidelines to 70.5 %. While Japanese-, Chinese-, and Vietnamese Americans residing in California are close to achieving this goal, it is uncertain that Korean- and Filipino Americans will achieve the 2020 goal, given the current screening rates and temporal trends. It should also be noted that screening rates in California are relatively high compared

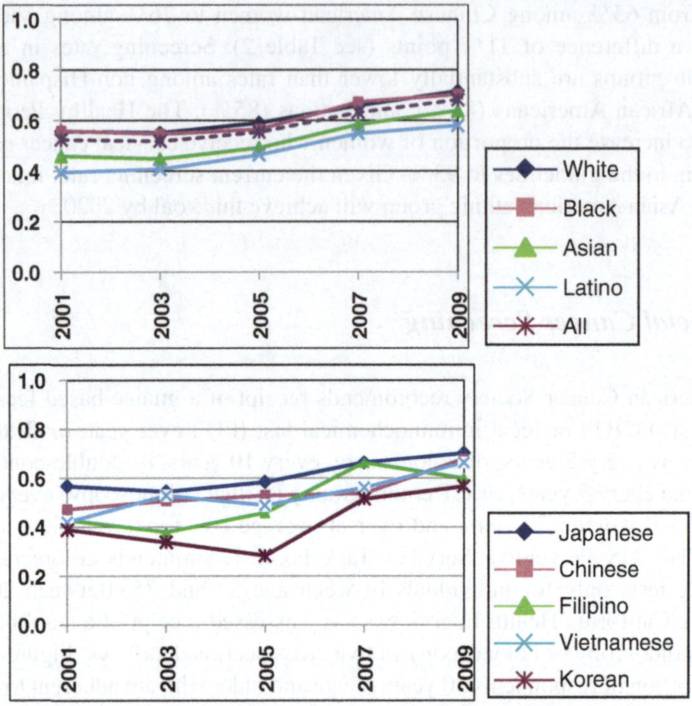

Fig. 1 Estimated age- and gender-standardized proportion of California residents aged 50 years and older who are adherent to colorectal cancer screening guidelines, California Health Interview Survey 2001–2009 (2001–2005 data were previously published in [18])

to other states. Based on data from the Behavioral Risk Factor Surveillance System, California ranks number 14 out of 51 states with regard to colorectal cancer screening prevalence [19]. According to the data from the 2010 National Health Interview Survey, only 46 % of Asians residing in the USA are up to date with colorectal cancer screening [19].

Hepatitis B Testing

Because Asian Americans are at increased risk for hepatitis B infection and resulting liver disease and liver cancer (see Chap. 10), the US Preventive Services Task Force and the American Association for the Study of Liver Diseases recommend screening for hepatitis B and subsequent vaccination, if appropriate [20, 21]. Screening is important because approximately 65% of those who are infected with hepatitis B do not know that they are infected [22]. Screening is an effective method of limiting the spread of hepatitis B by identifying uninfected individuals who will need vaccination to prevent future infection and by identifying infected individuals who will need monitoring or treatment and counseling to reduce vertical (from mother to child) and horizontal transmission to close contacts (e.g., household members). The standard test for hepatitis B infection involves the detection of the hepatitis B surface antigen, HBsAg [23].

Despite their elevated disease risk, hepatitis B testing rates among Asians in the USA are suboptimal with estimates ranging from 11 to 65 % based on self-reports in different Asian ethnic groups [9, 12, 24–31]. As shown in Table 3, only few studies have assessed hepatitis B testing rates in Asian American samples. The huge

Table 3 Hepatitis B screening rates among Asian American ethnic groups

Citation	Asian American population, study area	% ever screened for HBV	Study sample, age, source of study sample, survey method, and year(s) of study
Taylor et al. (2006) [28]	**Chinese immigrants** in Seattle	48	$N=395$, ages 20–64 years; identified through Chinese last names from a telephone directory; in-person interviews; survey cooperation rate 58 %; **2005**
Tanaka et al. (2014) [24]	**Chinese immigrants** in Washington, DC area	65	$N=252$, age>50 years; recruited from Chinese-speaking physicians' offices; patients had at least one doctor's visit in the past 2 years; telephone survey; response rate 49 **%; 2008–2011**
Bastani et al. (2007) [29]	**Korean** in Los Angeles, CA	56	$N=141$ adults; recruited at 5 Korean churches and one Korean-serving primary care clinic; in-person interviews, self-administered questionnaires or self-administered in a group setting; **2003**
Bastani et al. (2015)[31]	**Korean** in Los Angeles, CA	35	$N=866$ adults; recruited at 52 Korean churches**;** face-to-face survey; **2007–2010**
Strong et al. (2012) [25]	**Chinese, Korean, and Vietnamese** in Maryland	54, 46, and 39	303 Chinese, 294 Korean, and 280 Vietnamese adults; recruited at community organizations, faith-based organizations, language schools, grocery stores, and nail salons; self-administered survey; **2009–2010**
Ma et al. (2010) [12]	**Chinese, Korean, Vietnamese, and Cambodian** in Greater Philadelphia area, New Jersey, and New York City	38, 32, 20 and 11	718 Chinese, 289 Korean, 305 Vietnamese, and 291 Cambodian adults; recruited at Asian American community organizations; in-person interviews; **2005–2006**
Grytdal et al. (2009)[30]	**Cambodian** in Massachusetts; **Vietnamese** in California	49; 63	353 Cambodian adults, 1696 Vietnamese adults; CDC Racial and Ethnic Approaches to Community Health Risk Factor Survey; telephone survey; interview completion rate 25–31 %; **2010**
Nguyen et al. (2010) [26]	**Vietnamese** in Northern California and Washington, DC	62	$N=1704$ adults; identified through Vietnamese surnames; telephone survey; response rate 27.4 %; **2007–2008**
Taylor et al. (2011) [27]	**Cambodian** in Seattle	50	$N=667$, ages 18–64; identified through Cambodian last names from a telephone directory; in-person interviews; completion rate 70 %; **2010**
Chen et al. (2013) [9]	**Hmong** In Greater Sacramento CA area	18	$N=490$ adults; identified through Hmong surnames; telephone survey; **2007–2008**

variations in screening rates, even among different studies conducted in the same Asian ethnic group, are probably due to sample differences in demographic characteristics, as well as the variety of sampling and recruitment strategies and interviewing methods that were used.

Correlates of Screening Among Asian Americans

Individual health behaviors related to cancer screening are influenced by a complex myriad of individual, health system, community, and societal level factors. In the following section, we use a conceptual framework, the Health Behavior Framework, to systematically address the multiple determinants of cancer screening and to summarize some of the major findings among Asian Americans. The **Health Behavior Framework** (Fig. 2) is a multidimensional model derived from varying theoretical orientations [32]. It assumes that individual variables and provider and health-care system factors influence behavioral intentions which in turn influence health behavior. Intentions do not automatically translate into behavior. Rather, this connection depends on the absence of barriers and/or presence of supports which may function at the level of the individual (e.g., cultural beliefs), the health system (e.g., practice patterns), or society (e.g., impoverished neighborhood). Some model variables are mutable and are therefore potential targets for interventions (e.g., individual and provider and health-care system factors), while others are immutable, such as demographic factors. Despite some differences, the major drivers of behavior tend to be similar across populations. The Health Behavior Framework

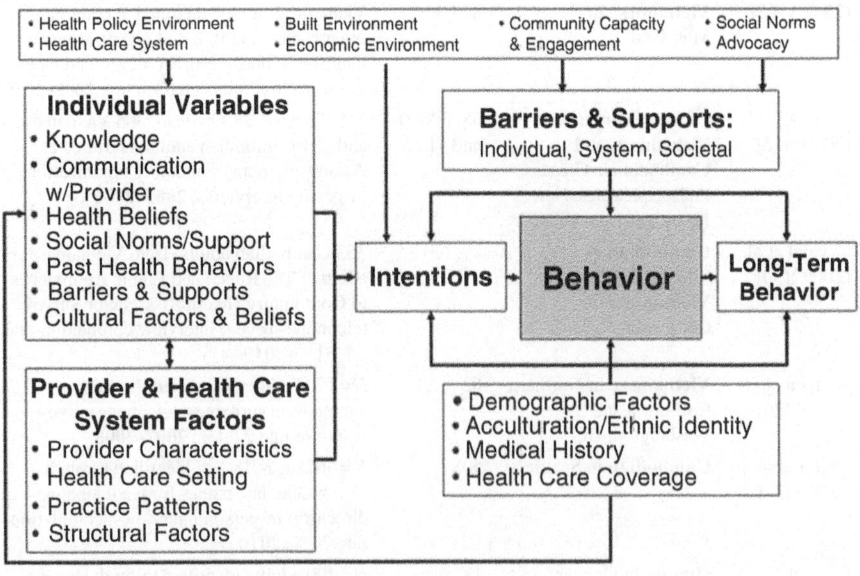

Fig. 2 The Health Behavior Framework

also recognizes the influence of broad socio-ecological factors on cancer screening such as health-care policy and social norms. These factors are theoretically mutable, for example, through health-care reform and long-term community engagement activities or campaigns.

Frequently, factors that have the potential to influence cancer screening and screening behaviors are identified at the same point in time through a survey [7, 11, 25]. This cross-sectional research design allows us to identify *correlates* of screening. Other studies examine the effects of factors identified at baseline on subsequent screening behaviors [33]. Such a longitudinal study design provides stronger evidence than cross-sectional data regarding *predictors* of cancer screening.

Demographic Factors, Acculturation, and Health-Care Coverage

Being married, higher level of income, being proficient in English, and having health insurance have been consistently associated with cancer screening among Asian American ethnic groups, including colorectal cancer screening [11, 34, 35], breast and cervical cancer screening [7, 11, 36], and hepatitis B testing [12, 37]. Several studies have examined the associations between acculturation and cancer screening using various measures of acculturation, such as length of residency in the USA, percent of lifetime in the USA, language proficiency, and language use. Generally, immigrants who have assimilated to the behaviors and beliefs of the host society are better able to obtain health care and have higher screening rates [11], but this is not always the case. A study among Vietnamese Americans found *lower* hepatitis B screening rates among those who had lived in the USA for more than 10 years and spoke Vietnamese less fluently compared to more recent immigrants. The authors suggest that efforts to promote testing in the USA have focused on more recent immigrants and that recent immigrants may be receiving medical care in immigrant and/or refugee clinics, where the providers may be more aware of the need for hepatitis B testing in Asian populations [26]. A study that examined the relative impact of access to care versus acculturation on breast and cervical cancer screening among Asian American women concluded that access explained more variation than acculturation alone for most Asian American ethnic groups that were studied [38]. Since demographic factors and acculturation are not mutable factors, they help to identify population groups with the lowest cancer screening rates that can then be targeted for screening promotion programs rather than inform the content of intervention programs to promote screening.

Individual Variables

Individual variables that influence cancer screening have been widely studied in many different Asian American ethnic groups. The most important variables that have emerged are not being aware of the screening test and the need for screening and lack of physician recommendation to receive screening [25, 26, 29, 33, 34, 39–41]. For cancer screening tests that require periodic retesting (breast, cervical, colorectal cancer screening), having had a test in the past is an important predictor of future testing [42]. Health beliefs are generally associated with cancer screening in the expected direction: screening is associated with high perceived susceptibility, high perceived severity of the disease, and low barriers to cancer screening [29, 37, 43].

Provider and Health-Care System Factors

The influence of provider and health-care system factors on cancer screening has not been comprehensively assessed among Asian Americans, although most cancer screening tests require a physician exam or referral, suggesting that these factors are extremely important. Strategies that fall into this category and have been shown to increase cancer screening include physician education, physician reminder systems, physician assessment and feedback regarding the proportion of patients that are up-to-date with cancer screening guidelines, and reminder mailings for patients [44–47]. Patient navigation is another strategy that has been shown to increase cancer screening in several Asian American ethnic groups [9, 47–49]. One study in an outpatient health-care organization serving a large number of Asian Americans in Northern California found that screening completion for breast and cervical cancer was positively associated with patient-provider gender concordance, i.e., female physicians had significantly higher breast and cervical cancer screening rates among their Asian American patients [16]. This finding corresponds well with the fact that many Asian American women prefer a female provider for these exams [50, 51].

Barriers to Cancer Screening

Many of the variables discussed above can be conceptualized as barriers, including lack of health insurance, lack of knowledge/awareness of specific screening tests and guidelines, lack of a physician recommendation to get tested, and health beliefs that do not support routine checkups in the absence of symptoms. These are common barriers for many ethnic groups, including Asian Americans. Other barriers that are frequently cited by Asian Americans are lack of time to obtain a screening test, not knowing where to obtain the test, lack of transportation, fear of finding a health problem, and embarrassment or shame [12, 29, 34]. A few studies have reported culturally specific attitudes and beliefs that may function as barriers to cancer screening in specific Asian American ethnic groups, such as the belief that illness is a matter of karma or fate [52, 53]. However, these barriers are less frequently assessed and are not endorsed by all Asian American ethnic groups and not for all cancer screening tests [29].

Overall, correlates of cancer screening among Asian American ethnic groups are similar to those of other US populations. In addition to barriers to screening that are faced by most ethnic groups, Asian Americans also experience culturally specific barriers to screening which need to be addressed in screening promotion efforts.

Intervention Research to Promote Cancer Screening Among Asian Americans

To address the low utilization of cancer-related screening tests among Asians Americans, many intervention studies have been implemented to test the most effective ways to increase screening participation. The majority of these studies have been conducted in metropolitan areas with relatively large Asian populations such as Los Angeles, San Francisco, Seattle, New York, and Washington, DC.

Study designs that involve concurrent comparison groups and prospective measurement of outcomes, and document actual receipt of screening tests, provide the strongest evidence for the effectiveness of cancer control interventions [54, 55]. This section focuses on studies that used experimental designs (i.e., randomized individuals or groups of people to experimental and control status) or quasi-experimental designs (i.e., compared an experimental group with a nonequivalent control group, no random assignment) and included screening test completion, assessed by self-report or provider report, as an outcome. Control groups for these studies either received no intervention, usual care, a minimal screening-related intervention (e.g., pamphlet), or a non-screening-related intervention (e.g., a physical activity program).

Cancer control interventions can be classified as provider directed (e.g., physician reminders) or client directed (e.g., health education). Client-directed interventions include one-on-one education (tailored or non-tailored), group education, small media (audiovisual and print), navigation (to reduce structural barriers to screening), and mass media [56]. Most previous cancer control initiatives for Asian Americans involved multiple intervention components [55].

Interventions to increase the use of cancer-related screening tests by Asian groups have been delivered in health-care settings, in community settings, and to entire communities. The interventions that were delivered in community settings can be broadly categorized as lay health worker (LHW) outreach or community-based group education. LHW outreach interventions have included one-on-one or group education combined with small media and/or peer navigation. Community-based group education interventions have been delivered by Asian health educators and usually included other components.

The following sections provide information about interventions that were delivered in health-care settings, LHW outreach and community-based group education interventions, one-on-one education and small media interventions, and community-level interventions. These studies focused on individuals who were nonadherent to breast, cervical, and colorectal cancer screening guidelines as well as individuals who had never been screened for HBV. As discussed previously, guidelines for cancer screening have changed over time. Eligibility criteria for cancer control intervention studies were based on the guidelines when they were conducted. Table 4 gives examples of individual and cluster-randomized controlled trials that evaluated cancer control inter-

Table 4 Examples of individual and cluster randomized trials that resulted in increased cancer screening rates

Intervention type(s) Publication	Participant characteristics Study location(s)	Experimental group intervention component(s) Control group intervention	Primary evaluation method(s) Sample size(s)	Key finding(s)
Breast cancer screening				
LHW outreach Nguyen et al. [61]	**Vietnamese** ≥40 years Santa Clara County, California	Group education Peer navigation Media-based education Mammography media-based education	Baseline survey Follow-up survey after an interval of 5 months 1,100 randomized 1,089 with follow-up data	Mammography in the previous 2 years increased significantly in the experimental group (65–82 %, $p<0.001$) but not in the control group (74–76 %, $p>0.05$)
Group education Lee et al. [67]	**Korean** immigrant ≥40 years No mammogram in past year Cook County, Illinois	Group education Couples discussion activity Nutrition group education	Follow-up survey 15 months after intervention 428 randomized 395 with follow-up data	56 % of the experimental group and 42 % of the control group reported mammography ($p=0.004$)
Group education Lee-Lin et al. [68]	**Chinese** immigrant ≥40 years No mammogram in past year Portland, Oregon	Group education Telephone counseling Navigation English language mammography brochure	Follow-up survey 12 months after intervention 300 randomized 280 with follow-up data	71 % of the experimental group and 43 % of the control group reported mammography ($p<0.001$)
Cervical cancer screening				
LHW outreach **Small media** Taylor et al. [64]	**Chinese** 20–69 years No Pap test in past 2 years or not intending to get Pap test in next 2 years Seattle, Washington Vancouver, British Columbia	*Experimental 1:* One-on-one education Chinese language video and print materials Peer navigation *Experimental 2*: Chinese language video and print materials None	Follow-up survey 6 months after randomization 482 randomized 402 with follow-up data	39 % of experimental group 1, 25 % of experimental group 2, and 15 % of the control group reported Pap testing (experimental group 1 versus control, $p<0.001$; experimental group 2 versus control, $p=0.03$; experimental group 1 versus experimental group 2, $p=0.02$)

LHW outreach Mock et al. [60]	**Vietnamese** ≥18 years Santa Clara County, California	Group education Peer navigation Media-based education Pap testing media-based education	Baseline survey Follow-up survey after an interval of 4 months 1,005 randomized 952 with follow-up data	Pap testing ever increased significantly in the experimental group (66–82 %, $p<0.001$) and the control group (70–76 %, $p<0.001$) but the experimental group increase was significantly greater than the control group increase ($p<0.001$)
LHW outreach Taylor et al. [62]	**Vietnamese** 20–79 years No Pap test in past 3 years (aged 20–69) Never had Pap test (aged 70–79) Seattle, Washington	One-on-one education Vietnamese language video and pamphlet Physical activity print materials	Follow-up survey 6 months after randomization 234 randomized 174 with follow-up data	33 % of the experimental group and 18 % of the control group reported Pap testing ($p=0.02$)
Colorectal cancer screening				
Health care system Tu et al. [57]	**Chinese** 50–78 years No FOBT in past year or colonoscopy in past 10 years Seattle, Washington	One-on-one education Chinese language video and print materials FOBT kit and instruction sheet Usual care	Medical records review 6 months after randomization 210 randomized	70 % of the experimental group and 28 % of the control group completed FOBT ($p<0.001$)
Group education Maxwell et al. [70]	**Filipino** 50–70 years No FOBT in past year, sigmoidoscopy in past 5 years or colonoscopy in past 10 years Los Angeles, California	*Experimental 1*: Group education Filipino language information packet and pamphlet FOBT kit Reminder letter *Experimental 2*: Same as experimental group 1 but no FOBT kit Physical activity group education	Follow-up survey 6 months after intervention 548 randomized 432 with follow-up data	30 % of experimental group 1, 25 % of experimental group 2, and 9 % of the control group completed colorectal cancer screening in an intent-to-treat analysis (experimental group 1 versus control, $p<0.001$; experimental 2 versus control, $p<0.001$; experimental group 1 versus experimental group 2, $p>0.05$)

(continued)

Table 4 (continued)

Intervention type(s) Publication	Participant characteristics Study location(s)	Experimental group intervention component(s) Control group intervention	Primary evaluation method(s) Sample size(s)	Key finding(s)
One-on-one education **Small media** Walsh et al. [80]	**Vietnamese** 50–79 years Santa Clara County, California	*Experimental 1*: Telephone counseling Vietnamese language brochure FOBT kit *Experimental 2*: Same as experimental group 1 but no telephone counseling Usual care	Baseline survey Follow-up survey after an interval of 12 months 793 with baseline data 640 with follow-up data	FOBT in the previous 12 months increased in experimental group 1 (53–79 %), experimental group 2 (56–65 %) and the control group (46–58 %) but the experimental group 1 increase was significantly greater than the control group increase (p=0.006) and the experimental group 2 increase (p<0.001)
Hepatitis B screening				
LHW outreach Chen et al. [9]	**Hmong** 18–64 years No previous HBV test Greater Sacramento, California	One-on-one education Peer navigation Nutrition LHW outreach	Follow-up survey 6 months after randomization 260 randomized 217 with follow-up data	24 % of the experimental group and 10 % of the control group reported HBV testing (p=0.006)
Health care system Hsu et al. [45]	**Chinese or Vietnamese** 18–64 years No record of HBV test Sacramento, California	Provider prompt Usual care	Medical records review 3 months after clinic visit 175 randomized	34 % of the experimental group and 0 % of the control group completed HBV testing (p<0.001)
LHW outreach Taylor et al. [63]	**Kampuchean (Cambodian)** 18–64 years No previous HBV test Greater Seattle, Washington	One-on-one education Khmer language video and pamphlet Physical activity LHW outreach	Follow-up survey 6 months after randomization 250 randomized 199 with follow-up data	22 % of the experimental group and 3 % of the control group reported HBV testing (p<0.001)
Group education Bastani et al. [31]	**Korean** 18–64 years No previous HBV test Los Angeles, California	Group education Korean language print materials Physical activity and nutrition group education	Follow-up survey 6 months after intervention 1123 randomized 961 with follow-up data	19 % of the experimental group and 6 % of the control group reported HBV testing (p<0.001)

ventions for Asian Americans. The tabulated examples are trials that demonstrated an intervention effect in primary analyses that included the whole study group. Quasi-experimental studies, negative trials, and trials that only demonstrated an intervention effect in secondary subgroup analyses are not included in the table.

Evaluations of Interventions Delivered in Health-Care Settings

Tu and colleagues have conducted two studies of colorectal cancer screening interventions for patients of a community clinic system serving Asian patients. Both interventions were delivered during routine clinic visits. In the first study, Chinese patients who were eligible for screening were randomized to a health educator intervention group or usual care control group. The intervention had a highly significant effect on fecal occult blood testing (FOBT) completion rates [57]. In the second study, trained medical assistants routinely provided Vietnamese language videos and pamphlets at an experimental clinic but not at a control clinic. Adherence to screening guidelines did not increase significantly in either clinic during the intervention period. However, subgroup analyses showed a significant intervention effect for guideline adherence among patients who were nonadherent at baseline [58].

Provider prompts about HBV testing were evaluated in a cluster-randomized trial, with primary care physician as the randomization unit. The study group included Chinese and Vietnamese patients of a primary care clinic network who had no record of HBV testing. Experimental group physicians received electronic health record prompts before scheduled appointments. Patients of experimental group physicians were significantly more likely to complete HBV testing than patients of control group physicians [45].

Lay Health Worker Outreach Trials

The Vietnamese Community Health Promotion Project in San Francisco has conducted one quasi-experimental study and two trials of LHW group education. The quasi-experimental study focused on both breast and cervical cancer screening. LHWs conducted over 200 small-group educational sessions and distributed small media in an experimental area (Tenderloin District of San Francisco). Mammography and Pap testing rates increased significantly in the Tenderloin District but not in the control area (Sacramento) [59]. One of the trials addressed breast cancer screening and the other trial addressed cervical cancer screening. Both trials compared LHW group education and peer navigation combined with media-based education to media-based education alone. The combined intervention was more effective in increasing mammography, as well as Pap testing levels [60, 61].

Multiple trials have evaluated LHW outreach interventions for Asian groups that included one-on-one education combined with small media and/or peer navigation. These trials focused on promoting Pap testing among women who underutilized Pap testing or HBV testing among men and women who had never been tested for HBV. All but one of these studies were conducted in the Pacific Northwest. The LHW interventions were effective in promoting Pap testing in Chinese and Vietnamese communities, as well as HBV testing in Kampuchean (Cambodian) and Hmong communities [9, 62–64]. However, they were not effective in promoting Pap testing among Kampuchean (Cambodian) women or HBV testing among Chinese men and women [65, 66].

Community-Based Group Education Studies

Two trials have documented that group education, delivered in community settings, can positively impact mammography completion rates among immigrant women who have not been recently screened. One of these studies evaluated group education for Korean immigrant women and their husbands combined with a couple discussion exercise that was subsequently completed at home [67]. The other study evaluated group education combined with telephone counseling and navigation for Chinese immigrant women [68].

Los Angeles researchers conducted cluster-randomized trials of breast and cervical cancer screening group education, as well as colorectal cancer screening group education (with or without the provision of FOBT kits) for Filipinos. Both trials involved group education by Filipino health professionals [69, 70]. In the breast and cervical cancer screening trial, equivalent increases in mammography and Pap testing rates were observed in experimental and control arms. However, mammography increased significantly more in the experimental arm than in the control arm among recent immigrants [69]. In the colorectal cancer screening trial, experimental arm participants were significantly more likely to be adherent to screening guidelines than control group participants at follow-up (regardless of whether or not they received FOBT kits) [70]. In another trial in the Korean community, this Los Angeles group found that small-group education and small media significantly increased HBV testing [31] .

Researchers from the Center for Asian Health in Philadelphia have evaluated group education combined with navigation, including arranging appointments with clinical partners, language translation, assisting with paperwork, and transportation. Their studies have focused on cervical cancer screening among Chinese women, recruited from four Asian community organizations (two experimental and two control), and colorectal cancer screening among older Koreans, recruited from six churches (three experimental and three control). At baseline, study participants were nonadherent to screening guidelines. While these studies had relatively small sample sizes, they both demonstrated a strong intervention effect ($p<0.001$) [48, 49].

One evaluation of group education included multiple Asian groups (Chinese, Koreans, and Vietnamese). This study focused on HBV testing. Experimental group participants were recruited through 15 community organizations in Baltimore, and control group participants were recruited through 12 community organizations in Washington, DC. Group education was provided by Asian health educators and included use of Asian language videos and photonovels. Control group participants received an English language brochure about HBV. The intervention had a significant effect on HBV testing rates among participants who were untested at baseline [15].

Trials of One-on-One Education and Small Media

Wu and colleagues examined the effect of telephone counseling about mammography for Chinese women who were nonadherent to screening guidelines. Control group participants received an English language mammography brochure. While mammography uptake after 4 months was equivalent in the experimental and control groups, there was a significant intervention effect among women with insurance coverage for breast cancer screening [71]. A comparative effectiveness trial tested two alternative mammography videos for Chinese women who had not received a mammogram in the previous year. Participants were randomized to receive a culturally targeted video, generic video, or fact sheet. All the small media were provided in Chinese. Primary analyses that included all randomized women found neither of the videos was effective. However, secondary analyses found the culturally targeted video was effective among a subgroup of women with low acculturation [72]. Another three-arm trial addressed approaches to promoting FOBT among Vietnamese patients of a primary care clinic network. Both experimental groups received a culturally and linguistically tailored brochure and FOBT kit by mail, and one of the experimental groups also received telephone counseling (provided by Vietnamese community health advisors). The trial findings indicated that telephone counseling was effective in increasing FOBT completion rates, but the culturally tailored brochure was not [73].

Quasi-experimental Studies of Community-Level Interventions

Four quasi-experimental studies evaluated breast and/or cervical cancer screening community interventions for Korean and Vietnamese women in California. The interventions included use of Asian language mass media combined with other components such as distribution of Asian language educational materials, workshops at Korean churches, and continuing medical education for Vietnamese physicians. Only one of these studies had positive findings [74–78].

Nguyen and colleagues assessed the impact of a community intervention to increase colorectal cancer screening levels among Vietnamese. Intervention components included a Vietnamese language media campaign, distribution of Vietnamese language educational materials, and continuing medical education for Vietnamese physicians. The proportions of participants who had never received a colonoscopy or sigmoidoscopy increased significantly in the experimental community (44 % at preintervention to 65 % postintervention) and a control community (37 % at preintervention to 47 % postintervention), but the increase was significantly greater in the experimental community. There was no intervention effect for FOBT [79].

Discussion

While intervention studies with positive findings are more likely to be published than intervention studies with negative findings, there is reasonably good evidence that LHW outreach and community-based group education (combined with other intervention components) can increase the use of cancer-related screening tests among Asian Americans [80]. However, trials of LHW outreach and community-based group education have not all demonstrated intervention effects. Since many Asian immigrant communities are relatively small and self-contained with strong social and extended family networks, it is possible that educational messages were disseminated to control groups in some of the negative trials [65, 66].

Researchers have reported relatively modest or no intervention effects from most quasi-experimental studies of community-level interventions to increase mammography and Pap testing levels among Asian women [55, 80]. Some of these interventions may have had insufficient reach, and their components may have lacked adequate intensity [75, 77]. Other factors that may have contributed to negative study results include the diffusion of intervention components from experimental to control communities, as well as the implementation of unanticipated and competing cancer screening programs in control communities [75, 77, 78].

The majority of cancer control intervention studies with Asian participants have used self-reports of screening test completion to measure outcomes [55]. There is some evidence that the reliability and validity of survey responses among Asians is relatively low, possibly because of a cultural tendency toward acquiescence [55, 81, 82]. While a few studies have attempted to verify self-reports with provider reports, Asian naming systems can result in the misfiling of test results, and health-care facilities that lack computerized technology can have difficulty locating medical records [62, 63, 83]. Recent initiatives to increase the use of electronic health records should facilitate the use of provider reports for outcome ascertainment in future studies [84].

Recommendations and Next Steps

In order to monitor cancer screening rates and to identify groups that underutilize cancer screening tests, it is important to continue to collect detailed information on ethnicity and acculturation among Asian Americans when assessing cancer screening. As many Asian Americans have limited English proficiency, it will be critical to provide linguistically appropriate access to health care to facilitate screening test use. In addition to promoting cancer screening in clinical settings, community venues can reach Asian Americans that may not have a regular health-care provider. Most cancer control interventions for Asian Americans have focused on Chinese, Koreans, and Vietnamese, and there is little information about evidence-based interventions for other large Asian groups (e.g., Indians) or for smaller groups such as the Hmong [5, 80]. Additionally, very few interventions have been tailored for use in more than one Asian group [55, 80]. More research is needed on how to balance the need for culturally appropriate interventions in settings that serve multiple ethnic groups, which is the case in most clinics. Finally, most interventions have sought to change individual factors (e.g., beliefs about screening tests) rather than factors related to health-care providers and systems [80]. Future cancer control research initiatives should develop and evaluate interventions for previously understudied Asian groups. They should also focus on the health-care system and other interventions that could be tailored to multiple Asian groups.

Financial Disclosure Authors' declaration of personal interests: none
Declaration of funding interests: none

References

1. Cox B, Sneyd MJ (2013) Bias in breast cancer research in the screening era. Breast 22(6):1041–1045
2. U.S. Preventive Services Task Force (2014) http://www.uspreventiveservicestaskforce.org/Page/Name/home
3. Centers for Disease Control and Prevention (2012) Cancer screening—United States, 2010. Morb Mortal Wkly Rep 61(3):41–45
4. California Health Interview Survey 2014. http://healthpolicy.ucla.edu/chis/Pages/default.aspx
5. Hoeffel EM, Rastogi S, Kim MO, Shahid H (2012) The Asian Population: 2010. 2010 Census Brief issued March 2012. US Census Bureau, Washington, DC
6. Ryu SY, Crespi CM, Maxwell AE (2013) Colorectal cancer among Koreans living in South Korea versus California: incidence, mortality, and screening rates. Ethnic Health 19:406–423
7. Lee HY, Ju E, Vang PD, Lundquist M (2010) Breast and cervical cancer screening disparity among Asian American women: does race/ethnicity matter [corrected]? J Womens Health 19(10):1877–1884
8. Lee HY, Lundquist M, Ju E, Luo X, Townsend A (2011) Colorectal cancer screening disparities in Asian Americans and pacific islanders: which groups are most vulnerable? Ethn Health 16(6):501–518
9. Chen MS Jr, Fang DM, Stewart SL, Ly MY, Lee S, Dang JH et al (2013) Increasing hepatitis B screening for hmong adults: results from a randomized controlled community-based study. Cancer Epidemiol Biomarkers Prev 22(5):782–791
10. Taylor VM, Bastani R, Burke N, Talbot J, Sos C, Liu Q et al (2011) Factors associated with hepatitis B testing among Cambodian American men and women. J Immigr Minor Health 14(1):30–38
11. Lee S, Chen L, Jung MY, Baezconde-Garbanati L, Juon HS (2014) Acculturation and cancer screening among Asian Americans: role of health insurance and having a regular physician. J Community Health 39(2):201–212
12. Ma GX, Tan Y, Wang MQ, Yuan Y, Chae WG (2010) Hepatitis B screening compliance and non-compliance among Chinese, Koreans, Vietnamese and Cambodians. Clin Med Insights Gastroenterol 3:1–10
13. Maxwell AE, Bastani R, Chen MS Jr, Nguyen TT, Stewart SL, Taylor VM (2010) Constructing a theoretically based set of measures for liver cancer control research studies. Prev Med 50(1–2):68–73
14. Stewart SL, Rakowski W, Pasick RJ (2009) Behavioral constructs and mammography in five ethnic groups. Health Educ Behav 36(5 Suppl):36S–54S

15. Juon HS, Lee S, Strong C, Rimal R, Kirk GD, Bowie J (2014) Effect of a liver cancer education program on hepatitis B screening among Asian Americans in the Baltimore-Washington metropolitan area, 2009-2010. Prev Chronic Dis 11:130258
16. Thompson CA, Gomez SL, Chan A, Chan JK, McClellan SR, Chung S et al (2014) Patient and provider characteristics associated with colorectal, breast, and cervical cancer screening among Asian Americans. Cancer Epidemiol Biomarkers Prev 23(11):2208–2217
17. Kandula NR, Wen M, Jacobs EA, Lauderdale DS (2006) Low rates of colorectal, cervical, and breast cancer screening in Asian Americans compared with non-Hispanic whites: cultural influences or access to care? Cancer 107(1):184–192
18. Maxwell AE, Crespi CM (2009) Trends in colorectal cancer screening utilization among ethnic groups in California: are we closing the gap? Cancer Epidemiol Biomarkers Prev 18(3): 752–759
19. American Cancer Society (2014) Colorectal Cancer Facts & Figures 2014-2016. American Cancer Society, Atlanta
20. Lok AS, McMahon BJ (2009) Chronic hepatitis B: update 2009. Hepatology 50(3):661–662
21. Chou R, Dana T, Bougatsos C, Blazina I, Khangura J, Zakher B (2014) Screening for hepatitis B virus infection in adolescents and adults: a systematic review to update the U.S. Preventive Services Task Force recommendation. Ann Intern Med 161(1):31–45
22. Colvin HM, Mitchell AE (2010) Hepatitis and liver cancer: A national strategy for prevention and control of hepatitis B and C. National Academic Press, Washington, DC
23. Khalili M, Burman B (2014) Liver disease. In: Hammer GD, McPhee SJ (eds) Pathophysiology of disease: An introduction to clinical medicine, 7th edn. Lange Medical Books/McGraw-Hill, New York
24. Tanaka M, Gehan E, Chen MY, Wang JH (2014) Hepatitis B screening practice among older Chinese in the Greater Washington, DC, area. South Med J 107(10):655–660
25. Strong C, Lee S, Tanaka M, Juon HS (2012) Ethnic differences in prevalence and barriers of HBV screening and vaccination among Asian Americans. J Community Health 37(5): 1071–1080
26. Nguyen TT, McPhee SJ, Stewart S, Gildengorin G, Zhang L, Wong C et al (2010) Factors associated with hepatitis B testing among Vietnamese Americans. J Gen Intern Med 25(7):694–700
27. Taylor VM, Talbot J, Do HH, Liu Q, Yasui Y, Jackson JC et al (2011) Hepatitis B knowledge and practices among Cambodian Americans. Asian Pac J Cancer Prev 12(4):957–961
28. Taylor VM, Tu SP, Woodall E, Acorda E, Chen H, Choe J et al (2006) Hepatitis B knowledge and practices among Chinese immigrants to the United States. Asian Pac J Cancer Prev 7(2):313–317
29. Bastani R, Glenn BA, Maxwell AE, Jo AM (2007) Hepatitis B testing for liver cancer control among Korean Americans. Ethn Dis 17(2):365–373
30. Grytdal SP, Liao Y, Chen R, Garvin CC, Grigg-Saito D, Kagawa-Singer M et al (2009) Hepatitis B testing and vaccination among Vietnamese- and Cambodian-Americans. J Community Health 34(3):173–180
31. Bastani R, Glenn BA, Maxwell AE, Jo AM, Herrmann AK, Crespi CM et al (2015) Cluster-randomized trial to increase hepatitis B testing among Koreans in Los Angeles. Cancer Epidemiol Biomarkers Prev 24(9):1341–1349
32. Bastani R, Glenn BA, Taylor VM, Chen MS Jr, Nguyen TT, Stewart SL et al (2010) Integrating theory into community interventions to reduce liver cancer disparities: the health behavior framework. Prev Med 50(1-2):63–67
33. Maxwell AE, Bastani R, Crespi CM, Danao LL, Cayetano RT (2011) Behavioral mediators of colorectal cancer screening in a randomized controlled intervention trial. Prev Med 52(2):167–173
34. Maxwell AE, Crespi CM, Antonio CM, Lu P (2010) Explaining disparities in colorectal cancer screening among five Asian ethnic groups: a population-based study in California. BMC Cancer 10:214
35. Beydoun HA, Beydoun MA (2008) Predictors of colorectal cancer screening behaviors among average-risk older adults in the United States. Cancer Causes Control 19(4):339–359

36. Wu TY, Guthrie BJ, Bancroft JM (2005) An integrative review on breast cancer screening practice and correlates among Chinese, Korean, Filipino, and Asian Indian American women. Health Care Women Int 26(3):225–246
37. Coronado GD, Taylor VM, Tu SP, Yasui Y, Acorda E, Woodall E et al (2007) Correlates of hepatitis B testing among Chinese Americans. J Community Health 32(6):379–390
38. Pourat N, Kagawa-Singer M, Breen N, Sripipatana A (2010) Access versus acculturation: identifying modifiable factors to promote cancer screening among Asian American women. Med Care 48(12):1088–1096
39. Nguyen TT, McPhee SJ, Nguyen T, Lam T, Mock J (2002) Predictors of cervical Pap smear screening awareness, intention, and receipt among Vietnamese-American women. Am J Prev Med 23(3):207–214
40. Taylor VM, Jackson JC, Tu SP, Yasui Y, Schwartz SM, Kuniyuki A et al (2002) Cervical cancer screening among Chinese Americans. Cancer Detect Prev 26(2):139–145
41. Ma GX, Fang CY, Feng Z, Tan Y, Gao W, Ge S et al (2012) Correlates of cervical cancer screening among Vietnamese American women. Infect Dis Obstet Gynecol 2012:617234
42. Bastani R, Maxwell AE, Bradford C, Das IP, Yan KX (1999) Tailored risk notification for women with a family history of breast cancer. Prev Med 29(5):355–364
43. Sun WY, Basch CE, Wolf RL, Li XJ (2004) Factors associated with colorectal cancer screening among Chinese-Americans. Prev Med 39(2):323–329
44. Anhang Price R, Zapka J, Edwards H, Taplin SH (2010) Organizational factors and the cancer screening process. J Natl Cancer Inst Monogr 2010(40):38–57
45. Hsu L, Bowlus CL, Stewart SL, Nguyen TT, Dang J, Chan B et al (2013) Electronic messages increase hepatitis B screening in at-risk Asian American patients: a randomized, controlled trial. Dig Dis Sci 58(3):807–814
46. Nguyen BH, Nguyen KP, McPhee SJ, Nguyen AT, Tran DQ, Jenkins CN (2000) Promoting cancer prevention activities among Vietnamese physicians in California. J Cancer Educ 15(2):82–85
47. Nguyen TT, McPhee SJ, Bui-Tong N, Luong TN, Ha-Iaconis T, Nguyen T et al (2006) Community-based participatory research increases cervical cancer screening among Vietnamese-Americans. J Health Care Poor Underserved 17(2 Suppl):31–54
48. Wang X, Fang C, Tan Y, Liu A, Ma GX (2010) Evidence-based intervention to reduce access barriers to cervical cancer screening among underserved Chinese American women. J Womens Health 19(3):463–469
49. Ma GX, Shive S, Tan Y, Gao W, Rhee J, Park M et al (2009) Community-based colorectal cancer intervention in underserved Korean Americans. Cancer Epidemiol 33(5):381–386
50. Tu SP, Yasui Y, Kuniyuki A, Thompson B, Schwartz SM, Jackson JC et al (2000) Breast cancer screening among Cambodian American women. Cancer Detect Prev 24(6):549–563
51. Wu TY, West B, Chen YW, Hergert C (2006) Health beliefs and practices related to breast cancer screening in Filipino, Chinese and Asian-Indian women. Cancer Detect Prev 30(1):58–66
52. Taylor VM, Schwartz SM, Jackson JC, Kuniyuki A, Fischer M, Yasui Y et al (1999) Cervical cancer screening among Cambodian-American women. Cancer Epidemiol Biomarkers Prev 8(6):541–546
53. Wang JH, Liang W, Chen MY, Cullen J, Feng S, Yi B et al (2006) The influence of culture and cancer worry on colon cancer screening among older Chinese-American women. Ethn Dis 16(2):404–411
54. Briss PA, Zaza S, Pappaioanou M, Fielding J, Wright-De Aguero L, Truman BI et al (2000) Developing an evidence-based Guide to Community Preventive Services--methods. The Task Force on Community Preventive Services. Am J Prev Med 18(1 Suppl):35–43
55. Lu M, Moritz S, Lorenzetti D, Sykes L, Straus S, Quan H (2012) A systematic review of interventions to increase breast and cervical cancer screening uptake among Asian women. BMC Public Health 12:413
56. Sabatino SA, Lawrence B, Elder R, Mercer SL, Wilson KM, DeVinney B et al (2012) Effectiveness of interventions to increase screening for breast, cervical, and colorectal cancers:

nine updated systematic reviews for the guide to community preventive services. Am J Prev Med 43(1):97–118
57. Tu SP, Taylor V, Yasui Y, Chun A, Yip MP, Acorda E et al (2006) Promoting culturally appropriate colorectal cancer screening through a health educator: a randomized controlled trial. Cancer 107(5):959–966
58. Tu SP, Chun A, Yasui Y, Kuniyuki A, Yip MP, Taylor V et al (2014) Adaptation of an evidence-based intervention to promote colorectal cancer screening: a quasi-experimental study. Implement Sci 9:85
59. Bird JA, McPhee SJ, Ha NT, Le B, Davis T, Jenkins CN (1998) Opening pathways to cancer screening for Vietnamese-American women: lay health workers hold a key. Prev Med 27(6):821–829
60. Mock J, McPhee SJ, Nguyen T, Wong C, Doan H, Lai KQ et al (2007) Effective lay health worker outreach and media-based education for promoting cervical cancer screening among Vietnamese American women. Am J Public Health 97(9):1693–1700
61. Nguyen TT, Le G, Nguyen T, Le K, Lai K, Gildengorin G et al (2009) Breast cancer screening among Vietnamese Americans: a randomized controlled trial of lay health worker outreach. Am J Prev Med 37(4):306–313
62. Taylor VM, Jackson JC, Yasui Y, Nguyen TT, Woodall E, Acorda E et al (2010) Evaluation of a cervical cancer control intervention using lay health workers for Vietnamese American women. Am J Public Health 100(10):1924–1929
63. Taylor VM, Bastani R, Burke N, Talbot J, Sos C, Liu Q et al (2013) Evaluation of a hepatitis B lay health worker intervention for Cambodian Americans. J Community Health 38(3):546–553
64. Taylor VM, Hislop TG, Jackson JC, Tu SP, Yasui Y, Schwartz SM et al (2002) A randomized controlled trial of interventions to promote cervical cancer screening among Chinese women in North America. J Natl Cancer Inst 94(9):670–677
65. Taylor VM, Jackson JC, Yasui Y, Kuniyuki A, Acorda E, Marchand A et al (2002) Evaluation of an outreach intervention to promote cervical cancer screening among Cambodian American women. Cancer Detect Prev 26(4):320–327
66. Taylor VM, Hislop TG, Tu SP, Teh C, Acorda E, Yip MP et al (2009) Evaluation of a hepatitis B lay health worker intervention for Chinese Americans and Canadians. J Community Health 34(3):165–172
67. Lee E, Menon U, Nandy K, Szalacha L, Kviz F, Cho Y et al (2014) The effect of a couples intervention to increase breast cancer screening among Korean Americans. Oncol Nurs Forum 41(3):E185–E193
68. Lee-Lin F, Nguyen T, Pedhiwala N, Dieckmann N, Menon U (2015) A breast health educational program for Chinese-American women: 3- to 12-month postintervention effect. Am J Health Promot 29(3):173–181
69. Maxwell AE, Bastani R, Vida P, Warda US (2003) Results of a randomized trial to increase breast and cervical cancer screening among Filipino American women. Prev Med 37(2):102–109
70. Maxwell AE, Bastani R, Danao LL, Antonio C, Garcia GM, Crespi CM (2010) Results of a community-based randomized trial to increase colorectal cancer screening among Filipino Americans. Am J Public Health 100(11):2228–2234
71. Wu TY, Lin C (2015) Developing and evaluating an individually tailored intervention to increase mammography adherence among Chinese American women. Cancer Nurs 38(1):40–49
72. Wang JH, Schwartz MD, Brown RL, Maxwell AE, Lee MM, Adams IF et al (2012) Results of a randomized controlled trial testing the efficacy of a culturally-targeted and a generic video on mammography screening among Chinese-American immigrants. Cancer Epidemiol Biomarkers Prev 21(11):1923–32
73. Walsh JM, Salazar R, Nguyen TT, Kaplan C, Nguyen LK, Hwang J et al (2010) Healthy colon, healthy life: a novel colorectal cancer screening intervention. Am J Prev Med 39(1):1–14
74. Jenkins CN, McPhee SJ, Bird JA, Pham GQ, Nguyen BH, Nguyen T et al (1999) Effect of a media-led education campaign on breast and cervical cancer screening among Vietnamese-American women. Prev Med 28(4):395–406

75. Nguyen T, Vo PH, McPhee SJ, Jenkins CN (2001) Promoting early detection of breast cancer among Vietnamese-American women. Results of a controlled trial. Cancer 91(1 Suppl): 267–273
76. Nguyen TT, McPhee SJ, Gildengorin G, Nguyen T, Wong C, Lai KQ et al (2006) Papanicolaou testing among Vietnamese Americans: results of a multifaceted intervention. Am J Prev Med 31(1):1–9
77. Moskowitz JM, Kazinets G, Wong JM, Tager IB (2007) "Health is strength": a community health education program to improve breast and cervical cancer screening among Korean American Women in Alameda County, California. Cancer Detect Prev 31(2):173–183
78. Wismer BA, Moskowitz JM, Min K, Chen AM, Ahn Y, Cho S et al (2001) Interim assessment of a community intervention to improve breast and cervical cancer screening among Korean American women. J Public Health Manag Pract 7(2):61–70
79. Nguyen BH, McPhee SJ, Stewart SL, Doan HT (2010) Effectiveness of a controlled trial to promote colorectal cancer screening in Vietnamese Americans. Am J Public Health 100(5): 870–876
80. Hou SI, Sealy DA, Kabiru CW (2011) Closing the disparity gap: cancer screening interventions among Asians--a systematic literature review. Asian Pac J Cancer Prev 12(11):3133–3139
81. McPhee SJ, Nguyen TT, Shema SJ, Nguyen B, Somkin C, Vo P et al (2002) Validation of recall of breast and cervical cancer screening by women in an ethnically diverse population. Prev Med 35(5):463–473
82. Pasick RJ, Stewart SL, Bird JA, D'Onofrio CN (2001) Quality of data in multiethnic health surveys. Public Health Rep 116(Suppl 1):223–243
83. Paskett ED, McLaughlin JM, Lehman AM, Katz ML, Tatum CM, Oliveri JM (2011) Evaluating the efficacy of lay health advisors for increasing risk-appropriate Pap test screening: a randomized controlled trial among Ohio Appalachian women. Cancer Epidemiol Biomarkers Prev 20(5):835–843
84. Pourat N, Hadler MW (2014) Ready for ACA? How community health centers are preparing for health care reform. Policy brief (UCLA Center for Health Policy Research (PB2014-4):1-6, appendix

Lung Cancer Among Asian Americans

S. Lani Park, Daniel O. Stram, Mindy C. De Rouen, Scarlett Lin Gomez, Anna H. Wu, and Iona Cheng

Abstract Among Asian-American men and women, lung cancer is the second most commonly occurring cancer and primary cause of cancer-related mortality. Collectively, Asian-American men and women have a lower incidence rate of lung cancer than their non-Hispanic white counterparts. However, there is considerable heterogeneity in incidence rates across Asian-American subgroups, some of whom experience increasing rates of lung cancer and/or rates similar to non-Hispanic Whites. Active cigarette smoking is the primary risk factor for lung cancer; cigarette smoking may be influenced by education, acculturation, and access to health care. Among never smokers, Asian-American women experience a higher risk of lung cancer in comparison to Asian-American men and non-Hispanic white women; and additional risk factors such as indoor- and outdoor air pollution, passive smoking, and lifestyle factors should be considered. In order to aid in disease prevention and improve survival through early stage diagnosis, further work towards understanding risk factors in never smokers as well as identifying at-risk individuals in this growing US population are needed.

Keywords Lung cancer • Asian Americans • Epidemiology • Smoking • Never smokers

S.L. Park, Ph.D., M.P.H. (✉) • D.O. Stram • A.H. Wu
Department of Preventive Medicine, Keck School of Medicine, University of Southern California, 1450 Biggy Street, Rm 1509G, Los Angeles, CA 90089-9234, USA
e-mail: sungship@med.usc.edu

M.C. De Rouen • S.L. Gomez • I. Cheng
Cancer Prevention Institute of California, Fremont, CA, USA

A.H. Wu, D.O. Stram (eds.), *Cancer Epidemiology Among Asian Americans*,
DOI 10.1007/978-3-319-41118-7_5

Introduction

Lung cancer is the second most commonly occurring cancer and the primary cause of cancer death in men and women in the United States (US). In 2015, approximately 221,200 Americans were diagnosed with lung cancer [1]. Asian Americans, defined as those who are ethnically East, South East, or South Asian, represented 5.6 % of the US population in 2010 with approximately two-thirds born outside of the US and a quarter who immigrated within the past decade [2]. It is estimated that by 2050, the Asian-American population will double and increase to 10.1 % of the US population [3]. Therefore, understanding the epidemiology of lung cancer in Asian Americans is a public health priority.

Trends

Incidence

Considered broadly, lung cancer incidence rates (IRs) among Asian American/Pacific Islanders (AAPI) are lower than that of their non-Hispanic White and non-Hispanic Black counterparts. Surveillance, Epidemiology, and End Results (SEER) data from 20 US geographical areas reported that in 2012, the lung cancer IRs among AAPI men and women were 46.7 and 27.9 per 100,000, respectively [4]. In comparison, IRs among non-Hispanic White men and women were 69.7 and 54.1 per 100,000, respectively.

However, specific Asian-American subgroups experience a higher burden of lung cancer. Table 1 presents the IRs of lung cancer across eight major Asian-American

Table 1 Incidence rates[a] of lung cancer (2004–2008)[b] for the eight largest Asian-American subgroups and non-Hispanic Whites, stratified by sex

	Lung cancer incidence rate IR (95 % CI)	
Asian-American subgroup	Men	Women
Asian Indians and Pakistanis	30.1 (26.0–34.6)	12.4 (10.3–14.9)
Chinese	52.0 (49.5–54.6)	29.9 (28.2–31.7)
Filipinos	68.4 (65.3–71.7)	30.1 (28.4–31.9)
Japanese	52.4 (49.1–55.7)	27.9 (26.1–29.9)
Kampucheans	51.7 (38.0–68.3)	26.7 (19.0–36.3)
Koreans	57.5 (52.1–63.1)	28.0 (25.2–31.1)
Laotians	70.6 (54.0–90.2)	27.1 (18.4–38.3)
Vietnamese	73.4 (67.4–79.7)	31.8 (28.5–35.4)
Non-Hispanic Whites	74.0 (73.5–74.6)	56.6 (56.2–57.1)

[a]IRs are presented as per 100,000 and adjusted to the US standard population
[b]Data abstracted from Gomez et al., JNCI, 2013 [5]

subgroups and non-Hispanic Whites from 2004 to 2008 [5]. In men, IRs for Filipinos, Vietnamese, and Laotians were comparable to non-Hispanic Whites (Table 1) (68.4, 73.4, and 70.6, respectively, compared to 74.0 per 100,000), while Asian Indians and Pakistanis had the lowest rate (30.1 per 100,000) [5]. In women, lung cancer IRs among subgroups of Asian Americans were about half that of non-Hispanic White women. Asian Indian and Pakistanis had the lowest IR (12.4 per 100,000) while Vietnamese had the highest IR (31.8 per 100,000) [5]. For the other Asian-American subgroups of women, IRs ranged from 26.7 in Kampucheans (Cambodians) to 30.1 in Filipinos (Table 1) [5]. While among all subgroups of Asian-American men the IRs for lung cancer from 1990 to 2008 were stable or decreasing, a 2.1 % annual increase was seen for both Filipina and Korean women, although this was only statistically significant in Filipina women [4, 5]. The increasing trends in Asian-American women may be due to their higher smoking rates among those more acculturated (see section "Smoking").

Lung cancer incidence varies by socioeconomic status (SES) among Asian Americans, but with a stronger correlation among men than women. In a study based on the California Cancer Registry (CCR), in which a neighborhood composite index of SES was used, AAPI men residing in the lowest neighborhood SES quintile had a higher risk of lung cancer than those residing in highest neighborhood SES quintile (relative index of inequality (RII) = 1.46, 95 % CI: 1.33–1.60) [6]. In AAPI women, this increased risk was less pronounced (RII = 1.16, 95 % CI: 1.02–1.33) between the lowest and highest SES neighborhoods [6]. These differences between AAPI men and women may be due to differences in smoking patterns and other risk factors associated with SES.

While collectively the lung cancer IRs are lower for Asian-American men and women compared to non-Hispanic White men and women, IRs by smoking status, the primary risk factor for lung cancer, and factors that influence smoking, -such as nativity, birth place, and acculturation, vary substantially. For example, among never smokers, lung cancer incidence has been found to be more common among women than men and this disparity may be greater in Asian Americans [7]. A pooled study of never smokers from 13 large cohort studies found that White men and women had IRs of 11.2 (95 % CI: 9.8–12.6) and 12.4 (95 % CI: 11.3–13.5) per 100,000, respectively, whereas IRs among Asian men and women were 12.9 (95 % CI: 6.7–19.1) and 15.0 (95 % CI: 10.4–19.7), respectively [8]. Furthermore, in a study utilizing CCR data (1998–2003), foreign-born Asian men and women had a 35 % higher rate of non-small cell lung cancers (NSCLCs) than US-born Asian men and women [9]. In Asian men, a higher rate of NSCLCs was consistent with the higher smoking prevalence in foreign-born Asian men (46 %) compared to US-born Asian men (35 %), but a higher rate of NSCLCs was not consistent with the lower smoking prevalence in foreign-born Asian women (11 %) than in US-born Asian women (22 %) [9]. These findings suggest that, particularly for Asian-American women, risk factors beyond smoking should be evaluated (see section "Risk Factors").

Stage of Disease, Survival, and Mortality

In the US, results from SEER showed that 5-year relative survival for lung cancer in all racial/ethnic groups was 17.4 %, and lower in men (15.6 %) than women (21.1 %) [4]. The 5-year relative survival was similar between AAPI women (21.9 %) and white women (21.2 %), but AAPI men had a slightly lower 5-year relative survival (15 %) than white men (16.1 %) [10].

Stage of disease is the most important prognostic indicator for lung cancer survival. Among White men and women, the 5-year relative survival (year of diagnosis 2005–2012) was 49.7 % and 60.3 %, respectively, for localized disease and 3.3 % and 4.8 %, respectively, for distant disease [10]. Compared to White men and women, AAPI men and women had better 5-year relative survival for both localized (52.9 % and 68.6 %, respectively) and distant (5.6 % and 6.4 %, respectively) disease [10]. However, all eight subgroups of AAPI men and women were more likely to be diagnosed with distant stage disease (men ranged from 45 to 60 %, women ranged from 48 to 59 %) than non-Hispanic white men (42 %) and women (40 %) [11].

The mortality and survival rates of lung cancer differ across Asian-American subgroups. Using data from 13 SEER registries (1991–2007) in a competing risk analysis, compared to non-Hispanic Whites, five of the seven Asian subgroups (Japanese and Koreans were the exceptions), had lower lung cancer-specific mortality (hazard ratios (HR) range = 0.71–0.88) [12]. When comparing within Asian subgroups, another study of NSCLC cases, using CCR data, found that most Asian American subgroups (with the exception of Indians/Pakistanis) presented with a poorer overall and disease-specific survival than Chinese [13].

Differences in survival can be also attributed to SES, access to healthcare, cancer treatment, as well as other environmental or biologic factors [13]. For instance, the lower survival observed among other AAPI and Vietnamese men may be related to more recent immigration to the US, lower SES, and less access to healthcare [2]. However, the SES differences do not explain the reported lower survival among Japanese Americans than other Asian groups [13]. Similar to Whites, 87–90 % of Asian Americans with stage 1 or 2 lung cancer received definitive treatment (surgical resection) for lung cancer, but three of the seven Asian-American groups (Chinese, Filipinos, and others) with stage 3 lung cancer were less likely to receive definitive treatment (54–55 %) compared to Whites (62 %) [12]. In a meta-analysis of randomized control trials (RCTs) to assess response to cytotoxic chemotherapy in NSCLC patients, Asians had a higher median overall survival (10.1 months vs. 8 months) and higher overall response rate (32.2 % vs. 25.9 %) than Whites [14]. The higher proportion of epidermal growth factor receptor (EGFR)-positive adenocarcinoma (see sections "Histopathology" and "Somatic Mutation") among Asian populations may play a role in improved survival among this population and additional studies are needed to investigate the contribution of genetic markers to clinical response rates and overall lung cancer survival.

Histopathology

The four major histologic cell-types of lung cancer are squamous cell carcinoma (SCC), large cell carcinoma (LCC), adenocarcinoma (AC), and small cell lung cancer (SCLC) [15]. SCC, LCC, and AC are classified under the group of NSCLC. The majority of SCCs and SCLCs occur in the central compartment of the lung, while the majority of ACs occurs in the periphery. Prior to the mid-1980s, SCC and AC were the most common histologic cell-type in US men and women, respectively [16]. However, since the 1990s, AC has become the predominant cell type in both US men and women [17–19]. This shift in histology has been attributed to the changing composition of the tobacco blend and the cigarette design over time, such as the introduction of cigarettes with filtered tips. This resulted in alterations in smoking behavior, such as greater smoking intensity (deeper inhalation) for the same delivery of nicotine, and more lung carcinogen exposures in the lung periphery [17, 20]. In the past 10 years, among non-Hispanic White men, IRs for the four main histologic-specific cell-types have been steadily declining. However, among non-Hispanic White women, during the same period, IRs declined for SCLC and LCC whereas the IRs for SCC and AC continued to increase and only have recently appeared to stabilize. This increase in non-Hispanic White women may be due in part to a cohort effect with their later adoption of smoking (started in 1920s and 1930s), roughly 20–30 years later than men [21].

Based on SEER data since the 1990s, lung cancer IRs showed a similar shift in histologic cell-type from SCC to AC in most Asian-American men [11]. In Asian-American women, AC remained the more common histologic cell-type. In a SEER report of registry data from 1990 through 2010, annual percent increases in AC were found in several Asian-American groups, including Chinese men (1.3 %, 95 % CI: 0–2.5), Filipino women (2.6 %, 95 % CI: 1.7–3.5), and Korean women (3.0 %, 95 % CI: 1.6–4.4) [11]. For most AAPI men and women, the other major histologic cell-types (SCC, SCLC, and LCC) were stable or decreased during this time period, similar to non-Hispanic White men and women. A noted exception was an annual percent increase in SCC (2.4 %; 95 % CI: 0.7–4.2) in Japanese women [11]. Better understanding of the risk factors influencing the rise in AC in some Asian-American subgroups is needed.

Somatic Mutations

While there is limited data on somatic mutations associated with lung cancer in Asian Americans, studies conducted in Asia suggest differences in the types and frequency of somatic mutations between Asians and Whites.

For example, K-Ras mutations have been found to occur in 15–25 % of AC among Whites in Western countries [22, 23], but it was generally found to be less common in Asian populations (range 3–10 %) [24–26]. In a study in Japan, KRAS mutations occurred in 6 % of females and 3 % of males; and in 5 % of never smokers and 4 % of ever smokers [24]. Similar low prevalence estimates were reported in studies of NSCLC in Taiwan and Hong Kong [25, 26].

P53 tumor suppressor mutations are common in lung cancer, especially smoking-related lung cancer, and has been found in approximately 33 % of AC and approximately 70 % of SCLC [27]. For lung cancer, common *p53* mutation hotspots occur in codons 157, 248, and 273 [28] and most frequently present as a GC to TA transversion. There is a correlation between GC to TA transversions and tobacco exposure, both in the quantity and duration of smoking [28, 29]. Among studies conducted in Asia, *p53* mutation frequencies varied widely from 1 to 70 %, but many of these studies were small and did not examine differences by sex, smoking status, or histologic cell-types [30–34]. In one of the larger studies in Asia (69 SCC and 67 AC), *p53* mutations were found in 70 % of smokers and 65 % of nonsmokers and 69 % of SCC cases and 67 % of AC cases [32].

EGFR gene mutations are commonly found in AC, but are virtually absent in other histologic cell-types [23]. They occur most frequently in AC of never smokers (51–68 %), women (42–62 %) and persons of East or Southeast Asian descent (>49 %) compared to persons from Western countries (≤26 %) [35–39]. Mutations in the human epidermal growth factor receptor II (*HER2)* gene, also a member of the EGFR family, are also more commonly found in AC, women, nonsmokers, and those of Asian descent [40]. *EGFR* mutations in AC are of particular importance as this mutation is particularly responsive to tyrosine kinase inhibitors (TKI) such as gefitinib and erlotinib for lung cancer treatment [38]. A meta-analyses of 14 RCTs found that in NSCLC patients, TKI therapy was particularly effective among never smokers but was less so for former/current smokers [41]. This study, however, did not evaluate the efficacy of TKI therapy in never smokers by EGFR mutation status.

Other common lung cancer mutations that differ in frequency across race/ethnicity include the liver kinase B1 (*LKB1*) and anaplastic lymphoma kinase (ALK) mutations. In a study of 144 lung tumors of primarily Whites, *LKB1* mutations were more common in AC (34 %) than in SCC (19 %) [42]. *LKB1* mutations have been reported to be less common in Asians (113 NSCLCs) than Whites (143 NSCLCs) for both AC (8 % and 19 %, respectively) and SCC (0 % and 13 %, respectively) [43]. Lastly, the fusion of echinoderm microtubule-associated protein-like 4 (EML4)-ALK genes has been found in 3–5 % of NSCLC, primarily AC. Patients with this fusion are more likely to be nonsmokers and younger than those without this fusion gene [44–47]. It has been suggested to be more frequently occurring in Asians (3–6.7 %) than Whites (~1 %) [44–47].

Reasons for differences in the frequency of tumor mutations between Asians and Whites remain unclear. Studies are needed to clarify the distribution of common lung cancer mutations by sex, and smoking status across Asian-American subgroups. This may provide additional insight into the relationships between somatic mutations, lung cancer histologic cell-types, etiology, and progression.

Risk Factors

Active Smoking

The primary risk factor for lung cancer is tobacco use, primarily from cigarette smoking [48]. Cigarette smoke is comprised of at least 4000 chemicals, of which over 70 are established carcinogens [48]. In the US, approximately 90 % of lung cancer deaths in men and 75–80 % of lung cancer deaths in women are caused by smoking [49, 50].

Cigarette smoking is associated with all lung cancer histologic cell-types but the association is weaker for AC. Results from a large pooled analysis (13,169 cases and 16,010 controls) from Europe and Canada [51] and a study from Japan [52] suggest differences in risk associated with current smoking by histology, sex, and by race/ethnicity (Table 2). These studies also showed that in all populations, greater quantity smoked (e.g., pack-years, duration of smoking, or cigarettes per day) were associated with an increasing trend in lung cancer risk for all groups by histology, sex, and race/ethnicity [51, 52].

Epidemiologic data suggests that, at least for some Asian-American subgroups, per smoking dose, the relative risk for lung cancer may be lower. In the Multiethnic Cohort study (MEC), the largest racially/ethnically diverse prospective US study with a focus on etiologies of cancer, it was found that Japanese Americans had a 75 % reduction in lung cancer risk (95 % CI: 0.18–0.36) for the stratum of ≤ 10 cigarettes per day (CPD) in comparison to African Americans, and for the heaviest smokers (≥ 31 CPD), Japanese-Americans had a 25 % reduction in risk (95 % CI: 0.57–1.00) in comparison to African Americans [53]. This is consistent with an earlier report from Le Marchand et al., who found that, compared to White men and women, respectively, for the same quantity smoked, Japanese American men and women had a lower risk of lung cancer (OR = 0.68, 95 % CI: 0.50–0.93 and OR = 0.36, 95 % CI: 0.11–1.2, respectively) [54]. For Japanese Americans, the difference in risk of disease may be partly explained by their slower metabolism of nicotine, thereby resulting in lower nicotine uptake and less exposure to tobacco carcinogens (see genetic risk factors) [55].

Table 2 Summary of the association between active smoking (current vs. never) and lung cancer risk in Whites[a] and Japanese[b] by sex and histologic cell-types

Lung cancer histologic cell-types	White men (pooled) OR (95 % CI)	White women (pooled) OR (95 % CI)	Japanese men OR (95 % CI)	Japanese women OR (95 % CI)
SCLC	45.7 (29.9–70.0)	21.7 (15.5–30.1)	13.1 (4.8–36.2)	85.7 (25.7–286)
SCC	45.6 (34.3–60.6)	13.6 (10.5–17.7)	10.4 (5.8–18.6)	15.0 (6.4–35.1)
AC	10.8 (8.7–13.3)	4.2 (3.5–5.0)	2.3 (1.7–3.2)	1.3 (0.9–1.3)

[a]Data abstracted from Pesch et al., IJC, 2012 [51]

[b]Data abstracted from Seki et al., Cancer Science, 2013 [52]

However, it is not known whether these differences in risk at a given level of smoking in Japanese Americans are applicable to other Asian-American subgroups. This was explored by Le Marchand et al. in a case–control study that also included Filipino and Chinese men and women. Although this study had limited statistical power to detect significant differences, results suggested that Japanese Americans may have lower risk of lung cancer at a given level of smoking than other Asian-American subgroups [54].

It is likely that overall lung cancer risk is lower in Asian Americans as a result of their lower prevalence of current smoking (9 %) compared to non-Hispanic Whites (19.4 %) [56]. On average within Asian-American subgroups, in both men and women, Chinese, Asian Indians, and Japanese had lower prevalence of being current and ever smokers compared to Koreans, Vietnamese, Cambodians, and Laotians [57]. In all Asian-American subgroups, the prevalence of ever smoking was higher in men than women. Although the lower prevalence of ever smoking in Asian Americans is somewhat consistent with their lower risk of disease, the variation within subgroups and particularly the risk in women cannot be entirely explained by the differences in smoking prevalence.

The prevalence of smoking in AAPI is influenced by nativity, education, English proficiency, duration of residence in the US, and ethnic enclave [58]. In particular, level of acculturation is strongly associated with smoking initiation, prevalence, and cessation but differs between Asian-American men and women. Asian-American men, with longer residence in the US (i.e., more acculturated) were found to be 53 % less likely to smoke than those with shorter residence [59]. The prevalence of smoking was also lower among English proficient Asian-American men (18 %) than non-English proficient Asian-American men (33 %) [60]. In contrast, smoking prevalence was five times higher in more acculturated than less acculturated Asian-American women [59] and smoking prevalence was higher among Asian-American women, who were English proficient than those who were less proficient in English [61]. In addition, early smoking initiation influences smoking addiction, resulting in difficulty in cessation, hence a greater likelihood of remaining a current smoker. While the risk of early smoking initiation among Asian-American adolescents is a third of that of Whites, there is marked variation across subgroups [62] and it has been found that tobacco companies currently market specifically to AAPI [63]. Therefore, an increase in smoking prevalence among Asian-American youth may be expected.

The benefits of smoking cessation are well known [64]. In a report from the Million Women Study in the UK, compared to never smokers, former smokers who permanently stopped smoking had higher risk of lung cancer-related mortality. However, those who stopped at 25–34 years of age were at lower risk of lung cancer mortality (rate ratio = 1.84, 95 % CI: 1.45–2.34) than those who quit at 35–44 years of age (rate ratio = 3.34, 95 % CI: 2.76–4.03) [65]. Similar patterns of results were found in an earlier study of men and women in Japan [66]. While the absolute risk of lung cancer in former smokers will not decrease to that of never smokers, the rate in which their absolute risk increases is lower than that of current smokers. Thus, among current smokers, smoking cessation remains the best preventable measure for lung cancer, reinforcing the importance of smoking cessation as a public health priority. Detailed data on the benefits of smoking cessation by Asian-American subgroups are lacking at this time.

Passive Smoking

Secondhand smoke is the complex mixture formed from the escaping smoke of a burning tobacco product and smoke exhaled by the smoker. Exposure to secondhand smoke is also referred to as involuntary smoking or passive smoking. Passive smoking is an established risk factor for lung cancer in never smokers. In a large international study that pooled data from 18 case–control studies including 2504 never smoking lung cancer cases (men and women), passive smoking was associated with a 31 % increased risk of overall lung cancer (95 % CI: 1.17–1.45) [67]. This study found that in never smoking Asians, passive smoking was associated with a 20 % increase in lung cancer risk (95 % CI: 0.98–1.45). This lower risk estimate in Asians may be due to a greater proportion of AC in never smoking Asians compared to never smoking Whites, with a lower passive smoking risk association seen in AC than the other histologic cell-types. The proportion of lung cancers in never smokers attributable to passive smoking has been estimated to range from 20 to 25 % [68] to 37 % [69]. Passive smoking may be more relevant to lung cancer risk in Asian American women than men, as there is a greater proportion of never smoking lung cancer cases among women than men, but its contribution to the burden of lung cancer in these never smoking women is unclear [70–74].

Indoor and Outdoor Air Pollution

Indoor Air Pollution

Indoor air pollution may originate from outdoor or indoor air pollution exposures such as radon from soil and/or water and combustion, passive smoking, and burning coal, wood or cooking fumes.

Radon is a decay product from radium. Residential radon has been found to be associated with lung cancer in smokers due to the interaction between smoking and radon [48, 75]. In studies from Western countries, residential radon has been associated with an increase in lung cancer risk in never smokers [76]. A meta-analysis of 13 European case–control studies in never smokers found that >100 Bq/m^3 cumulative radon exposure during 5–30 years before lung cancer diagnosis or death was associated with an increase in lung cancer risk (100–199 Bq/m^3: OR = 1.23, 95 % CI: 1.02–1.48) [77]. There have been a few studies of residential radon exposure and lung cancer risk in Asia. In a large pooled study of residential radon and lung cancer in China that included both men and women never and ever smokers, exposure to >100 Bq/m^3 radon was associated with a 33 % increase in risk (95 % CI: 1.01–1.36) [78]. Results by smoking status were not presented for this study in China. Little has been done in the study of residential radon and lung cancer risk among never smokers in Asia. Also, it has been suggested that there may be a potential synergism between radon exposure and passive smoking in relation to lung cancer risk in never smokers, which has not been thoroughly explored in either Western or Asian countries [76].

In Asia, indoor air pollution from solid fuel combustion (from coal and wood) as well as cooking oil vapors have been found to be risk factors for lung cancer, particularly among never smoking women [79, 80]. Smoky coal and wood have been classified as a human carcinogen (group 1) and probable human carcinogen (group 2a), respectively, by the International Agency for Research on Cancer (IARC) [81]. In China and other regions in Asia, smoky coal and wood in unventilated homes are the primary heating source for both heating and cooking. One pooled study and two meta-analyses consistently found that indoor air pollution from solid fuel was associated with an approximately two-fold increase in lung cancer risk in Asian men and women, and ever and never smokers [82–84]. As coal use is more common in Asia, in a meta-analysis of three studies, household coal use in never smoking Asian women was associated with an almost three-fold increase in lung cancer risk (1.40–6.12), a risk estimate was not available for never smoking Asian men [84]. Only one meta-analysis presented the associations by histologic cell-type and found that in primarily Asian men and women, ever and never smokers, coal use was associated with a significant two- to three-fold increase in risk for both AC and SCC lung cancers [83].

In China, it is also common practice to cook with rapeseed and soybean oil at extremely hot temperatures, resulting in oil vapors that are genotoxic and a source of indoor air pollution [85]. Nonsmoking Chinese women who reported exposure to cooking oil fumes ("high" exposure measured by greater cooking frequency) compared to those with "no to little" exposure have shown significantly elevated lung cancer risk, ranging from ORs = 1.4–3.8 [86–88]. Furthermore, Taiwanese nonsmoking housewives who did not use fume extractors in the kitchens when they stir-fried, fried, or deep fried had significantly higher lung cancer risk (OR ranges of 3.2–12.2) [89]. In the US, there have been no studies of fumes from extremely hot cooking oil and lung cancer risk, although studies assessing indoor air quality in the US have reported harmful levels of both ultrafine particle and other air pollutant emissions associated with this method of cooking [90, 91].

Household coal combustion and cooking oils at high temperatures may be important risk factors for Asian Americans as many are foreign-born with potential exposure to indoor air pollution prior to migration to the US. Additionally, this exposure may continue even after immigration, among the Asian Americans who continue to cook with oils at high temperatures in the US.

Outdoor Air Pollution

In 2013, IARC classified outdoor air pollution and particulate matter (PM) as carcinogenic to humans (Group 1) and a cause of lung cancer [92]. In a meta-analysis of 14 studies, the risk for lung cancer per 10 μg/m^3 increase of $PM_{2.5}$ and PM_{10} was 1.09 (95 % CI: 1.04–1.14) and 1.08 (95 % CI: 1.00–1.17), respectively [93]. The $PM_{2.5}$ and lung cancer association was more pronounced for former smokers (HR = 1.44, 95 % CI: 1.04–2.01), intermediate for never smokers (HR = 1.18, 95 % CI: 1.00–1.39), and weaker for current smokers (HR = 1.06, 95 % CI: 0.97–1.15) [93]. In a Japanese cohort study, lung cancer risk increased significantly in relation to $PM_{2.5}$ among women who never smoked (RR = 1.16; 95 % CI: 1.02–1.33) [94].

Air pollution and risk of lung cancer has not been studied in Asian Americans but may be particularly important as Asians Americans are more likely to live in areas with high levels of ambient air pollution exposures [95–105], including high traffic volume [95] and $PM_{2.5}$ [96, 97], and in US counties that exceed the U.S. Environmental Protection Agency (EPA) health standards for $PM_{2.5}$ [106].

Occupational Exposures

Occupational exposures to radon, asbestos, metals, polycyclic aromatic compounds, vinyl chloride, volatile organic compounds, dust, and particulates have been associated with an increased risk of lung cancer [107]. Many of these compounds have been classified by the IARC as known carcinogens [108]. These compounds may induce lung cancer through a carcinogenic mechanism and/or an inflammatory mechanism, that may involve the development of chronic obstructive pulmonary disease (COPD), a known risk factor for lung cancer [109]. The occupational risks for lung cancer in Asians remain unclear, particularly among never smokers as there are few published studies in this population that were adequately powered [110, 111]. Also, we are not aware of studies that have investigated the role of specific occupational exposures and risk of lung cancer in Asian Americans.

Previous Lung Diseases

Numerous studies have investigated the role of previous lung diseases and risk of lung cancer [71, 112–118]. Brenner et al. conducted a comprehensive meta-analysis of studies in Asian and Western populations. Subgroup analysis of studies in Asia found an increased risk of lung cancer in men and women associated with a history of chronic bronchitis (RR = 2.01; 95 % CI: 1.43–2.81), pneumonia (RR = 1.84; 95 % CI: 1.37–2.46), and tuberculosis (TB) (RR = 1.96; 95 % CI: 1.54–2.50) [113]. However, smoking status was only considered in the individual studies and thus residual confounding from smoking quantity cannot be ruled out. In a subgroup analysis restricted to never smokers in Asian and Western populations (results were not presented for Asians only), the association was not significant for chronic bronchitis (RR = 1.18; 95 % CI: 0.88–1.58) and emphysema (RR = 1.22; 95 % CI: 0.97–2.81), but remained significant for pneumonia (RR = 1.36; 95 % CI: 1.10–1.69), and TB (RR = 1.90; 95 % CI: 1.45–2.50) [113]. This study also found that TB was associated with increased lung cancer risk among Asian never smoking women (RR = 2.23; 95 % CI: 1.38–3.61) [113]. Meta-analyses for the other lung diseases (aside from TB) and lung cancer risk in Asian never smoking men or women were not presented. In 2008, the incidence rate of TB was 23 times higher among Asian Americans (25.6 per 100,000) than non-Hispanic Whites (1.1) [119]; accordingly, TB infections may be a relevant risk factor among never smoking Asian Americans. Although asthma was not investigated in the above meta-analysis [113], a meta-analysis of US studies, consisting of primarily Whites, found that never smokers with a history of asthma had an elevated risk of lung cancer risk (RR = 1.8; 95 % CI: 1.3–2.3) [120]. These findings suggest that in never smokers, a prior history of lung diseases may play a role in lung carcinogenesis. However, there is no prospective study that systematically examines previous lung diseases in relation to lung cancer risk in never smoking Asian Americans.

Infectious Disease

Infection with *Chlamydia pneumonia* (*C. pneumoniae*) and human papillomavirus virus (HPV) have been implicated in the development of lung cancer. In a nested case–control study from the Alpha-Tocopherol, Beta-Carotene Cancer Prevention (ATBC) Study, a higher prevalence of antibody markers for *C. pneumoniae* (Chlamydia IgA titers) was associated with an increased risk of lung cancer (OR = 1.6; 95 % CI: 1.0–2.3) [121]. Subsequently, a meta-analysis of four prospective and eight case–control studies (four in Asia), reported an association of seropositive Chlamydia IgA titers with lung cancer risk (OR = 1.48, 95 % CI: 1.32–1.67) [122]. This association was detected in both prospective (OR = 1.16, 95 % CI: 1.00–1.36) and retrospective (OR = 2.17, 95 % CI: 1.79–2.63) studies. However, not all studies accounted for smoking status [123] and the largest of the four Asian studies, in nonsmoking women, found no association [124]. This study used IgG and IgA assays, which has been shown to have modest reliability [125]. In fact, in a nested case–control study in the Prostate, Lung, Colorectal, and Ovarian (PLCO) cancer screening trial, the *C. pneumoniae* IgG or IgA antibodies assay were not associated with lung cancer risk, but the Chlamydia heat shock protein-60 (CHSP-60) IgG antibodies, possibly a more reliable assay, was associated with lung cancer (OR = 1.30, 95 % CI: 1.02–1.67) and this association remained even for seropositivity detected at 2–5 years prior to lung cancer diagnosis [126]. Such studies in Asian Americans have not been conducted.

HPV, particularly HPV 16/18, is a well-established risk factor for cervical, penile, anal, and squamous cell skin cancers [127]. HPV can activate carcinogenesis via the E6/E7 proteins of HPV by inactivating p53 and RB [128]. HPV infection in lung cancer may be of particular importance in Asian Americans. In an extensive review of 53 studies, HPV positivity was higher in lung cancer cases from Asia (36 %) than from Europe (17 %) or from the US (15 %) [129]. A higher HPV prevalence in Asians was found in another comprehensive analysis that considered histologic cell-type, showing significantly higher HPV positivity in Asian than in European populations for SCC (33.2 vs. 9.5 %, respectively) but not for AC (9.8 vs. 6.8 %, respectively) [130]. In a subset of studies with information on smoking status, HPV positivity was significantly higher in never smokers from East Asia (33.9 %) than those in Europe (14.8 %) [130]. The prospective investigations of these infections in relation to lung cancer risk are needed to better understand the prevalence of infectious exposure and risk in ever and never smoking Asian Americans.

Reproductive History and Hormone Exposure

The association of reproductive history with risk of lung cancer is unclear. Estrogen receptors (ER-alpha and ER-beta) are expressed in normal and tumor lung tissues but it is unclear whether the expression of these receptors differs by sex and/or smoking status. In a study of resected NSCLC tumors from Taiwan, significantly higher ER-beta expression was found in tumors from never smokers (53.5 %) than in smokers (36.6 %), and also higher in never smoking women (58.3 %) than never smoking men (40.9 %) [131]. In cohort studies of never smoking Chinese women in Shanghai and Singapore, there were suggestive lower risks of lung cancer associated with later age of menopause and higher parity [132], but higher risk associated with later age at menarche [133]. However, these findings were not seen in never smoking Japanese women [134]. The use of hormone replacement therapy (HRT) in Asia has been reported to be low [135] and not associated with lung cancer risk in these Asian studies [132–134]. However, in the Women Health Initiative study and a pooled international study, HRT use was more prevalent and was associated with a lower risk of lung cancer [136, 137].

Body Size

The role of body mass index (BMI, kg/m^2) and risk of lung cancer is best considered in never smokers because of the confounding effects of active smoking and preexisting lung disease [138–140]. In a meta-analysis of five prospective studies among never smoking men and women, primarily of European descent, BMI was not associated with lung cancer risk [141]. However, BMI is an interesting risk factor to explore among Asian Americans given that adverse BMI-related outcomes, such as cardio-metabolic diseases, manifest in this population at lower BMI measures than in Whites [142, 143]. To date, studies of never smokers from Korea [144], China [145], and a meta-analysis of cancer mortality in the Asia-Pacific Cohort Studies Collaboration [146] have not found consistent results.

Diet

Fruit and Vegetables

A review by the IARC concluded that diets high in fruits and vegetables are inversely associated with lung cancer risk, particularly in current smokers [147]. In a large meta-analysis of prospective studies, a 100 g/day increase in fruit and vegetable intake was associated with a 4 % decrease in lung cancer risk (95 % CI: 0.94–0.98) [148]. For smoking status-specific findings, the highest intake of fruits and vegetables compared to the lowest intake was inversely associated with lung cancer risk in current smokers (RR: 0.90; 95 % CI: 0.81–1.00), but not in never (RR: 0.94; 95 % CI: 0.70–1.27) or former smokers (RR: 0.95; 95 % CI: 0.83–1.10) [148]. The associations did not appear specific to a histologic cell-type, but data stratified by histologic cell-types were available in only a few studies. When restricting studies to those conducted in Asia, the inverse association for vegetables (five studies, RR = 0.98, 95 % CI: 0.93–1.04) or fruits (six studies, RR = 0.94, 95 % CI: 0.83–1.06) was not detected, although inverse associations for cruciferous (two studies, RR = 0.94, 95 % CI: 0.88–1.00) or leafy green vegetables (three studies, RR = 0.90, 95 % CI: 0.82–0.99) were found [148].

Cruciferous vegetables are rich in isothiocyanates. Isothiocyanates have been found in animal studies to reduce the formation of the carcinogenic metabolites from polycyclic aromatic hydrocarbons (PAHs), found in tobacco smoke, through the inhibition and induction of xenobiotic metabolizing pathways, cytochrome P450s (phase I enzymes) and glutathione S-transferase (phase II enzymes), respectively [149, 150]. A meta-analysis of ten studies in women found an inverse association between cruciferous vegetables and risk of lung cancer after adjusting for active smoking (RR = 0.75; 95 % CI: 0.63–0.89) [151]. This association was statistically significant in never smokers (RR = 0.70; 95 % CI: 0.58–0.85) but not in current smokers (RR = 0.77; 95 % CI: 0.41–1.46), and also stronger in studies conducted in Asia (RR = 0.66; 95 % CI: 0.55–0.81) [151]. Results from another meta-analysis of studies in men and women confirmed a significant inverse association between cruciferous vegetables and lung cancer risk in never smokers (OR = 0.78; 95 % CI: 0.64–0.95), which was more pronounced among those with the glutathione S-transferase theta 1 (*GSTT1*) null genotype (OR = 0.41; 95 % CI, 0.26–0.65; *P* for interaction was 0.01) [152]. The frequencies for *GSTT1* null genotype are higher in Asians (37–63 %) than those of European descent (10–28 %) [153].

Supplements

Specific antioxidant micronutrients, such as beta-carotene, vitamins C and E, selenium, that are commonly found in fruits and vegetables have been extensively studied for their role in lung cancer. Early epidemiologic studies and animal studies suggested that beta-carotene may have anticarcinogenic effects and was inversely associated with lung cancer risk [154]. However, RCTs to evaluate the effect of beta-carotene supplementation on lung cancer incidence in primarily White smokers found either no effect [155, 156] or an increased incidence of lung cancer at high doses of beta-carotene (≥20 mg/day) [157–159], including a meta-analysis of eight RCTs in men and women combined [160] and among current smokers [160, 161]. Prospective epidemiologic studies of lung cancer risk have reported neither benefit nor harm associated with beta-carotene supplementation or dietary consumption of beta-carotene [154, 162, 163]. Results from trials on selenium supplementation also showed no benefit [164, 165]. Similarly, a large prospective study in the US that investigated supplement use and lung cancer risk found no association between vitamins C and E use and risk of disease [166]. In contrast, a large prospective study of nonsmoking women in Shanghai found dietary intake of foods containing vitamin E was associated with a reduced risk (≥14 mg/day of vitamin E vs. less: HR=0.78; 95 % CI: 0.60–0.99), yet vitamin E supplement use was associated with an increase in risk (HR=1.33; 95 % CI: 1.01–1.73), with a stronger association for AC (HR=1.79; 95 % CI: 1.23–2.60) [167]. Chemoprevention trials of lung cancer found that beta-carotene, alpha-tocopherol, or selenium have not demonstrated reproducible associations [168]. In 2013, the U.S. Prevention Services Task Force (USPSTF) concluded that beta-carotene supplementation increases risk of lung cancer among high risk individuals, such as heavy smokers and/or asbestos workers and that neither vitamins C nor E were associated with risk of lung cancer [169]. Given the large number of null results mostly from studies in Whites, there is little motivation for additional studies of dietary supplementation and lung cancer risk among less-studied groups such as Asian Americans.

Alcohol

Studies on alcohol and lung cancer risk have yielded inconsistent results by type of alcohol and in men and women [170, 171]. In a meta-analysis of never smokers (n=1913 lung cancer cases), lung cancer risk was not associated with alcohol intake (per 10 g/day, RR=1.01; 95 % CI: 0.92–1.10) [172], suggesting that confounding or effect modification by smoking likely occurred in prior studies reporting positive associations between alcohol and lung cancer risk [170, 171]. In a meta-analysis restricted to Chinese men and women, including smokers and nonsmokers, alcohol was not associated with risk of lung cancer (four case–control and two cohort studies, OR=1.39; 95 % CI: 0.93–2.07) [173].

Soy

Soy foods are rich in phytoestrogens, namely isoflavones, and have been found to have anticarcinogenic effects, particularly in hormone-related cancers by binding competitively to estrogen receptors [174]; they also have antioxidative and anti-inflammatory properties [175]. Three meta-analyses of overlapping studies found a significant inverse association (17–41 %) between the highest quantile of soy intake and risk of lung cancer [176–178]. In stratified analyses, the inverse association was seen in nonsmokers (high vs. low intake RR=0.59; 95 % CI: 0.49–0.71); in women (RR=0.79; 95 % CI: 0.67–0.94); and in Asians (RR=0.83; 95 % CI: 0.70–0.99) [177]. The risk for per gram of soy protein intake per day was 0.98 (95 % CI: 0.96–1.00) [178]. It is of note that the inverse association was present when restricted to a meta-analysis of the four cohort studies (RR=0.85; 95 % CI: 0.74–0.97) [177, 178].

Tea

Tea may have anticarcinogenic effects due to its antioxidant components including catechins, flavonols, lignans, and phenolic acids. In a meta-analysis of 26 case–control studies and 12 cohort studies (59,041 lung cancer cases and 396,664 controls) from China, Japan, and Western countries, any tea consumption (green or black or the two combined), compared to nondrinkers, was inversely associated with risk of lung cancer (RR=0.78, 95 % CI: 0.70–0.87) [179]. Stratified analyses showed that this association was found for both green and black tea consumption. Also, the association for any tea consumption was significant only in women (RR=0.76; 95 % CI: 0.62–0.93) and not in men (RR=0.88, 95 % CI: 0.72–1.07) [179]. This association did not differ by smoking status (in smokers RR=0.79, 95 % CI: 0.59–1.07 and in nonsmokers RR=0.88, 95 % CI: 0.72–1.07). However, the inverse association for green and black tea consumption and lung cancer risk was primarily seen in case–control studies (OR=0.72, 95 % CI: 0.63–0.83), but not in prospective studies (RR=0.91, 95 % CI: 0.77–1.08). Tea consumption is greater in some Asian-American subgroups and may be a protective factor against lung cancer.

Other Dietary Factors

Other dietary risk factors that have been considered include red meats, processed meats, saturated fat and cholesterol, which have been associated with increase in lung cancer risk in some studies [180, 181]. However, the findings from prospective studies have been conflicting, and therefore the lung cancer associations for these factors are inconclusive [182–185]. These dietary factors have not been systematically studied in Asian-American populations.

Genetic Susceptibility

Globally, approximately 15 % of men and 53 % of women diagnosed with lung cancer are never smokers [186]. An estimate of 15–20 % of smokers will develop lung cancer over their lifetime [187]. Individuals with a first-degree relative with lung cancer have been found to have a 1.51-fold increased risk of lung cancer, accounting for smoking and other potential confounders (95 % CI: 1.39–1.63) [188]. Furthermore, among never smokers, family history of lung cancer has been associated with an increased risk of disease (OR=1.25; 95 % CI: 1.03–1.52). These findings suggest that genetic susceptibility and gene–environment interactions play a role in lung cancer risk. Single nucleotide polymorphisms (SNPs) associated with lung cancer risk in Asians will be reviewed in three categories: those identified through genome-wide association studies (GWAS), xenobiotic metabolic genes, and DNA repair genes.

GWAS of Lung Cancer

The majority of GWAS of lung cancer have been conducted in populations of European descent. The identified genomic regions include variants at 15q25, *TERT-CLPTM1L* at 5p15.33 and at 6p21.33 [189–191]. The susceptibility region on 15q25 encodes for the cholinergic nicotine receptor genes in *CHRNA5-CHRNA3-CHRNA4* [192–194]. These genes are likely involved in nicotine addiction, and influence smoking initiation and the amount smoked; thereby, increasing an individual's risk of lung cancer. However, three large studies have reported conflicting findings, where it is unclear whether the association between SNPs in *CHRNA5-CHRNA3-CHRNA4* and lung cancer risk are independent or dependent on active smoking [192, 193, 195]. Smaller studies in Japan, China, and Korea did not replicate, at a genome-wide significance level ($p<5x10^{-8}$), the risk associations for SNPs in *CHRNA5-CHRNA3-CHRNA4* that were previously identified by GWAS of lung cancer in European populations; the frequency of these risk variants were considerably lower in Asians than in Europeans [196–198]. However, other variants in the same region were strongly associated with lung cancer risk in GWAS of lung cancer in Asian populations, especially among ever smokers and those with SCC [198], indicating the importance of this region for lung cancer in Asians and population-specific risk variants.

GWAS in Asians have not confirmed associations found in populations of European descent in 6p21.33, which contains the *BAT3-MSH5* genes. However again, there are indications that population-specific variants may play a role, in particular a low-frequency missense (protein changing) allele in the *BAT3* coding region (also in the same cluster of genes) was associated with lung cancer in a Chinese population [199].

The 5p15.33 region near the telomerase reverse transcriptase (*TERT*) and cleft lip and palate transmembrane 1-like protein (*CLPTM1L*) genes has been identified as a lung cancer susceptibility locus. *TERT* encodes for the catalytic subunit of telomerase, which maintains telomeres, the chromosomal ends. *CLPTM1L* has been found to resist apoptosis caused by genotoxic agents. Two SNPs in *TERT* have been reported to be associated with lung cancer in both European and Asian populations, for both smokers and nonsmokers [198, 200]. Also, a study showed that a genetic risk score of seven *TERT* SNPs, identified to be associated with longer telomeric length, was associated with risk of lung cancer in never smoking women in Asia (OR = 1.51, 95 % CI: 1.34–1.69) [201].

GWAS in populations of Asian descent (Chinese, Japanese, and Korean) have identified several other additional risk variants including: rs12296850 (in 12q23.1, genes: SLC17A8-NR1H4), which was associated with SCC [202], rs7216064 (17q24.3) and rs3817963 (6p21.3) [200], which were associated with AC, and rs2131877 (3q29), which was associated with NSCLC [203]. These four lung cancer risk variants did not appear to be specific by smoking status.

Xenobiotic Metabolic Genes

Candidate gene studies of a number of variants (e.g., deletions) not necessarily well captured in GWAS studies have identified associations between xenobiotic genes (e.g., *GSTT1*, *GSTM1*, *GSTP1*) and lung cancer risk. Some of these associations have been found to be population-specific such as the *GSTM1* null genotype, which appears as a risk factor for the major histology types in Asians but not in Europeans [204]. The *GSTT1* null genotype was found to be predictive of risk in Asian ever smokers but not in never smokers [205].

The cytochrome P450 (CYP) enzymes play a role in the metabolism of nicotine and in many other compounds commonly found in cigarettes. Associations with variants in these genes have been found in Asians and Europeans [206, 207]. Cytochrome P450 2A6 (*CYP2A6*) catalyzed C-oxidation accounts for >75% of nicotine metabolism [208]. Variations in the rate of nicotine metabolism have been found to influence smoking behavior [55]. Studies have found that internal smoking dose, measured by nicotine equivalents per cigarette, is lower in Asian Americans than in non-Hispanic Whites. This has been attributed to Asians having a larger proportion of *CYP2A6* alleles that correlate with poor or no CYP2A6 enzymatic activity [209–211]; this may contribute to their lower risk of lung cancer [53, 55, 212, 213].

DNA Repair Genes

The carcinogens from cigarette smoke results in DNA damage. Therefore, it is possible that variants in the DNA repair pathway may be associated with lung cancer risk, especially in smokers or in cell-types with greater associations with smoking. A meta-analysis of genetic variants for lung cancer susceptibility in East Asians ($n=6287$ cases) found variants in DNA repair genes, *APE1*, *ERCC2*, and *XRCC1*, were associated with the risk of lung cancer [207]. There is some indication that the effects of these variants may be stronger in the cell types more strongly associated with smoking.

GWAS in Never Smokers

It has been suggested that lung cancer in never smokers may be a different disease. In GWAS of lung cancer among never smoking Asian women (5510 cases and 4544 controls from 14 studies from mainland China, South Korea, Japan, Singapore, Taiwan, and Hong Kong), susceptibility loci have been identified at 10q25.2 (rs7086803, OR = 1.28, 95 % CI: 1.21–1.35, $P=3.54\times10^{-18}$), 6q22.2 (rs9387478, OR = 0.85, 95 % CI: 0.81–0.90, $P=4.14\times10^{-10}$), and 6p21.32 (rs2395185, OR = 1.17, 95 % CI: 1.11–1.23, $P=9.51\times10^{-9}$) [214]. In a study of Korean never smoking men and women (434 cases and 1000 controls), 18p11.22 rs11080466 (OR = 0.68, 95 % CI: 0.58–0.79, $P=1.1\times10^{-6}$) was inversely associated with risk of NSCLC [215].

Another GWAS of never smoking Japanese and Korean men and women (2098 AC cases and 11,048 controls) found that rs10937405 in the tumor protein 63 (*TP63*) gene at 3q28 was associated with lung cancer risk (OR = 0.76; $P = 7.26 \times 10^{-12}$) [216]. This association was replicated in a study restricted to never smoking women from 10 studies conducted in Taiwan, mainland China, South Korea, and Singapore (3467 cases and 3787 controls; OR = 0.82, per allelic increase, 95 % CI: 0.76–0.86). This study found that the association was present for both AC ($n = 2529$ cases, OR = 0.80, 95 % CI: 0.74–0.87) and SCC ($n = 302$ cases, OR = 0.82, 95 % CI: 0.67–0.99) [217].

Also, a recent meta-analysis of four imputed GWAS of lung cancer in never smoking Asian women (6877 cases and 6277 controls) found three novel loci to be associated with lung cancer risk: rs7741164 at 6p21.1 (OR = 1.17; $P = 5.8 \times 10^{-13}$), rs72658409 at 9p21.3 (OR = 0.77; $P = 1.41 \times 10^{-10}$), and rs11610143 at 12q13.13 (OR = 0.89; $P = 4.96 \times 10^{-9}$) [218]. Findings by histologic site were not presented; however, >80 % of the cases in this study were AC.

The majority of GWAS of lung cancer in Asians have been conducted in East Asian populations; additional work in South and Southeast Asians are needed to determine whether these variants found in populations of East Asian or European descent are generalizable to other Asian populations. Also, tests for gene and environmental interactions are needed to determine whether lifestyle factors may modify these genetic effects. Lastly, many of the associated variants do not directly alter protein coding and further mechanistic studies are needed to understand how these variants influence gene activity and risk.

Lung Cancer Screening

In 2013, the U.S. National Lung Screening Trial (NLST) of ever heavy smokers reported low-dose thoracic Computed Tomography (CT) scans reduced the mortality from lung cancer by 20 % [219]. Subsequently, the USPSTF recommended that "adults aged 55–80 years who have a 30 pack-year smoking history and currently smoke or have quit within the past 15 years [NLST criteria] should be screened by low-dose CT annually" [220]. It was estimated that at a 75 % screening rate by low dose CT could prevent more than 8000 premature lung cancer deaths at an annual cost of $240,000 per prevented death [221]. Low-dose CT screening was also found to prevent an even greater proportion of lung cancer deaths when screening was conducted in populations at highest risk of lung cancer death, those who were identified using a lung cancer death risk model, as opposed to only the USPSTF recommendation [222]. On the other hand, this screening may be overly sensitive, as at least 20 % of NLST participants who underwent low-dose CT screening required further follow-up that may have included invasive procedures such as surgical lung biopsies [223].

While this screening recommendation can improve lung cancer survival by detecting lung cancer at an earlier stage, many Asian Americans may not meet the screening criteria of heavy smoking (a 30 pack-year smoking history and currently smoke or have quit within the past 15 years). On average this population has a smoking history of less than 30 pack-years, and the majority of Asian-American women diagnosed with lung cancer are never smokers. However, in the only published study of lung cancer screening using the USPSTF recommendation in Asian Americans, it was found that the percentage of Asian Americans eligible for screening was similar to the general US population [224]. In conclusion, while low-dose CT screening for lung cancer under the NLST criteria has been shown to have many benefits, additional work should be conducted to better identify at risk individuals for lung cancer screening. This will help to reduce the proportion of unnecessary invasive follow-up procedures as well as address populations that are at risk of non-tobacco-related lung cancer.

Conclusions

Lung cancer is the second most common cancer in Asian-American men and women. While incidence is lower for Asian Americans compared to non-Hispanic Whites, in some Asian-American populations the incidence is increasing and smoking rates are rising. The Asian-American population is particularly heterogeneous, and comprises many different ethnicities and a range in the levels of SES and acculturation, all of which influences smoking status as well as the exposure to other known lung cancer risk factors. Further research understanding how these risk factors impact the Asian-American community is essential as this population rapidly grows in the US and lung cancer is a highly preventable and survivable with the respective smoking cessation strategies and early stage diagnostic technologies.

References

1. Siegel RL, Miller KD, Jemal A (2015) Cancer statistics, 2015. CA Cancer J Clin 65(1): 5–29
2. Reeves TJ, Bennett CE. United States Census Bureau. American Community Survey. Census 2000 Special Reports. https://www.census.gov/prod/2004pubs/censr-17.pdf
3. Department of Health and Human Services (1998) Tobacco use among US racial/ethnic minority groups—African–Americans, American–Indians and Alaska Natives, Asian-Americans and Pacific Islanders, and Hispanics: a report of the Surgeon General. Centers for Disease Control and Prevention, Atlanta
4. Fast Stats: an interactive tool for access to SEER cancer statistics. http://seer.cancer.gov/faststats
5. Gomez SL, Noone A-M, Lichtensztajn DY et al (2013) Cancer incidence trends among Asian American populations in the United States, 1990–2008. J Natl Cancer Inst 105(15): 1096–1110
6. Yin D, Morris C, Allen M et al (2010) Does socioeconomic disparity in cancer incidence vary across racial/ethnic groups? Cancer Causes Control 21(10):1721–1730

7. Gomez SL, Chang ET, Shema SJ et al (2011) Survival following non–small cell lung cancer among Asian/Pacific Islander, Latina, and non-Hispanic White women who have never smoked. Cancer Epidemiol Biomarkers Prev 20(3):545–554
8. Thun MJ, Hannan LM, Adams-Campbell LL et al (2008) Lung cancer occurrence in never-smokers: an analysis of 13 cohorts and 22 cancer registry studies. PLoS Med 5(9):e185
9. Raz DJ, Gomez SL, Chang ET et al (2008) Epidemiology of non-small cell lung cancer in Asian Americans: incidence patterns among six subgroups by nativity. J Thorac Oncol 3(12):1391–1397
10. Howlader N, Noone A, Krapcho M, et al (2015) SEER Cancer Statistics Review, 1975–2012. http://seer.cancer.gov/csr/1975_2012, based on November 2014 SEER data submission, posted to the SEER web site, April 2015
11. Cheng I, Le GM, Noone A-M et al (2014) Lung cancer incidence trends by histology type among Asian American, native Hawaiian, and Pacific Islander populations in the United States, 1990–2010. Cancer Epidemiol Biomarkers Prev 23(11):2250–2265
12. Trinh Q-D, Nguyen PL, Leow JJ et al (2015) Cancer-specific mortality of Asian Americans diagnosed with cancer: a nationwide population-based assessment. J Natl Cancer Inst 107(6):djv054
13. Chang ET, Shema SJ, Wakelee HA et al (2009) Uncovering disparities in survival after non–small–cell lung cancer among Asian/Pacific Islander ethnic populations in California. Cancer Epidemiol Biomarkers Prev 18(8):2248–2255
14. Soo RA, Loh M, Mok TS et al (2011) Ethnic differences in survival outcome in patients with advanced stage non-small cell lung cancer: results of a meta-analysis of randomized controlled trials. J Thorac Oncol 6(6):1030–1038
15. Janssen-Heijnen MLG, Coebergh J-WW (2001) Trends in incidence and prognosis of the histological subtypes of lung cancer in North America, Australia, New Zealand and Europe. Lung Cancer 31(2–3):123–137
16. Travis WD, Travis LB, Devesa SS (1995) Lung cancer. Cancer 75(1 Suppl):191–202
17. Wynder EL, Muscat JE (1995) The changing epidemiology of smoking and lung cancer histology. Environ Health Perspect 103(Suppl 8):143–148
18. Lewis DR, Check DP, Caporaso NE et al (2014) US lung cancer trends by histologic type. Cancer 120(18):2883–2892
19. Meza R, Meernik C, Jeon J et al (2015) Lung cancer incidence trends by gender, race and histology in the United States, 1973–2010. PLoS One 10(3):e0121323
20. Burns DM, Anderson CM, Gray N (2011) Do changes in cigarette design influence the rise in adenocarcinoma of the lung? Cancer Causes Control 22(1):13–22
21. CDC (2001) Women and smoking: a report of the Surgeon General. Centers for Disease Control and Prevention, Atlanta
22. Riely GJ, Kris MG, Rosenbaum D et al (2008) Frequency and distinctive spectrum of KRAS mutations in never smokers with lung adenocarcinoma. Clin Cancer Res 14(18):5731–5734
23. Corvalan A, Witstuba II (2010) Molecular pathology of lung cancer. In: Stewart DJ (ed) Lung cancer. Springer, Berlin, pp 1–25
24. Suzuki M, Shigematsu H, Iizasa T et al (2006) Exclusive mutation in epidermal growth factor receptor gene, HER-2, and KRAS, and synchronous methylation of nonsmall cell lung cancer. Cancer 106(10):2200–2207
25. Lung ML, Wong M, Lam WK et al (1992) Incidence of ras oncogene activation in lung carcinomas in Hong Kong. Cancer 70(4):760–763
26. Wang YC, Lee HS, Chen SK et al (1998) Analysis of K-ras gene mutations in lung carcinomas: correlation with gender, histological subtypes, and clinical outcome. J Cancer Res Clin Oncol 124(9):517–522
27. Soussi T. The TP53 website. http://p53.free.fr/index.html
28. Toyooka S, Tsuda T, Gazdar AF (2003) The TP53 gene, tobacco exposure, and lung cancer. Hum Mutat 21(3):229–239
29. Hainaut P, Pfeifer GP (2001) Patterns of p53 G→T transversions in lung cancers reflect the primary mutagenic signature of DNA-damage by tobacco smoke. Carcinogenesis 22(3):367–374

30. Wang Y-C, Chen C-Y, Chen S-K et al (1998) High frequency of deletion mutations in p53 gene from squamous cell lung cancer patients in Taiwan. Cancer Res 58(2):328–333
31. Lung ML, Wong MP, Skaanild MT et al (1996) P53 mutations in non-small cell lung carcinomas in Hong Kong. Chest 109(3):718–726
32. Gao HG, Chen JK, Stewart J et al (1997) Distribution of p53 and K-ras mutations in human lung cancer tissues. Carcinogenesis 18(3):473–478
33. Krishnan VG, Ebert PJ, Ting JC et al (2014) Whole-genome sequencing of Asian lung cancers: second-hand smoke unlikely to be responsible for higher incidence of lung cancer among Asian never-smokers. Cancer Res 74(21):6071–6081
34. Takagi Y, Osada H, Kuroishi T et al (1998) p53 mutations in non-small-cell lung cancers occurring in individuals without a past history of active smoking. Br J Cancer 77(10): 1568–1572
35. Mitsudomi T (2014) Molecular epidemiology of lung cancer and geographic variations with special reference to EGFR mutations. Transl Lung Cancer Res 3(4):205–211
36. Shigematsu S (2005) Clinical and biological features associated with epidermal growth factor receptor gene mutations in lung cancers. J Natl Cancer Inst 97:339–346
37. Paez JG (2004) EGFR mutations in lung cancer: correlation with clinical response to gefitinib therapy. Science 304:1497–1500
38. Lynch TJ (2004) Activating mutations in the epidermal growth factor receptor underlying responsiveness of non-small-cell lung cancer to gefitinib. N Engl J Med 350:2129–2139
39. Kosaka T (2004) Mutations of the epidermal growth factor receptor gene in lung cancer: biological and clinical implications. Cancer Res 64:8919–8923
40. Shigematsu H, Takahashi T, Nomura M et al (2005) Somatic mutations of the HER2 kinase domain in lung adenocarcinomas. Cancer Res 65(5):1642–1646
41. Sohn HS, Kwon JW, Shin S et al (2015) Effect of smoking status on progression-free and overall survival in non-small cell lung cancer patients receiving erlotinib or gefitinib: a meta-analysis. J Clin Pharm Ther 40(6):661–671. doi:10.1111/jcpt.12332:n/a-n/a
42. Ji H, Ramsey MR, Hayes DN et al (2007) LKB1 modulates lung cancer differentiation and metastasis. Nature 448(7155):807–810
43. Koivunen JP, Kim J, Lee J et al (2008) Mutations in the LKB1 tumour suppressor are frequently detected in tumours from Caucasian but not Asian lung cancer patients. Br J Cancer 99(2):245–252
44. Inamura K, Takeuchi K, Togashi Y et al (2008) EML4-ALK fusion is linked to histological characteristics in a subset of lung cancers. J Thorac Oncol 3(1):13–17
45. Wong DW-S, Leung EL-H, So KK-T et al (2009) The EML4-ALK fusion gene is involved in various histologic types of lung cancers from nonsmokers with wild-type EGFR and KRAS. Cancer 115(8):1723–1733
46. Soda M, Choi YL, Enomoto M et al (2007) Identification of the transforming EML4-ALK fusion gene in non-small-cell lung cancer. Nature 448(7153):561–566
47. Koivunen JP, Mermel C, Zejnullahu K et al (2008) EML4-ALK fusion gene and efficacy of an ALK kinase inhibitor in lung cancer. Clin Cancer Res 14(13):4275–4283
48. IARC (2004) Monographs on the evaluation of carcinogenic risks to humans. Tobacco smoke and involuntary smoking. IARC, Lyon
49. Centers for Disease Control (1989) The Surgeon General's 1989 report on reducing the health consequences of smoking: 25 years of progress. U.S. Department of Health and Human Services, Atlanta
50. Shopland DR (1995) Tobacco use and its contribution to early cancer mortality with a special emphasis on cigarette smoking. Environ Health Perspect 103(Suppl 8):131–142
51. Pesch B, Kendzia B, Gustavsson P et al (2012) Cigarette smoking and lung cancer—relative risk estimates for the major histological types from a pooled analysis of case–control studies. Int J Cancer 131(5):1210–1219
52. Seki T, Nishino Y, Tanji F et al (2013) Cigarette smoking and lung cancer risk according to histologic type in Japanese men and women. Cancer Sci 104(11):1515–1522

53. Haiman CA, Stram DO, Wilkens LR et al (2006) Ethnic and racial differences in the smoking-related risk of lung cancer. N Engl J Med 354(4):333–342
54. Le Marchand L, Wilkens LR, Kolonel LN (1992) Ethnic differences in the lung cancer risk associated with smoking. Cancer Epidemiol Biomarkers Prev 1(2):103–107
55. Derby KS, Cuthrell K, Caberto C et al (2008) Nicotine metabolism in three ethnic/racial groups with different risks of lung cancer. Cancer Epidemiol Biomarkers Prev 17(12): 3526–3535
56. Centers for Disease Control and Prevention (2015) Current cigarette smoking among adults—United States, 2005–2014. Morb Mortal Wkly Rep 64(44):1233–1240
57. Asian American Smoking Prevalence Ranges. http://www.appealforcommunities.org/wp-content/uploads/2014/06/1653_AsianAmericanprevalenceranges2013.pdf
58. Chae DH, Gavin AR, Takeuchi DT (2006) Smoking prevalence among Asian Americans: findings from the National Latino and Asian American Study (NLAAS). Public Health Rep 121(6):755–763
59. Choi S, Rankin S, Stewart A et al (2008) Effects of acculturation on smoking behavior in Asian Americans: a meta-analysis. J Cardiovasc Nurs 23(1):67–73
60. Fu SS, Ma GX, Tu XM et al (2003) Cigarette smoking among Chinese Americans and the influence of linguistic acculturation. Nicotine Tob Res 5(6):803–811
61. Tang H, Shimizu R, Chen MS (2005) English language proficiency and smoking prevalence among California's Asian Americans. Cancer 104(S12):2982–2988
62. Chen X, Unger JB (1999) Hazards of smoking initiation among Asian American and non-Asian adolescents in California: a survival model analysis. Prev Med 28(6):589–599
63. Muggli ME, Pollay RW, Lew R et al (2002) Targeting of Asian Americans and Pacific Islanders by the tobacco industry: results from the Minnesota Tobacco Document Depository. Tob Control 11(3):201–209
64. Jha P, Ramasundarahettige C, Landsman V et al (2013) 21st-century hazards of smoking and benefits of cessation in the United States. N Engl J Med 368(4):341–350
65. Pirie K, Peto R, Reeves GK et al (2013) The 21st century hazards of smoking and benefits of stopping: a prospective study of one million women in the UK. Lancet 381(9861):133–141
66. Sakata R, McGale P, Grant EJ et al (2012) Impact of smoking on mortality and life expectancy in Japanese smokers: a prospective cohort study. BMJ 345:e7093
67. Kim CH, Lee Y-CA, Hung RJ et al (2014) Exposure to secondhand tobacco smoke and lung cancer by histological type: a pooled analysis of the International Lung Cancer Consortium (ILCCO). Int J Cancer 135(8):1918–1930
68. Sun S, Schiller JH, Gazdar AF (2007) Lung cancer in never smokers—a different disease. Nat Rev Cancer 7(10):778–790
69. Lee CH, Ko YC, Goggins W et al (2000) Lifetime environmental exposure to tobacco smoke and primary lung cancer of non-smoking Taiwanese women. Int J Epidemiol 29(2):224–231
70. Clement-Duchene C, Vignaud JM, Stoufflet A et al (2010) Characteristics of never smoker lung cancer including environmental and occupational risk factors. Lung Cancer 67(2): 144–150
71. Brenner DR, Hung RJ, Tsao MS et al (2010) Lung cancer risk in never-smokers: a population-based case-control study of epidemiologic risk factors. BMC Cancer 10:285
72. Kurahashi N, Inoue M, Liu Y et al (2008) Passive smoking and lung cancer in Japanese non-smoking women: a prospective study. Int J Cancer 122(3):653–657
73. Veglia F, Vineis P, Overvad K et al (2007) Occupational exposures, environmental tobacco smoke, and lung cancer. Epidemiology 18(6):769–775
74. Taylor R, Najafi F, Dobson A (2007) Meta-analysis of studies of passive smoking and lung cancer: effects of study type and continent. Int J Epidemiol 36(5):1048–1059
75. Darby S (2005) Radon in homes and risk of lung cancer: collaborative analysis of individual data from 13 European case–control studies. BMJ 330:223
76. Torres-Durán M, Barros-Dios JM, Fernández-Villar A et al (2014) Residential radon and lung cancer in never smokers. A systematic review. Cancer Lett 345(1):21–26

77. Darby S, Hill D, Deo H et al (2006) Residential radon and lung cancer—detailed results of a collaborative analysis of individual data on 7148 persons with lung cancer and 14,208 persons without lung cancer from 13 epidemiologic studies in Europe. Scand J Work Environ Health 32(Suppl 1):1–83
78. Lubin JH, Wang ZY, Boice JD et al (2004) Risk of lung cancer and residential radon in China: pooled results of two studies. Int J Cancer 109(1):132–137
79. Lee T, Gany F (2013) Cooking oil fumes and lung cancer: a review of the literature in the context of the U.S. population. J Immigr Minor Health 15(3):646–652
80. Lam WK (2005) Lung cancer in Asian women—the environment and genes*. Respirology 10(4):408–417
81. IARC Working Group on the Evaluation of Carcinogenic Risks to Humans (2010) Household use of solid fuels and high-temperature frying. IARC Monogr Eval Carcinog Risks Hum 95:1–430
82. Hosgood HD 3rd, Boffetta P, Greenland S et al (2010) In-home coal and wood use and lung cancer risk: a pooled analysis of the International Lung Cancer Consortium. Environ Health Perspect 118(12):1743–1747
83. Kurmi OP, Arya PH, Lam KB et al (2012) Lung cancer risk and solid fuel smoke exposure: a systematic review and meta-analysis. Eur Respir J 40(5):1228–1237
84. Hosgood HD, Wei H, Sapkota A et al (2011) Household coal use and lung cancer: systematic review and meta-analysis of case–control studies, with an emphasis on geographic variation. Int J Epidemiol 40(3):719–728
85. Shields PG, Xu GX, Blot WJ et al (1995) Mutagens from heated Chinese and U.S. cooking oils. J Natl Cancer Inst 87(11):836–841
86. Gao Y-T, Blot WJ, Zheng W et al (1987) Lung cancer among Chinese women. Int J Cancer 40(5):604–609
87. Metayer C, Wang Z, Kleinerman RA et al (2002) Cooking oil fumes and risk of lung cancer in women in rural Gansu, China. Lung Cancer 35(2):111–117
88. Wang TJ, Zhou BS, Shi JP (1996) Lung cancer in nonsmoking Chinese women: a case–control study. Lung Cancer 14(Suppl 1):S93–S98
89. Ko Y-C, Cheng LS-C, Lee C-H et al (2000) Chinese food cooking and lung cancer in women nonsmokers. Am J Epidemiol 151(2):140–147
90. Bhangar S, Mullen NA, Hering SV et al (2011) Ultrafine particle concentrations and exposures in seven residences in northern California. Indoor Air 21(2):132–144
91. Evans GJ, Peers A, Sabaliauskas K (2008) Particle dose estimation from frying in residential settings. Indoor Air 18(6):499–510
92. Loomis D, Huang W, Chen G (2014) The International Agency for Research on Cancer (IARC) evaluation of the carcinogenicity of outdoor air pollution: focus on China. Chin J Cancer 33(4):189–196
93. Hamra GB, Guha N, Cohen A et al (2014) Outdoor particulate matter exposure and lung cancer: a systematic review and meta-analysis. Environ Health Perspect 122(9):906–911
94. Katanoda K, Sobue T, Satoh H et al (2011) An association between long-term exposure to ambient air pollution and mortality from lung cancer and respiratory diseases in Japan. J Epidemiol 21(2):132–143
95. Gunier RB, Reynolds P, Hurley SE et al (2006) Estimating exposure to polycyclic aromatic hydrocarbons: a comparison of survey, biological monitoring, and geographic information system-based methods. Cancer Epidemiol Biomarkers Prev 15(7):1376–1381
96. Bell ML, Ebisu K (2012) Environmental inequality in exposures to airborne particulate matter components in the United States. Environ Health Perspect 120(12):1699–1704
97. Payne-Sturges D, Gee GC (2006) National environmental health measures for minority and low-income populations: Tracking social disparities in environmental health. Environ Res 102(2):154–171
98. Brooks N, Sethi R (1997) The distribution of pollution: community characteristics and exposure to air toxics. J Environ Econ Manag 32(2):233–250

99. Clark LP, Millet DB, Marshall JD (2014) National patterns in environmental injustice and inequality: outdoor NO_2 air pollution in the United States. PLoS One 9(4):e94431
100. Downey L, Dubois S, Hawkins B et al (2008) Environmental inequality in metropolitan America. Organ Environ 21(3):270–294
101. Morello-Frosch R, Jesdale BM (2006) Separate and unequal: residential segregation and estimated cancer risks associated with ambient air toxics in U.S. metropolitan areas. Environ Health Perspect 114(3):386–393
102. Morello-Frosch R, Pastor M Jr, Porras C et al (2002) Environmental justice and regional inequality in southern California: implications for future research. Environ Health Perspect 110(Suppl 2):149–154
103. Quach T, Liu R, Nelson DO et al (2014) Disaggregating data on Asian American and Pacific Islander women to provide new insights on potential exposures to hazardous air pollutants in California. Cancer Epidemiol Biomarkers Prev 23(11):2218–2228
104. Woodruff TJ, Parker JD, Kyle AD et al (2003) Disparities in exposure to air pollution during pregnancy. Environ Health Perspect 111(7):942–946
105. Zou B, Peng F, Wan N et al (2014) Spatial cluster detection of air pollution exposure inequities across the United States. PLoS One 9(3):e91917
106. Yip FY, Pearcy JN, Garbe PL et al (2011) Unhealthy air quality—United States, 2006–2009. MMWR Suppl 60(1):28–32
107. Purdue MP, Hutchings SJ, Rushton L et al (2015) The proportion of cancer attributable to occupational exposures. Ann Epidemiol 25(3):188–192
108. International Agency for Research on Cancer (IARC) (2010) Agents classified by the IARC Monographs, vols 1–100. http://monographs.iarc.fr/ENG/Classification/index.php
109. Houghton AM (2013) Mechanistic links between COPD and lung cancer. Nat Rev Cancer 13(4):233–245
110. Pronk A, Coble J, Ji B-T et al (2009) Occupational risk of lung cancer among lifetime nonsmoking women in Shanghai, China. Occup Environ Med 66(10):672–678
111. Tse LA, Yu IT, Qiu H et al (2012) Occupational risks and lung cancer burden for Chinese men: a population-based case-referent study. Cancer Causes Control 23(1):121–131
112. Brenner DR, Boffetta P, Duell EJ et al (2012) Previous lung diseases and lung cancer risk: a pooled analysis from the international lung cancer consortium. Am J Epidemiol 176(7): 573–585
113. Brenner DR, McLaughlin JR, Hung RJ (2011) Previous lung diseases and lung cancer risk: a systematic review and meta-analysis. PLoS One 6(3):e17479
114. Wang XR, Yu IT, Chiu YL et al (2009) Previous pulmonary disease and family cancer history increase the risk of lung cancer among Hong Kong women. Cancer Causes Control 20(5): 757–763
115. Mayne ST, Buenconsejo J, Janerich DT (1999) Previous lung disease and risk of lung cancer among men and women nonsmokers. Am J Epidemiol 149(1):13–20
116. Gorlova OY, Zhang Y, Schabath MB et al (2006) Never smokers and lung cancer risk: a case–control study of epidemiological factors. Int J Cancer 118(7):1798–1804
117. Kreuzer M, Heinrich J, Kreienbrock L et al (2002) Risk factors for lung cancer among nonsmoking women. Int J Cancer 100(6):706–713
118. Wu AH, Fontham ET, Reynolds P et al (1995) Previous lung disease and risk of lung cancer among lifetime nonsmoking women in the United States. Am J Epidemiol 141(11):1023–1032
119. American Lung Association (2010) State of lung disease in diverse communities. American Lung Association, Washington, DC
120. Santillan AA, Camargo CA Jr, Colditz GA (2003) A meta-analysis of asthma and risk of lung cancer (United States). Cancer Causes Control 14(4):327–334
121. Laurila AL, Anttila T, Läärä E et al (1997) Serological evidence of an association between Chlamydia pneumoniae infection and lung cancer. Int J Cancer 74(1):31–34
122. Zhan P, Suo L-j, Qian Q et al (2011) Chlamydia pneumoniae infection and lung cancer risk: a meta-analysis. Eur J Cancer 47(5):742–747

123. Littman AJ, Jackson LA, Vaughan TL (2005) Chlamydia pneumoniae and lung cancer: epidemiologic evidence. Cancer Epidemiol Biomarkers Prev 14(4):773–778
124. Koh W-P, Chow VTK, Phoon M-C et al (2005) Lack of association between chronic Chlamydophila pneumoniae infection and lung cancer among nonsmoking Chinese women in Singapore. Int J Cancer 114(3):502–504
125. Littman AJ, Jackson LA, White E et al (2004) Interlaboratory reliability of microimmunofluorescence test for measurement of Chlamydia pneumoniae-specific immunoglobulin A and G antibody titers. Clin Diagn Lab Immunol 11(3):615–617
126. Chaturvedi AK, Gaydos CA, Agreda P et al (2010) Chlamydia pneumoniae infection and risk for lung cancer. Cancer Epidemiol Biomarkers Prev 19(6):1498–1505
127. zur Hausen H (1999) Papillomaviruses in human cancers. Proc Assoc Am Physicians 111:581–587
128. Ishiji T (2000) Molecular mechanism of carcinogenesis by human papillomavirus-16. J Dermatol 27(2):73–86
129. Klein F, Amin Kotb WFM, Petersen I (2009) Incidence of human papilloma virus in lung cancer. Lung Cancer 65(1):13–18
130. Hasegawa Y, Ando M, Kubo A et al (2014) Human papilloma virus in non-small cell lung cancer in never smokers: a systematic review of the literature. Lung Cancer 83(1):8–13
131. Wu CT, Chang YL, Shih JY et al (2005) The significance of estrogen receptor beta in 301 surgically treated non-small cell lung cancers. J Thorac Cardiovasc Surg 130:979–986
132. Weiss JM, Lacey JV, Shu X-O et al (2008) Menstrual and reproductive factors in association with lung cancer in female lifetime nonsmokers. Am J Epidemiol 168(11):1319–1325
133. Seow A, Koh W-P, Wang R et al (2009) Reproductive variables, soy intake, and lung cancer risk among nonsmoking women in the Singapore Chinese Health Study. Cancer Epidemiol Biomarkers Prev 18(3):821–827
134. Liu Y, Inoue M, Sobue T et al (2005) Reproductive factors, hormone use and the risk of lung cancer among middle-aged never-smoking Japanese women: a large-scale population-based cohort study. Int J Cancer 117(4):662–666
135. Huang KE, Xu L, I NN et al (2010) The Asian menopause survey: knowledge, perceptions, hormone treatment and sexual function. Maturitas 65(3):276–283
136. Schwartz AG, Ray RM, Cote ML et al (2015) Hormone use, reproductive history, and risk of lung cancer: the women's health initiative studies. J Thorac Oncol 10(7):1004–1013
137. Pesatori AC, Carugno M, Consonni D et al (2013) Hormone use and risk for lung cancer: a pooled analysis from the International Lung Cancer Consortium (ILCCO). Br J Cancer 109(7):1954–1964
138. Cornfield J, Haenszel W, Hammond EC et al (2009) Smoking and lung cancer: recent evidence and a discussion of some questions. Int J Epidemiol 38(5):1175–1191
139. Chiolero A, Faeh D, Paccaud F et al (2008) Consequences of smoking for body weight, body fat distribution, and insulin resistance. Am J Clin Nutr 87(4):801–809
140. Akbartabartoori M, Lean ME, Hankey CR (2005) Relationships between cigarette smoking, body size and body shape. Int J Obes (Lond) 29(2):236–243
141. Renehan AG, Tyson M, Egger M et al (2008) Body-mass index and incidence of cancer: a systematic review and meta-analysis of prospective observational studies. Lancet 371(9612):569–578
142. Jih J, Mukherjea A, Vittinghoff E et al (2014) Using appropriate body mass index cut points for overweight and obesity among Asian Americans. Prev Med 65:1–6
143. Araneta MR, Kanaya AM, Hsu WC et al (2015) Optimum BMI cut points to screen Asian Americans for type 2 diabetes. Diabetes Care 38(5):814–820
144. Jee SH, Yun JE, Park EJ et al (2008) Body mass index and cancer risk in Korean men and women. Int J Cancer 123(8):1892–1896
145. Yang L, Yang G, Zhou M et al (2009) Body mass index and mortality from lung cancer in smokers and nonsmokers: a nationally representative prospective study of 220,000 men in China. Int J Cancer 125(9):2136–2143

146. Parr CL, Batty GD, Lam TH et al (2010) Body-mass index and cancer mortality in the Asia-Pacific cohort studies collaboration: pooled analyses of 424 519 participants. Lancet Oncol 11(8):741–752
147. International Agency for Research on Cancer, World Health Organization (2003). In: IARC Handbooks of Cancer Prevention. Fruit and vegetables, vol 8. IARC Press, Lyon
148. Vieira AR, Abar L, Vingeliene S et al (2015) Fruits, vegetables and lung cancer risk: a systematic review and meta-analysis. Ann Oncol 27(1):81–96. doi:10.1093/annonc/mdv381
149. Conaway CC, Yang YM, Chung FL (2002) Isothiocyanates as cancer chemopreventive agents: their biological activities and metabolism in rodents and humans. Curr Drug Metab 3(3):233–255
150. Hecht SS (2000) Inhibition of carcinogenesis by isothiocyanates. Drug Metab Rev 32(3–4): 395–411
151. Wu QJ, Xie L, Zheng W et al (2013) Cruciferous vegetables consumption and the risk of female lung cancer: a prospective study and a meta-analysis. Ann Oncol 24(7):1918–1924
152. Lam TK, Gallicchio L, Lindsley K et al (2009) Cruciferous vegetable consumption and lung cancer risk: a systematic review. Cancer Epidemiol Biomarkers Prev 18(1):184–195
153. Kurose K, Sugiyama E, Saito Y (2012) Population differences in major functional polymorphisms of pharmacokinetics/pharmacodynamics-related genes in Eastern Asians and Europeans: implications in the clinical trials for novel drug development. Drug Metab Pharmacokinet 27(1):9–54
154. Goralczyk R (2009) Beta-carotene and lung cancer in smokers: review of hypotheses and status of research. Nutr Cancer 61(6):767–774
155. Virtamo J, Taylor PR, Kontto J et al (2014) Effects of α-tocopherol and β-carotene supplementation on cancer incidence and mortality: 18-year postintervention follow-up of the alpha-tocopherol, beta-carotene cancer prevention study. Int J Cancer 135(1):178–185
156. Cook NR, Le IM, Manson JE et al (2000) Effects of beta-carotene supplementation on cancer incidence by baseline characteristics in the Physicians' Health Study (United States). Cancer Causes Control 11(7):617–626
157. The ATBC Cancer Prevention Study Group (1994) The alpha-tocopherol, beta-carotene lung cancer prevention study: design, methods, participant characteristics, and compliance. Ann Epidemiol 4(1):1–10
158. Rautalahti M, Albanes D, Virtamo J et al (1997) Beta-carotene did not work: aftermath of the ATBC study. Cancer Lett 114(1–2):235–236
159. Omenn GS, Goodman G, Thornquist M et al (1994) The β-carotene and retinol efficacy trial (CARET) for chemoprevention of lung cancer in high risk populations: smokers and asbestos-exposed workers. Cancer Res 54(7 Supplement):2038s–2043s
160. Druesne-Pecollo N, Latino-Martel P, Norat T et al (2010) Beta-carotene supplementation and cancer risk: a systematic review and metaanalysis of randomized controlled trials. Int J Cancer 127(1):172–184
161. Tanvetyanon T, Bepler G (2008) Beta-carotene in multivitamins and the possible risk of lung cancer among smokers versus former smokers. Cancer 113(1):150–157
162. Gallicchio L, Boyd K, Matanoski G et al (2008) Carotenoids and the risk of developing lung cancer: a systematic review. Am J Clin Nutr 88(2):372–383
163. Männistö S, Smith-Warner SA, Spiegelman D et al (2004) Dietary carotenoids and risk of lung cancer in a pooled analysis of seven cohort studies. Cancer Epidemiol Biomarkers Prev 13(1):40–48
164. Reid ME, Duffield-Lillico AJ, Garland L et al (2002) Selenium supplementation and lung cancer incidence: an update of the nutritional prevention of cancer trial. Cancer Epidemiol Biomarkers Prev 11(11):1285–1291
165. Fritz H, Kennedy D, Fergusson D et al (2011) Selenium and lung cancer: a systematic review and meta analysis. PLoS One 6(11):e26259
166. Slatore CG, Littman AJ, Au DH et al (2008) Long-term use of supplemental multivitamins, vitamin C, vitamin E, and folate does not reduce the risk of lung cancer. Am J Respir Crit Care Med 177(5):524–530

167. Wu Q-J, Xiang Y-B, Yang G et al (2015) Vitamin E intake and the lung cancer risk among female nonsmokers: a report from the Shanghai Women's Health Study. Int J Cancer 136(3): 610–617
168. Szabo E, Mao JT, Lam S et al (2013) Chemoprevention of lung cancer: diagnosis and management of lung cancer, 3rd ed: American college of chest physicians evidence-based clinical practice guidelines. Chest 143(5 Suppl):e40S–e60S
169. Fortmann SP, Burda BU, Senger CA, et al (2013) Vitamin, mineral, and multivitamin supplements for the primary prevention of cardiovascular disease and cancer: a systematic evidence review for the U.S. Preventive Services Task Force. Rockville, MD
170. Freudenheim JL, Ritz J, Smith-Warner SA et al (2005) Alcohol consumption and risk of lung cancer: a pooled analysis of cohort studies. Am J Clin Nutr 82(3):657–667
171. Chao C (2007) Associations between beer, wine, and liquor consumption and lung cancer risk: a meta-analysis. Cancer Epidemiol Biomarkers Prev 16(11):2436–2447
172. Bagnardi V, Rota M, Botteri E et al (2011) Alcohol consumption and lung cancer risk in never smokers: a meta-analysis. Ann Oncol 22(12):2631–2639
173. Li Y, Yang H, Cao J (2011) Association between alcohol consumption and cancers in the Chinese population—a systematic review and meta-analysis. PLoS One 6(4):e18776
174. Xu X, Duncan AM, Merz BE et al (1998) Effects of soy isoflavones on estrogen and phytoestrogen metabolism in premenopausal women. Cancer Epidemiol Biomarkers Prev 7(12): 1101–1108
175. Masilamani M, Wei J, Sampson H (2012) Regulation of the immune response by soybean isoflavones. Immunol Res 54(1–3):95–110
176. Yang W-S, Va P, Wong M-Y et al (2011) Soy intake is associated with lower lung cancer risk: results from a meta-analysis of epidemiologic studies. Am J Clin Nutr 94(6):1575–1583
177. Yang G, Shu XO, Chow W-H et al (2012) Soy food intake and risk of lung cancer: evidence from the Shanghai women's health study and a meta-analysis. Am J Epidemiol 176(10): 846–855
178. Wu SH, Liu Z (2013) Soy food consumption and lung cancer risk: a meta-analysis using a common measure across studies. Nutr Cancer 65(5):625–632
179. Wang L, Zhang X, Liu J et al (2014) Tea consumption and lung cancer risk: a meta-analysis of case–control and cohort studies. Nutrition 30(10):1122–1127
180. Yang WS, Wong MY, Vogtmann E et al (2012) Meat consumption and risk of lung cancer: evidence from observational studies. Ann Oncol 23(12):3163–3170. doi:10.1093/annonc/mds207
181. Smith-Warner SA, Ritz J, Hunter DJ et al (2002) Dietary fat and risk of lung cancer in a pooled analysis of prospective studies. Cancer Epidemiol Biomarkers Prev 11(10):987–992
182. Tasevska N, Cross AJ, Dodd KW et al (2011) No effect of meat, meat cooking preferences, meat mutagens or heme iron on lung cancer risk in the prostate, lung, colorectal and ovarian cancer screening trial. Int J Cancer 128(2):402–411
183. Tasevska N, Sinha R, Kipnis V et al (2009) A prospective study of meat, cooking methods, meat mutagens, heme iron, and lung cancer risks. Am J Clin Nutr 89(6):1884–1894
184. Linseisen J, Rohrmann S, Bueno-de-Mesquita B et al (2011) Consumption of meat and fish and risk of lung cancer: results from the European Prospective Investigation into Cancer and Nutrition. Cancer Causes Control 22(6):909–918
185. American Institute for Cancer Research/World Cancer Research Fund (2007) Food, nutrition, physical activity, and the prevention of cancer: a global perspective. AICR, Washington, DC
186. Parkin DM, Bray F, Ferlay J et al (2005) Global cancer statistics, 2002. CA Cancer J Clin 55(2):74–108
187. U.S. Department of Health and Human Services (2004) The health consequences of smoking: a report of the Surgeon General
188. Coté ML, Liu M, Bonassi S et al (2012) Increased risk of lung cancer in individuals with a family history of the disease: a pooled analysis from the International Lung Cancer Consortium. Eur J Cancer 48(13):1957–1968

189. McKay JD, Hung RJ, Gaborieau V et al (2008) Lung cancer susceptibility locus at 5p15.33. Nat Genet 40(12):1404–1406
190. Wang Y, Broderick P, Webb E et al (2008) Common 5p15.33 and 6p21.33 variants influence lung cancer risk. Nat Genet 40(12):1407–1409
191. Broderick P, Wang Y, Vijayakrishnan J et al (2009) Deciphering the impact of common genetic variation on lung cancer risk: a genome-wide association study. Cancer Res 69(16):6633–6641
192. Hung RJ, McKay JD, Gaborieau V et al (2008) A susceptibility locus for lung cancer maps to nicotinic acetylcholine receptor subunit genes on 15q25. Nature 452(7187):633–637
193. Thorgeirsson TE, Geller F, Sulem P et al (2008) A variant associated with nicotine dependence, lung cancer and peripheral arterial disease. Nature 452(7187):638–642
194. Thorgeirsson TE, Gudbjartsson DF, Surakka I et al (2010) Sequence variants at CHRNB3-CHRNA6 and CYP2A6 affect smoking behavior. Nat Genet 42(5):448–453
195. Amos CI, Wu X, Broderick P et al (2008) Genome-wide association scan of tag SNPs identifies a susceptibility locus for lung cancer at 15q25.1. Nat Genet 40(5):616–622
196. Ito H, McKay JD, Hosono S et al (2012) Association between a genome-wide association study-identified locus and the risk of lung cancer in Japanese population. J Thorac Oncol 7(5):790–798
197. Wu C, Hu Z, Yu D et al (2009) Genetic variants on chromosome 15q25 associated with lung cancer risk in Chinese populations. Cancer Res 69(12):5065–5072
198. Bae EY, Lee SY, Kang BK et al (2012) Replication of results of genome-wide association studies on lung cancer susceptibility loci in a Korean population. Respirology 17(4):699–706
199. Jin G, Zhu M, Yin R et al (2015) Low-frequency coding variants at 6p21.33 and 20q11.21 are associated with lung cancer risk in Chinese populations. Am J Hum Genet 96(5):832–840
200. Shiraishi K, Kunitoh H, Daigo Y et al (2012) A genome-wide association study identifies two new susceptibility loci for lung adenocarcinoma in the Japanese population. Nat Genet 44(8):900–903
201. Machiela MJ, Hsiung CA, Shu X-O et al (2015) Genetic variants associated with longer telomere length are associated with increased lung cancer risk among never-smoking women in Asia: a report from the female lung cancer consortium in Asia. Int J Cancer 137(2):311–319
202. Dong J, Jin G, Wu C et al (2013) Genome-wide association study identifies a novel susceptibility locus at 12q23.1 for lung squamous cell carcinoma in Han Chinese. PLoS Genet 9(1):e1003190
203. Yoon K-A, Park JH, Han J et al (2010) A genome-wide association study reveals susceptibility variants for non-small cell lung cancer in the Korean population. Hum Mol Genet 19(24):4948–4954
204. Carlsten C, Sagoo GS, Frodsham AJ et al (2008) Glutathione S-Transferase M1 (GSTM1) polymorphisms and lung cancer: a literature-based systematic HuGE review and meta-analysis. Am J Epidemiol 167(7):759–774
205. Yang X, Qiu M-T, Hu J-W et al (2013) GSTT1 null genotype contributes to lung cancer risk in Asian populations: a meta-analysis of 23 studies. PLoS One 8(4):e62181
206. Ji Y-N, Wang Q, Suo L-J (2012) CYP1A1 Ile462Val polymorphism contributes to lung cancer susceptibility among lung squamous carcinoma and smokers: a meta-analysis. PLoS One 7(8):e43397
207. Zhang Q, Jin H, Wang L et al (2014) Lung cancer risk and genetic variants in East Asians: a meta-analysis. Tumour Biol 35(6):5173–5179
208. Benowitz NL, Jacob P, Fong I et al (1994) Nicotine metabolic profile in man: comparison of cigarette smoking and transdermal nicotine. J Pharmacol Exp Ther 268(1):296–303
209. Nakajima M, Yokoi T (2005) Interindividual variability in nicotine metabolism: C-oxidation and glucuronidation. Drug Metab Pharmacokinet 20(4):227–235
210. Nakajima M, Fukami T, Yamanaka H et al (2006) Comprehensive evaluation of variability in nicotine metabolism and CYP2A6 polymorphic alleles in four ethnic populations. Clin Pharmacol Ther 80(3):282–297

211. Park SL, Tiirikainen MI, Patel YM et al (2016) Genetic determinants of CYP2A6 activity across racial/ethnic groups with different risks of lung cancer and effect on their smoking intensity. Carcinogenesis 37(3):269–279
212. Liu Y-l, Xu Y, Li F et al (2013) CYP2A6 deletion polymorphism is associated with decreased susceptibility of lung cancer in Asian smokers: a meta-analysis. Tumour Biol 34(5): 2651–2657
213. Park SL, Carmella SG, Ming X et al (2015) Variation in levels of the lung carcinogen NNAL and its glucuronides in the urine of cigarette smokers from five ethnic groups with differing risks for lung cancer. Cancer Epidemiol Biomarkers Prev 24(3):561–569
214. Lan Q, Hsiung CA, Matsuo K et al (2012) Genome-wide association analysis identifies new lung cancer susceptibility loci in never-smoking women in Asia. Nat Genet 44(12):1330–1335
215. Ahn M-J, Won H-H, Lee J et al (2012) The 18p11.22 locus is associated with never smoker non-small cell lung cancer susceptibility in Korean populations. Hum Genet 131(3):365–372
216. Miki D, Kubo M, Takahashi A et al (2010) Variation in TP63 is associated with lung adenocarcinoma susceptibility in Japanese and Korean populations. Nat Genet 42(10):893–896
217. Hosgood HD III, Wang W-C, Hong Y-C et al (2012) Genetic variant in TP63 on locus 3q28 is associated with risk of lung adenocarcinoma among never-smoking females in Asia. Hum Genet 131(7):1197–1203
218. Wang Z, Seow WJ, Shiraishi K et al (2016) Meta-analysis of genome-wide association studies identifies multiple lung cancer susceptibility loci in never-smoking Asian women. Hum Mol Genet 25(3):620–629
219. National Lung Screening Trial Research Team (2011) Reduced lung-cancer mortality with low-dose computed tomographic screening. N Engl J Med 365(5):395–409
220. U.S. Preventive Services Task Force. Screening for Lung Cancer, Topic Page. http://www.uspreventiveservicestaskforce.org/uspstf/uspslung.htm
221. Goulart BHL, Bensink ME, Mummy DG et al (2012) Lung cancer screening with low-dose computed tomography: costs, national expenditures, and cost-effectiveness. J Natl Compr Canc Netw 10(2):267–275
222. Kovalchik SA, Tammemagi M, Berg CD et al (2013) Targeting of low-dose CT screening according to the risk of lung-cancer death. N Engl J Med 369(3):245–254
223. Bach PB, Mirkin JN, Oliver TK et al (2012) Benefits and harms of ct screening for lung cancer: a systematic review. JAMA 307(22):2418–2429
224. Kumar V, Becker K, Zheng HX et al (2015) The performance of NLST screening criteria in Asian lung cancer patients. BMC Cancer 15(1):1–6

Colorectal Cancer Among Asian Americans

Song-Yi Park and Loïc Le Marchand

Abstract The Asian ethnic subgroups that migrated to the USA are experiencing an increase in colorectal cancer (CRC) rates. This is in contrast to the decline in invasive CRC incidence reported for non-Hispanic whites in the USA, which has been widely attributed to an increase in screening rates. Studies have shown that at least some of the Asian ethnic subgroups are less likely to undergo screening. A number of lifestyle-related factors have been associated with CRC. Indeed, the evidence for a causal link between certain types of dietary factors (e.g., dietary fiber, folate, calcium, vitamin D, red meat, processed meats), alcohol, medications, obesity and physical inactivity and CRC is stronger than for any other common types of cancer. However, it has been suggested that differences in the distribution of known/suspected lifestyle risk factors account for only a portion of the excess risk in Asian Americans for CRC and that other factors, possibly including genetic susceptibility (in particular, gene–environment interactions), are important contributors to the observed disparities in incidence. Based on the available evidence, it is unlikely that risk factors for CRC in Asians differ markedly from those in non-Hispanic whites and other ethnic/racial groups. Further research is warranted to better understand the relationship between genetic and environmental factors that increase the CRC risk of Asians when they migrate to the USA. Most importantly, utilization of screening services should be further promoted to reduce the incidence of this disease in Asian Americans.

Keywords Asian Americans • Colorectal cancer • Diet • Epidemiology • Genetics • Physical activity • Screening • Smoking

---

S.-Y. Park • L. Le Marchand, M.D., Ph.D. (✉)
Epidemiology Program, University of Hawaii Cancer Center,
701 Ilalo Street, Honolulu, HI 96813, USA
e-mail: loic@cc.hawaii.edu

A.H. Wu, D.O. Stram (eds.), *Cancer Epidemiology Among Asian Americans*,
DOI 10.1007/978-3-319-41118-7_6

Introduction

Colorectal cancer (CRC) is a common cancer among Asians who migrated to the USA, particularly for those populations that migrated several generations ago. For example, Japanese Americans who migrated to Hawaii and California between 1886 and 1924 have had one of the highest incidence rates in the world for this cancer starting in the early 1980s [1]. Similarly, Asian migrant subgroups that more recently migrated to the USA are now also experiencing an increase in CRC rates. Importantly, a similar pattern of raising rates has taken place for this cancer in recent decades in Asian countries (e.g., Japan, Korea) where lifestyle and diet have become more westernized (Fig. 1). In this chapter, we briefly review CRC rates in USA Asians and focus on what is known of the risk factors that may explain this alarming pattern. Cancer epidemiological research in Asian-American populations often involves several types of comparisons: (1) among different Asian ethnic subgroups and with non-Hispanic whites or other racial/ethnic groups; (2) with the population of their home country; or (3) by duration of residence in the USA or between migrants themselves and subsequent generations. We report on these types of comparisons, when available.

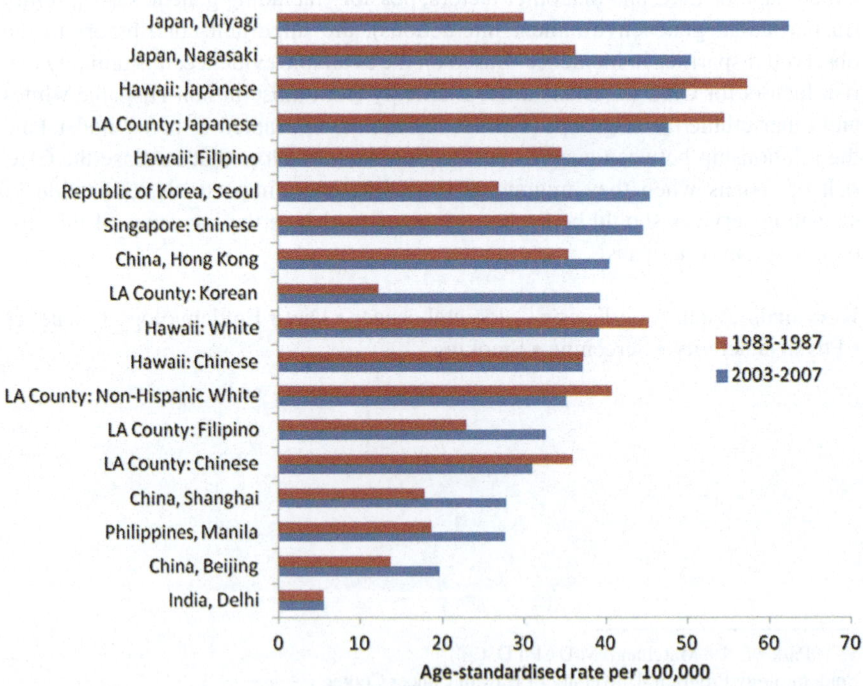

Fig. 1 Male colorectal cancer incidence in selected countries for the periods 1983–1987 and 2003–2007 [2, 3]

Rates and Characteristics of CRC in US Asians

In a recent analysis of the Surveillance, Epidemiology, and End Results (SEER) data for 2004–2008 that included eight Asian subgroups (Asian Indians/Pakistanis, Chinese, Filipinos, Japanese, Kampucheans (Cambodians), Koreans, Laotians, and Vietnamese), Japanese (66.6 per 100,000 for men and 43.0 per 100,000 for women) and Koreans (58.2 for men and 40.9 for women) had the highest CRC incidence rates, higher than or comparable to non-Hispanic whites (54.0 for men and 40.6 for women), as illustrated in Fig. 2 [4]. When comparing incidence trends across three time-periods, 1990–1994, 1998–2002, and 2004–2008, trends varied across the eight Asian subgroups [4]. Sharp increases in incidence were observed for Korean, Kampuchean (Cambodians), Laotian, and Vietnamese men and women and among South Asian and Filipina women. This is in contrast to the decreasing trend in incidence observed for non-Hispanic white men and women in the USA. Similar trends were reported in an analysis of the 1988–2007 California Cancer Registry data [5]. Although decreasing trends in CRC incidence were observed in California among all major racial/ethnic groups, including Asians/Pacific Islanders as a whole, CRC incidence was actually increasing among some Asian subgroups, namely, Korean males and females, as well as South Asian and Filipino females.

Consistent with the incidence patterns, Japanese Americans have been reported to experience the highest mortality rate from CRC, compared to the other Asian subgroups (Chinese, Filipinos, Vietnamese, and Koreans) and non-Hispanic whites in the USA [6] and in California [7, 8]. Based on the 1988–2007 SEER data, 5-year CRC-specific mortality was lower in Asian-American patients (hazard ratio, HR=0.90; 95% confidence interval, CI: 0.87–0.94), compared to non-Hispanic

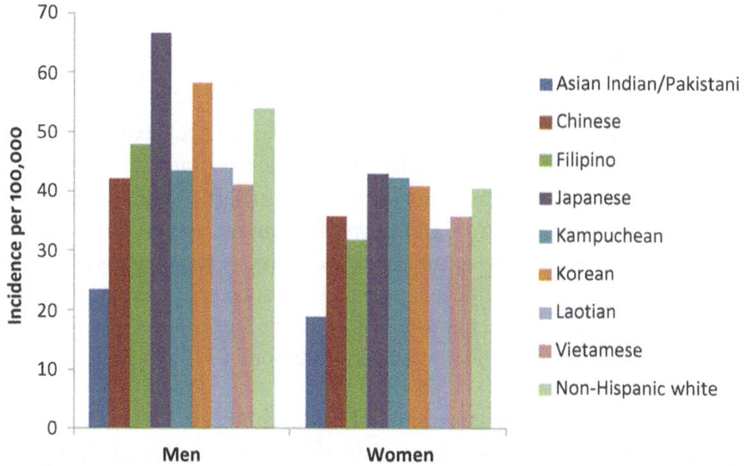

Fig. 2 Age-adjusted incidence rates of colorectal cancer among Asian-American populations, 2004–2008 [4]

white patients after adjustment for demographic factors, stage at diagnosis and other factors [9]. In analyses stratified by Asian-American ethnic groups, CRC-specific mortality was lower in each of the Asian ethnic subgroups of patients (Chinese, Filipino, Japanese, Korean, other Asian, South Asian, and Vietnamese), compared to non-Hispanic white patients but this difference was statistically significant only in Japanese (HR=0.84; 95 % CI: 0.77–0.92) and South Asian-American patients (HR=0.72; 95 % CI: 0.56–0.92) (1991-2007 SEER) [10].

In a study comparing Japanese CRC patients living in Hawaii and in Japan (1996–2002), there were significant differences in age distribution, with Japanese American patients (n=410) being older, and more often female, with normal preoperative carcinoembryonic antigen levels, and with a tumor located in the cecum or transverse colon, compared to patients in Japan (n=621). However, tumor characteristics (stage, tumor size, and grade) of Japanese American patients were similar to those for the general American population in SEER [11]. In Massachusetts during 1997–2001, Asian/Pacific Islanders had over two times the incidence rate of the left colon cancer (28.1 per 100,000) compared with right colon cancer (13.6 per 100,000), whereas non-Hispanic whites had a 1.3 times higher incidence rate for the left colon (32.7 per 100,000) than the right colon (24.6 per 100,000) [12]. The North American Association of Central Cancer Registries (NAACCR) data for 1995–1999 showed that among Asians/Pacific Islanders, the rate of distal colon cancer (17.7 per 100,000) was higher than the rate of proximal colon cancer (15.2 per 100,000) in male, with little variation in rates across subsites in female (12.3 per 100,000 and 13.1 per 100,000, respectively) [13]. In contrast, among white males and females, proximal colon cancer rates were over 25 % higher than the rate of distal colon cancer. Chinese patients in China were more likely to have distal CRC and developed the disease at a significantly earlier stage than non-Hispanic white patients in the USA [14].

Migrant Studies

Like other migrant populations, Asians immigrants to the USA experienced changes in lifestyle and often have substantially different cancer rates from those in their home country. These differences often become more marked after two or three generations. Therefore, studies in migrants provide unique research opportunities to understand cancer etiology by comparing cancer risk in populations with a similar genetic background living in different physical and social environments, or in populations of different genetic background living in the same environment [1, 15, 16] (see Hamilton et al., chapter "Resources and Methods for Studying Cancer among Asian Americans").

Like for other cancers, the general trend has been for the CRC rates of migrants to move to an intermediate level between the risks of their home and host countries. However, several groups have exhibited a rapid and complete transition to the risk of the host country [15]. Among migrant groups displaying this complete transition, Japanese Americans have been studied the most extensively [1]. In a study of

Japanese migrants to Hawaii during the period from 1973 to 1977, the incidence of colon cancer in Japan was 25 % that of whites in Hawaii, whereas the incidence rates for first generation migrants and their descendants were the same as, or slightly higher than, that of non-Hispanic whites [17]. A study of Chinese migrants to the USA for 1968–1972 showed that the colon cancer mortality rate among first generation also exceeded that of non-Hispanic whites [18, 19]. These early studies showed that the increase in CRC risk occurred rapidly in the first generation migrants; however, these studies included limited numbers of second generation migrants. A later study of CRC incidence rates (per 100,000) during 1973–1986 among Asian Americans in Hawaii, San Francisco/Oakland SMSA, and western Washington state showed that US-born Japanese (142.5 for men and 90.1 for women) had a higher incidence rate of CRC compared to Japan-born Japanese (69.3 for men and 63.5 for women) or US-born non-Hispanic whites (89.9 for men and 64.3 for women) [20]. This is in contrast to US-born Chinese (66.9 for men and 40.9 for women) who had a lower rate compared to China-born Chinese (87.8 for men and 44.7 for women) [20].

Colorectal Cancer Screening

Wide spread screening is critical to reducing the public health burden posed by CRC since it results in a decrease in incidence (by the removal of precursor lesions) and in improved survival (through the diagnosis of tumors at an earlier stage). The nationally reported decline in invasive CRC incidence in non-Hispanic whites in the USA has been widely attributed to an increase in screening rates; however, some Asian-American groups are less likely to undergo screening [4] (see chapter "Cancer Screening among Asian Americans").

The percentage of adults (≥40 years) who receive CRC screening was 64.8 % overall and 52.5 % in Asian Americans in 2010 in the National Health Interview Survey [21]. In an analysis of the 2010 Behavioral Risk Factor Surveillance System (BRFSS) data that included adults aged 50–75 years, the rate of self-reported CRC screening [by fecal occult blood test (FOBT), sigmoidoscopy, or colonoscopy] was 59.6 % overall [22]. The rate was highest in non-Hispanic whites (62.0 %), followed by African Americans (59.0 %), Native Hawaiian/Pacific Islanders (54.6 %), Hispanic-English (52.5 %), American Indians/Alaska Natives (49.5 %), Asians (47.2 %), and Hispanic-Spanish (30.6 %). Similarly in the California Health Interview Survey data for 2001, 2003, and 2005, the CRC screening rate (46.8 %) for Asian Americans (Chinese, Japanese, Koreans, Filipinos, South Asians, and Vietnamese) and Pacific Islanders (AAPIs) considered as an aggregated group (≥ 50 years) was lower than that of non-Hispanic whites (57.7 %) [23]. When the AAPI group was disaggregated, further disparity was noted: Koreans showed the lowest CRC screening rate (32.7 %), whereas Japanese had the highest (59.8 %). Over the 5-year period, CRC screening rates increased slightly for most AAPI subgroups, except for Koreans who showed a decreasing trend from 2001 to 2005 (Fig. 3).

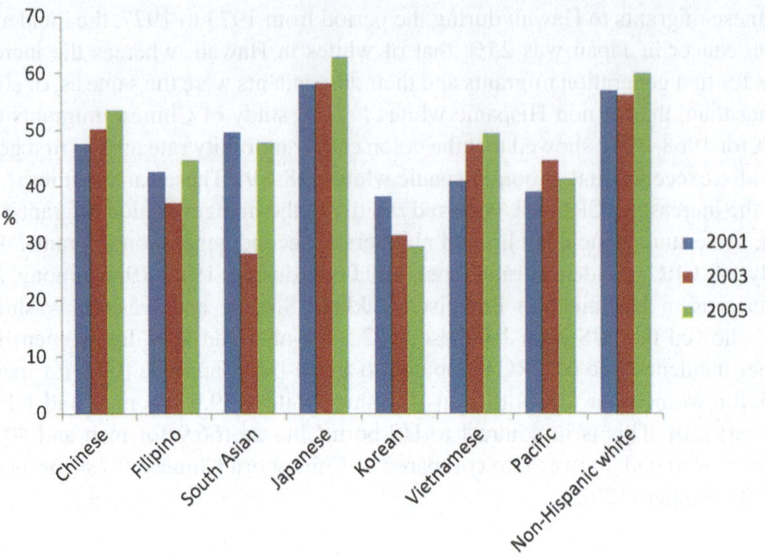

Fig. 3 Colorectal cancer screening rates in California in 2001, 2003, and 2005 [23]

In an analysis of electronic health records in Northern California among adults aged 50–75 years [24], Asian Indians had the lowest rate (45.6 %) of CRC screening among Asian subgroups (Japanese: 63.8 %; Chinese: 66.7 %; Filipinos: 59.0 %; Koreans: 66.2 %; Vietnamese: 65.8 %; Native Hawaiians/Pacific Islanders: 53.8 %), well below that of non-Hispanic whites (63.7 %).

The length of time spent in the USA has been shown to be a significant predictor of CRC screening in different Asian-American subgroups. In the 2001 California Health Interview Survey, Asian-American immigrants who have lived in the USA for less than 15 years were less likely to undergo CRC screening (odds ratio, OR=0.48; 95 % CI: 0.32–0.71) compared to those born in the USA [25]. In addition to the length of residency in the USA, various factors were shown to affect CRC screening in Asian Americans, including socioeconomic status, English fluency, cancer knowledge, social support, access to health care services, and comorbidity [26–35].

Intervention trials in Asian Americans found that culturally tailored approaches are effective in improving screening rates [36–42]. For instance, among Vietnamese Americans, a controlled trial of a public education and provider intervention was conducted including a Vietnamese-language CRC screening media campaign from 2004 to 2006 in one community vs. no intervention in a control community [39]. The post- to pre-intervention OR for having ever had a CRC screening was 44 % greater (95 % CI: 1.03–1.99) in the intervention community than in the control community. In an educational intervention conducted in Michigan to promote CRC awareness using Asian-language media throughout local Asian Indian, Chinese, Filipino, Hmong, Japanese, Korean, and Vietnamese American communities, 78 %

of those receiving the educational intervention reported to have been screened in the last 12 months, compared with the 37 % who said to have ever been screened prior to the study [42].

Lifestyle-Related Risk Factors

A number of lifestyle-related factors have been associated with CRC risk. Indeed, the evidence for a causal link between certain types of diet, obesity, diabetes, alcohol, medications and physical inactivity and CRC is stronger than for any other common types of cancer.

Obesity

Obesity increases risk of developing CRC in both men and women. The 2007 World Cancer Research Fund (WCRF)/American Institute for Cancer Research (AICR) Second Expert Report based on the most comprehensive systematic literature reviews concluded that there was convincing evidence that body fatness and abdominal fatness, and adult attained height as a marker for genetic, environmental, hormonal, and nutrition factors affecting growth, are causes of CRC [43]. A meta-analysis also suggested that central obesity, as measured by waist-to-hip ratio, may be particularly important in increasing risk of CRC compared to overall obesity measured by body mass index (BMI, kg/m^2) [44]. It has been noted that Asians have a higher percentage of body fat and, especially, visceral adiposity for the same BMI compared with European-origin populations [45–49].

In a cohort of Japanese-American men in Hawaii initiated in 1965, a BMI of ≥ 25.8 kg/m^2 was associated with an increased risk of colon cancer (relative risk, RR = 1.38; 95 % CI: 1.01–1.90), compared to a BMI < 21.7 kg/m^2 [50]. Several cohort studies conducted in Asia have also reported an increased risk of CRC with obesity. In cohort studies in Shanghai, China, both a measure of general adiposity (BMI) and measures of central adiposity (elevated waist-to-hip ratio (WHR) and waist circumference (WC)) were significantly associated with an increased risk of colon cancer in men but not in women [51]. HRs for colon cancer in men in the highest compared with the lowest quintiles were 2.15 (95 % CI: 1.35–3.43; P for trend < 0.001) for BMI, 1.97 (95 % CI: 1.19–3.24; P for trend < 0.001) for WHR, and 2.00 (95 % CI: 1.21–3.29; P for trend < 0.001) for WC. A cohort study in South Korea reported that obese men (BMI $\geq$ 30 kg/m^2) were at increased risk for colon cancer (RR = 1.42; 95 % CI: 1.02–1.98), but not obese women (RR = 1.01; 95 % CI: 0.72–1.42); the average ages of men and women in this cohort was 45.0 and 49.4 years old [52]. In another Korean cohort of postmenopausal women (mean age 55.9), BMI was related to an increased colon cancer risk (HR for a one unit BMI increase = 1.05; 95 % CI: 1.02–1.08) [53]. A pooled analysis of eight prospective cohort studies in Japan found that the risk of CRC increased with increasing BMI; the adjusted HRs for a one unit BMI increase were 1.03 (95 % CI: 1.02–1.04) for males and 1.02 (95 % CI: 1.00–1.03) for females [54]. In a Chinese cohort in Singapore, a significant increase in CRC risk was observed in subjects with BMI ≥ 27.5 kg/m^2, compared to those with BMI 21.5–24.4 kg/m^2 (HR = 1.25; 95 % CI: 1.01–1.55). The BMI-cancer association was similar in men and women. However, this association was more pronounced in never smokers (HR = 1.35; 95 % CI: 1.04–1.76) than in ever smokers (HR = 1.08; 95 % CI: 0.74–1.58) [55]. Although data are limited for Asian Americans, the evidence suggests that obesity is a modifiable risk factor for CRC in Asians, especially in men and irrespective of where they live.

Diabetes

Type 2 diabetes has been associated with an increased risk of cancer at several sites including colorectum [56]. A recent meta-analysis of observational studies found that diabetes was related to a 27 % increased risk of CRC (summary RR = 1.27; 95 % CI: 1.21–1.34) [57]. The observed associations between diabetes and cancer could be either causal (e.g., caused by hyperglycemia or hyperinsulinemia) or because of confounding from common risk factors such as adiposity [57]. However, studies showed that diabetes is a risk factor of CRC independently of obesity. In the Multiethnic Cohort Study (MEC) that was established to study lifestyle and genetic factors and cancer in African American, Native Hawaiian, Japanese American, Latino, and non-Hispanic white older adults living in Hawaii and Los Angeles in 1993–1996 [58], participants with a history of diabetes had a significantly greater risk of CRC than those without such a history with adjustment for BMI in the entire cohort (RR = 1.19; 95 % CI: 1.09–1.29) and in Japanese Americans (RR = 1.27; 95 % CI: 1.09–1.47) [59]. A later study in the MEC showed that despite their lower BMI, Asian Americans had a higher diabetes risk than whites [60]. Similarly, in a cohort study in Korea, elevated fasting serum glucose levels and a diagnosis of diabetes were independent risk factors for CRC [61].

Smoking

The association between cigarette smoking and CRC was recently reevaluated by an expert panel assembled by the International Agency for Research on Cancer (IARC), with the conclusion that smoking is a risk factor for both colon and rectal cancer [62]. Although IARC and the American College of Gastroenterology CRC screening guidelines highlight cigarette smoking as a risk factor, cigarette smoking is still an arguably underappreciated risk factor for the disease in the USA [63].

In a meta-analysis of 25 prospective cohort studies, the risk of CRC was higher in current (RR = 1.20; 95 % CI: 1.10–1.30) and former smokers (RR = 1.18; 95 % CI: 1.12–1.25), compared to never smokers [64]. In a subset analysis limited to five studies in Asian countries, the RRs were similar: 1.21 (95 % CI: 1.07–1.36) for current smokers and 1.17 (95 % CI: 1.02–1.35) for former smokers. Other meta-analyses in populations of European ancestry have all shown an increased CRC risk associated with smoking, with possibly a greater risk for rectal cancer [63, 65]. Smoking has also been related to a poor survival among CRC patients. In a meta-analyses of 62,278 CRC patients from 16 studies, HR for all-cause mortality was 1.26 (95 % CI: 1.15–1.37) for current smokers and 1.11 (95 % CI: 0.93–1.33) for former smokers, compared with never smokers [66]. In the Seattle Colon Cancer Family Registry, current smokers had a significantly elevated risk of CRC-specific (HR = 1.30; 95 % CI: 1.09–1.74) and all-cause (HR = 1.51; 95 % CI: 1.24–1.83) mortality compared to never smokers [67].

In the cohort study of Japanese American men in Hawaii, current smokers had a higher risk of colon (RR = 1.42; 95 % CI: 1.09–1.85) and rectal (RR = 1.95; 95 % CI: 1.25–3.04) cancer, compared to never smokers [50]. In a population-based case–control study conducted among Caucasians, Japanese, Native Hawaiians, Filipinos, and Chinese in Hawaii, ever smokers were at an increased risk of CRC compared with never smokers (OR = 1.23; 95 % CI: 0.99–1.52 for men and OR = 1.27; 95 % CI: 1.01–1.59 for women). ORs for the highest quartile of pack-years vs. never smokers was 1.48 (95 % CI: 1.12–1.96) in men and 1.38 (95 % CI: 0.91–1.95) in women [68]. In ethnic-specific analyses, the positive association was observed in all of the three largest ethnic groups (Japanese, Caucasians, and Native Hawaiians). The evidence indicates that smoking is a risk factor for CRC in Asia and among Asian Americans.

Diet and Alcohol

In the 2011 WCRF/AICR report [43], the evidence that food containing dietary fiber decreases CRC risk and that red and processed meat, and alcohol (in men), increase risk, was considered to be convincing. The report also concluded that consumption of garlic, milk, and calcium probably protects against this cancer. Only a limited number of studies have been performed in Asian Americans and have examined the diet–CRC relationship.

In the MEC that measured dietary intake by a quantitative food frequency questionnaire, dietary fiber consumption was associated with a lower risk of CRC in men (RR = 0.62; 95 % CI: 0.48–0.79 for the highest vs. lowest quintile) but not in women (RR = 0.88; 95 % CI: 0.67–1.14) after multivariate adjustment that included age, ethnicity, and other lifestyle and dietary factors. This inverse association was observed in Japanese-American men but not in Japanese-American women [69]. The association with dietary fiber was recently reevaluated in the MEC with a larger number of cases ($n = 4388$) and an inverse association was observed in women who never used menopausal hormone therapy (MHT) [70]. The magnitude of this association was similar to that found in men, and was suggested to be present in each ethnic group. There was also evidence that dietary fiber did not exert an additional protective effect against CRC among woman who ever used MHT over that afforded by MHT alone. In a large, multicenter, case–control study of Chinese residing in North America, consumption of non-fiber carbohydrate, i.e., the digestible non-fiber portion of carbohydrates that stimulates insulin release, was associated with an increased risk of CRC in North-American Chinese men (OR=1.7; 95% CI: 1.1–2.7 for the highest vs. lowest tertile) and women (OR=2.7; 95% CI: 1.5–4.8) [71]. In contrast, in the MEC, carbohydrate intake was inversely associated with CRC risk in women (RR=0.71; 95% CI: 0.53–0.95 for the highest vs. lowest quintile) but not in men (RR=1.09; 95% CI: 0.84–1.40) [72]. A meta-analysis of 12 cohort studies (including the MEC) found no significant association between CRC risk and carbohydrate intake (summary RR=0.93; 95% CI: 0.84–1.04 for high vs. low intake) [73].

Intake of fruits and vegetables, rich sources of dietary fiber and bioactive phytochemicals, among the MEC participants was reported to be related to a decreased CRC risk in all men combined and in Japanese American men specifically, but not in all women combined or in Japanese American women [74]. A cohort study of Chinese men in Shanghai found an inverse association with fruit intake but not with vegetable consumption [75]. However, a cohort study of Singapore Chinese men and women reported no significant association of CRC risk with dietary isothiocyanates from cruciferous vegetables [76] or a dietary pattern characterized by a high vegetable, fruit, and soy food intake [77].

In the MEC, no association with CRC risk was detected for total meat, red meat, or processed meat intake or for total or specific heterocyclic amine intake either overall or in Japanese Americans [78]. Neither total nor specific types of fats were associated with CRC risk. However, individuals consuming a dietary pattern rich in meat and fat were at increased risk of CRC (RR=1.20; 95% CI: 1.08–1.35 for the highest vs. lowest quartile; *P* for trend <0.001) but the association was attenuated in multivariable models adjusting for other risk factors (*P* for trend=0.10) [78]. A cohort of Chinese women in Shanghai, China, reported a decreased risk of CRC with intake of polyunsaturated fatty acids [79] and an increase risk with cholesterol intake [80]. In the case–control study of Chinese residing in North America and China, saturated fat intake was significantly associated with CRC risk; ORs per 100 kcal from saturated fat were 1.8–2.9 (*P*<0.001) in North America and 1.1–1.6 in China depending on sex and anatomic site [81]. The association between saturated fat and CRC was stronger among the sedentary than among the physically active participants. Risk among sedentary Chinese Americans increased more than fourfold from the lowest to the highest category of saturated fat intake.

In a meta-analysis of 6 cohort studies and 13 case–control studies conducted in Japan, the summary RR (95% CIs) for the highest vs. lowest categories of red meat consumption was 1.16 (1.001–1.34) and 1.21 (1.03–1.43) for colorectal and colon cancer, respectively, and that for processed meat consumption was 1.17 (1.02–1.35) and 1.23 (1.03–1.47) for colorectal and colon cancer, respectively. Poultry consumption was associated with a lower risk of rectal cancer, with a summary RR (95% CI) of 0.80 (0.67–0.96) [82]. The corresponding pooled OR for fish was 1.03

(0.89–1.18) and 0.84 (0.75–0.94) for cohort and case–control studies, respectively [83]. A meta-analysis of three Asian cohort studies (from Japan and Singapore) found that dietary fat was not associated with CRC risk [84].

In the prospective cohort of Japanese-American men in Hawaii initiated in the 1960s, saturated fat intake was associated with a lower risk of colon cancer (RR = 0.44; 95 % CI: 0.23–0.83 for the highest vs. lowest quintile) [85]. Serum triglycerides and glucose levels were not associated with CRC [86]. Serum cholesterol levels were associated with a decrease in risk for colon cancer (*P* for trend = 0.01) but not for rectal cancer [87]. These findings were not consistent with those from a meta-analysis of prospective studies mostly performed in Europe and North America showing that serum triglycerides (summary RR = 1.18; 95 % CI: 1.04–1.34 for high vs. low concentrations) and cholesterol levels (summary RR = 1.11; 95 % CI: 1.01–1.21) were related to an increased risk of CRC [88].

Calcium intake was found to be inversely associated with CRC risk in the MEC and this association was strongest among Japanese Americans (RR = 0.69; 95 % CI: 0.52–0.91 for the highest vs. lowest quartile; *P* for trend = 0.008) [89]. However, calcium intake was not related to the risk of colon cancer in the Japanese men cohort in Hawaii, regardless of whether it came from dairy or nondairy sources [90]. While vitamin D intake was not related to risk overall or in any ethnic/racial group in the MEC [89], pre-diagnostic plasma 25-hydroxyvitamin D levels in a case–control study nested within the MEC were associated with a lower risk of CRC overall (OR = 0.60; 95 % CI: 0.33–1.07; *P* for trend = 0.01) and, in an ethnic-specific analysis, the inverse trend was only significant in Japanese Americans (*P* for trend = 0.03) [91]. In a case–control study of plasma levels of B vitamins nested in the MEC, folate levels were inversely associated with CRC risk among nondrinkers (OR for > median vs. ≤ median = 0.55; 95 % CI: 0.31–0.95). PLP (pyridoxal-5′-phosphate, the active form of vitamin B6) levels were related to a lower risk overall (OR = 0.49 for the highest vs. lowest quartile; 95 % CI: 0.29–0.83; *P* for trend = 0.009) [92]. Ethnic-specific analysis did not show any heterogeneity in the association of CRC with plasma PLP. However, in Chinese cohorts in Shanghai, plasma folate levels were not associated with CRC risk in both men [93] and women [94].

Calories from alcohol (≥ 14 %) was associated with a higher risk of colon (RR = 1.88; 95 % CI: 1.38–2.56) and rectal (RR = 2.51; 95 % CI: 1.59–3.97) cancer, compared to nondrinkers in the Japanese American men cohort in Hawaii [50]. Alcohol intake in the MEC was also related to an increased risk of CRC in Japanese American men (HR = 1.54; 95 % CI: 1.19–2.01 for ≥ 40 g/day of alcohol vs. nondrinkers) but not in women (unpublished data). Although a meta-analysis of ten case–control studies in Chinese populations found no significant association between alcohol consumption and CRC risk (pooled OR = 1.58; 95 % CI: 0.90–2.76) [95], another meta-analysis of 19 studies in Asia reported an increased risk of CRC with a pooled RR of 1.21 (95 % CI: 1.03–1.43) for all drinkers and 1.81 (95 % CI: 1.33–2.46) for heavy drinkers compared to non-/occasional drinkers [96].

The Shanghai cohorts reported a decreased risk of CRC with intake of green tea both in men [97] and women [98], whereas the Singapore Chinese cohort found an increased risk with green tea consumption [99]. Coffee consumption was related to a decreased risk of CRC in the Singapore Chinese cohort [100].

The evidence to date suggests that red meat and alcohol increase risk and that dietary fiber and calcium decrease risk of CRC in Asian Americans. The evidence for the association of CRC with other dietary factors (e.g., soy or green tea) is still inconclusive for this population.

Physical Activity

The evidence that physical activity protects against colon cancer was considered as convincing by the WCRF expert panel [43]. In a dose–response meta-analyses, total physical activity (expressed as METs-hour/day) was associated with a significant decreased risk for colorectal (RR=0.97 for an increase of five METs-hour/day; 95 % CI: 0.94–0.99), as well as for colon cancer (RR=0.92; 95 % CI: 0.86–0.99) but not rectal cancer.

In the cohort of Japanese American men in Hawaii, physical activity was found to be associated with a lower risk of colon cancer; RRs were 0.56 (95 % CI: 0.39–0.80) and 0.71 (95 % CI: 0.51–0.99) for the middle and upper tertiles of a physical activity index, respectively, compared to the lower tertile [101]. In the population-based case–control study of Chinese in North America and China, on both continents and in both sexes, CRC risks increased with increasing time spent sitting [81]. ORs for CRC among Chinese American men were 2.4 ($P<0.05$) for 5–9 h sitting and 3.9 ($P<0.001$) for ten or more hours sitting, compared with less than 5 h sitting.

Two cohort studies in Japan reported an inverse association between physical activity and CRC. In the Japan Public Health Center-based Prospective Study (JPHC study), men in the highest quartiles of MET hours per day had a 31 % lower risk (95 % CI: 0.49–0.97), compared to those in the lowest quartile [102]. In the Miyagi Cohort Study, time spent walking was inversely associated with CRC risk in men. Men who walked 1 h or more per day had a 43 % lower risk (95 % CI: 0.38–0.83), compared to those who walked 0.5 h or less (P for trend=0.003) [103].

Overall Effect of Lifestyle on CRC Risk

A study in the MEC investigated whether the higher age-adjusted CRC risk of Japanese Americans (RR=1.40; 95 % CI: 1.21–1.61 in men and RR=1.38; 95 % CI: 1.17–1.62 in women), compared to non-Hispanic whites, may be explained by the effects of lifestyle risk factors. After accounting for obesity, cigarette smoking, physical activity, alcohol consumption, and dietary intakes of red meat, dietary fiber, calcium, folate, and vitamin D, CRC risk still remained significantly elevated in Japanese Americans (RR=1.27; 95 % CI: 1.09–1.48 in men; RR=1.49; 95 % CI: 1.24–1.78 in women), relative to non-Hispanic whites [104]. These findings suggest that differences in the distribution of known/suspected lifestyle risk factors account for only a modest proportion of the excess risk in Japanese Americans for CRC and that other factors, possibly including genetic susceptibility, are important contributors to the observed disparities in incidence.

Medications

Although conclusive evidence is still lacking, epidemiologic studies and randomized trials [105] suggest that long-term use of nonsteroidal anti-inflammatory drugs (NSAIDs) exerts chemopreventive properties against CRC [106, 107]. In a meta-analysis of 12 cohort studies (Europe and USA), an inverse association between aspirin use and CRC was observed both overall (RR = 0.74; 95 % CI: 0.64–0.83 for aspirin dose; RR = 0.80; 95 % CI: 0.75–0.85 for frequency of aspirin use; RR = 0.75; 95 % CI: 0.68–0.81 for years of aspirin use) and in subgroups stratified by sex and cancer site [108]. A meta-analysis of 19 case–control studies also reported that regular use of aspirin or NSAID was associated with a reduced risk of CRC [109]. No study of NSAIDs and CRC risk has been published for Asian-American populations. In a cohort of CRC patients in Singapore, the risk of CRC relapse or death from CRC was approximately 60 % lower compared to patients who were not postoperative aspirin users (HR=0.38; 95 % CI: 0.17–0.84) [110]. In the MEC, NSAID user had a lower risk of CRC (HR=0.82; 95 % CI: 0.70–0.95) among Japanese American men but not among Japanese American women (HR=0.93; 95 % CI: 0.78–1.11) (unpublished data).

Epidemiological evidence suggests that estrogen is probably involved in the physiology of the large bowel and the etiology of CRC [111]. While initially protective against CRC, once the tumor has developed, estrogens are thought to increase proliferation. Consequently, oral contraceptives and MHT may be effective against CRC development. However, further data on the risk-benefit profile of short-term MHT use are needed and will determine whether there is any role for estrogens in the chemoprevention of CRC [112]. In the MEC, MHT users at baseline had a 25 % lower risk of CRC compared to never users among Japanese American women (Park et al., under review), while oral contraceptive use was not associated with CRC risk (HR=0.98; 95 % CI: 0.78–1.23) (unpublished data).

Genetic Susceptibility

Genetics may explain a sizable portion of CRC incidence through the direct effects of susceptibility genes, as well as their possible interactions with environmental and lifestyle factors [113, 114]. It is currently believed that even sporadic CRC cases, i.e., those occurring outside familial syndromes (e.g., Familial Adenomatous Polyposis, Lynch Syndrome), are influenced by low-penetrance genes or gene combinations. These susceptibility loci have very modest effect sizes, with ORs for developing CRC in risk allele carriers usually from 1.1 to 1.3 [115].

In early years, genetic studies for CRC were limited to examining genetic polymorphisms in candidate genes. Genes involved in mutagenesis (carcinogen metabolism, DNA repair and synthesis and maintenance of genome integrity) were naturally prime candidates, alongside a few genes involved in cell signaling and transcriptional control [114]. With rapid technological advances in genotyping, a global interrogation of the genome became possible through genome-wide association studies (GWAS). These studies identified a greater number of variants related to CRC risk [116, 117].

Family History

A history of CRC among one's first-degree relatives is known to confer an increased risk of the disease. A meta-analysis of 47 studies, including eight studies conducted in Asian countries, reported a risk estimate of 2.24 (95 % CI: 2.06–2.43) for one affected first-degree relative, rising to 3.97 (95 % CI: 2.60–6.06) for two or more [118].

In a population-based multiethnic case–control study in Hawaii, which was included in the above meta-analysis, first-degree relatives of cases were found to have a 2.5-fold increased risk of CRC compared with relatives of controls (95 % CI: 1.8–3.4). This increase in risk was stronger in Japanese American (OR = 3.0; 95 % CI: 2.1–4.6) than in Caucasians (OR = 1.8; 95 % CI: 1.2–2.9) (*P* for interaction = 0.07) [119].

Candidate Gene Studies

A meta-analysis of the literature for 267 genetic variants in 150 candidate genes found that 62 variants in 50 genes showed a nominally significant association with CRC risk ($P<0.05$) [120]. In this analysis, epidemiological evidence for a significant association with CRC risk was considered to be "strong" for eight variants in five genes (*APC*, *CHEK2*, *DNMT3B*, *MLH1*, and *MUTYH*), "moderate" for two variants in two genes (*GSTM1* and *TERT*), and "weak" for 52 variants in 45 genes. Although this meta-analysis reported that genetic variants in *MTHFR*, involved in one-carbon metabolism, showed no relation to CRC risk [120], another meta-analysis of 21 Asian studies found a significant association of the *MTHFR* 677T allele with a decreased risk of CRC (OR = 0.91; 95 % CI: 0.85–0.98) [121]. In a study of the *MTHFR* C677T polymorphism [122] in the MEC, OR for the TT vs. CC genotype was 0.77 (95 % CI: 0.58–1.03) overall. This inverse association was statistically significant in Japanese Americans (OR = 0.59; 95 % CI: 0.36–0.95), suggested for whites (OR = 0.62; 95 % CI: 0.34–1.15) and not observed in Latinos (OR = 0.96; 95 % CI: 0.56–1.15). This association was also similar in both sexes, stronger at high levels of folate intake, and limited to light and nondrinkers (*P* for interaction with ethanol = 0.02).

A number of interactions between genetic variants and diet have been suggested to play a role in CRC etiology [123]. Interactions have been reported in prospective studies for meat with *NAT1*, *NAT2*, *ABCB1*, and *NFKB1*, cruciferous vegetables with *GSTM1*, *GSTT1*, and *CCND1*, calcium with *VDR*, vitamins C and E and carotene with *MGTM*, dietary fiber with *IL10*, and alcohol with *PPARG*, *ADH*, and *ALDH* [123, 124]. However, these findings need replication in independent, well-characterized cohort studies before conclusions regarding these interactions and the underlying biological mechanisms can be reached [123, 125].

In a Korean population, subjects with low-methyl diets (as defined by a combined low intake of folate and high intake of alcohol) had higher risk of CRC (OR = 2.32; 95 % CI: 1.18–4.56) than did those with high-methyl diets among *MTHFR* CC/CT carriers, whereas the amount of dietary methyl did not affect the CRC risk among carriers with the TT homozygous variant (*P* for interaction = 0.65) [126].

A Chinese case–control study found that the *NQO1* 609 CT and TT genotypes were associated with an increased risk of CRC (CT: OR = 2.02, 95 % CI: 1.55–2.57; TT: OR = 2.51, 95 % CI: 1.82–3.47), compared with the CC genotype. Moreover, NQO1 609C>T appeared to have a multiplicative joint effect with both tobacco smoking and alcoholic drinking (*P* for multiplicative interactions were 0.0001 and 0.013, respectively) on CRC risk [127].

In a Singapore Chinese population, individuals with both the *GSTM1* and *GSTT1* null genotypes were reported to have a 57 % reduction in CRC risk among high vs. low consumers of isothiocyanates-rich cruciferous vegetables (OR = 0.43; 95 % CI: 0.20–0.96), in particular for colon cancer (OR = 0.31; 95 % CI: 0.12–0.84) [76]. However, no statistical interactions were detected between cruciferous vegetable intake and *GST* gene variants on the odds of CRC in a case–control study in Shanghai, China [128].

GWAS

Studies in twins have suggested that heredity is responsible for approximately one-third of the susceptibility to CRC [129]. This is in contrast to the known familial forms that account for less than 6 % of all CRC cases [130]. This has led to the suspicion that there may be other genes that, when mutated, predispose to CRC with or without polyposis [115]. To date, more than 50 chromosome regions harboring common variants conferring altered CRC risk have been identified using the GWAS approach [116, 117, 131]. Although these CRC susceptibility SNPs have been shown to only explain a small proportion of the genetic risk, it is not clear how much of the heritability remains to be explained by other, yet unidentified, rarer SNPs that would have a greater penetrance [132].

While most GWAS have been conducted in European-ancestry populations [133], multiple GWAS have identified novel loci associated with CRC risk in Asian populations.

A trans-ethnic GWAS of CRC conducted in two populations (Japanese and African Americans) identified a new susceptibility locus in *VTI1A* and replicated this association in cases and controls of European ancestry [134]. This variant was associated with risk in all three populations.

In a GWAS of 7456 CRC cases and 11,671 controls conducted as part of the Asian Colorectal Cancer Consortium [135], three new loci at 5q31.1 (near *PITX1*), 12p13.32 (near *CCND2*), and 20p12.3 (near *HAO1*) were associated with CRC risk. Also, a new CRC risk variant was identified in the *SMAD7* gene among East Asians [136]. Further, a large-scale GWAS in East Asians (14,963 CRC cases and 31,945 controls) identified 6 new loci associated with CRC risk at 10q22.3, 10q25.2, 11q12.2, 12p13.31, 17p13.3, and 19q13.2 [137].

A GWAS in a Japanese population identified a novel locus (rs7758229 in *SLC22A3*) in the 6q26-q27 region associated with distal colon cancer and replicated this association in a Korean population [138].

A number of studies have also tested whether CRC risk variants identified in CRC GWAS conducted in European-ancestry populations are generalizable to Asians. In the five ethnic/racial groups of the MEC, among 11 risk variants for CRC identified by GWAS in populations of European ancestry, an increased risk of CRC/adenoma was confirmed for the 8q24, 11q23, and 15q13 loci in whites, and for the 8q24 and 20p12 loci in African Americans [139]. Statistically significant cumulative effects of risk alleles on CRC/adenoma risk were found in every population (OR per allele = 1.07–1.09, $P \leq 0.039$), except in Japanese Americans (OR = 1.01, $P = 0.52$).

GWAS-identified variants for diseases related to CRC (e.g., diabetes, obesity) were also tested for association with CRC in various populations, including Asians. In a case–control study within the MEC, the risk variants (24 SNPs in 15 loci) identified in GWAS of BMI and waist size were also examined in relation to CRC risk [140]. Risk alleles for two obesity SNPs were associated with CRC risk: *KCTD15* rs29941 (OR for C allele = 0.90; 95 % CI: 0.83–0.98) and *MC4R* rs17782313 (OR for C allele = 1.12; 95 % CI: 1.02–1.22) without heterogeneity observed across race/ethnic groups. Nineteen Type 2 diabetes GWAS SNPs were tested in the MEC for association with CRC [141]. Four SNPs were associated with CRC: rs7578597 (*THADA*), rs864745 (*JAZF1*), rs5219 (*KCNJ11*), and rs7961581 (*TSPAN8*, *LGR5*). For rs7578597 (*THADA*), a significant inverse association with the diabetes risk (T) allele was observed overall (OR = 0.84; 95 % CI: 0.75–0.95), with the strongest effect seen among Japanese Americans (OR = 0.52; 95 % CI: 0.36–0.75).

A genetic variant on chromosome 10p14, first identified to be associated with CRC risk in a GWAS in Europeans, was tested in a Chinese population [142]. OR per A allele was 0.71 (95 % CI: 0.54–0.94). A meta-analysis by the same authors further confirmed the significant association, reporting an OR per A allele of 0.91 (95 % CI: 0.89–0.93) in European-descent populations and 0.86 (95 % CI: 0.78–0.96) in Chinese. A common SNP, rs3802842 at 11q23 identified in CRC GWAS, was also tested in a Chinese population and found to be significantly associated with CRC risk [143]. A meta-analysis of 25 studies, including four conducted in Asian populations, also provided convincing evidence that the same SNP, rs3802842 at 11q23, significantly contributed to CRC risk [143]. Whether 7 SNPs associated with gastric cancer were also associated with CRC was tested in a Chinese population [144]. Two of the five SNPs located at 10q23 (rs3765524 and rs2274223) were found to have significant protective effects against CRC, with equal OR per allele (OR=0.31). Two other gastric cancer risk SNPs located on 1q22 (rs4072037 and rs4460629) similarly showed a weak association with CRC.

The GWAS SNP, rs961253 in 20p12.3, associated with increased risk of CRC in Europeans was also found to be related to CRC (OR per A allele=1.60; 95 % CI: 1.26–2.02) in a Chinese population. This association was confirmed with an OR of 1.34 (95 % CI:1.20–1.50) for the Asian studies included in a meta-analysis of the published literature [145]. The association of rs7758229 in 6q26-q27 with distal colon cancer, identified in a GWAS in Japan, was not found to be associated with CRC risk in a Chinese population [146]. This inability to replicate the Japanese GWAS findings among Chinese might be partly due to inadequate power (>75 %).

Eleven GWAS risk loci identified in European-ancestry populations were investigated in a Singapore Chinese population [147]. Only SNPs at 1q41, 8q23.3, 11q23.1, 16q22.1, and 18q21.1 showed evidence of associations with CRC risk, with ORs ranging from 1.13 to 1.40. Half of the loci did not show any evidence for association with CRC in Singapore Chinese, which could be due to different linkage disequilibrium patterns and allelic frequencies or genetic heterogeneity. Two CRC risk SNPs in the 8q24 region were assessed in Japan [148]. An increased risk of CRC was observed with rs6983267 but not with rs10090154.

Overall, these studies indicate that fine-mapping studies of the CRC GWAS risk loci are needed to identify the variants responsible for a potential association with CRC in Asians. For instance, a fine-mapping study of the 21 known risk loci in African Americans in the MEC identified two markers at two known loci that may better predict CRC risk in that population than the previous index SNPs [149].

Conclusion

Among Asian Americans, increased susceptibility to CRC in some groups (Japanese, Koreans) and upward incidence trends for other groups have been documented. The available data suggest that it is unlikely that risk factors for CRC in Asians differ markedly from those in other ethnic/racial groups. However, it remains unclear why some Asian groups in the USA have a clearly elevated risk for CRC, compared to whites. It is conceivable that they may experience increased exposure to some risk factors (e.g., central obesity, hyperinsulinemia), or a greater risk associated with a given exposure (e.g., smoking, alcohol, red meat). These effects may reflect specific genetic susceptibilities. Further research is warranted to better understand the interplay of genetic and environmental factors that increase CRC risk in Asians when they migrate to the USA. Utilization of screening services should be further promoted to reduce the incidence of this disease in Asian Americans.

Acknowledgments Financial Disclosure: This work was in part supported by the National Cancer Institute grants U01CA164973 and 1R01CA126895.

Authors' declaration of personal interests: None declared.

Declaration of funding interests: None declared.

References

1. Le Marchand L (1999) Combined influence of genetic and dietary factors on colorectal cancer incidence in Japanese Americans. J Natl Cancer Inst Monogr:101–105
2. Forman D, Bray F, Brewster DH et al (2014) Cancer incidence in five continents, vol 10. International Agency for Research on Cancer, Lyon
3. Parkin DM, Muri CS, Whelan SL et al (1992) Cancer incidence in five continents, vol 6. International Agency for Research on Cancer, Lyon
4. Gomez SL, Noone AM, Lichtensztajn DY et al (2013) Cancer incidence trends among Asian American populations in the United States, 1990–2008. J Natl Cancer Inst 105:1096–1110
5. Giddings BH, Kwong SL, Parikh-Patel A et al (2012) Going against the tide: increasing incidence of colorectal cancer among Koreans, Filipinos, and South Asians in California, 1988–2007. Cancer Causes Control 23:691–702
6. Miller BA, Chu KC, Hankey BF et al (2008) Cancer incidence and mortality patterns among specific Asian and Pacific Islander populations in the U.S. Cancer Causes Control 19:227–256
7. Kwong SL, Chen MS Jr, Snipes KP et al (2005) Asian subgroups and cancer incidence and mortality rates in California. Cancer 104:2975–2981
8. Mccracken M, Olsen M, Chen MS Jr et al (2007) Cancer incidence, mortality, and associated risk factors among Asian Americans of Chinese, Filipino, Vietnamese, Korean, and Japanese ethnicities. CA Cancer J Clin 57:190–205
9. Aizer AA, Wilhite TJ, Chen MH et al (2014) Lack of reduction in racial disparities in cancer-specific mortality over a 20-year period. Cancer 120:1532–1539
10. Trinh QD, Nguyen PL, Leow JJ et al (2015) Cancer-specific mortality of Asian Americans diagnosed with cancer: a nationwide population-based assessment. J Natl Cancer Inst 107(6):djv054
11. Sakamoto K, Machi J, Prygrocki M et al (2006) Comparison of characteristics and survival of colorectal cancer between Japanese-Americans in Hawaii and native Japanese in Japan. Dis Colon Rectum 49:50–57
12. The Massachusetts Cancer Registry (2005) Data report on colorectal cancer in Massachusetts. Harvard Center for Cancer Prevention, Massachusetts Department of Public Health, Boston, MA
13. Wu X, Chen VW, Martin J et al (2004) Subsite-specific colorectal cancer incidence rates and stage distributions among Asians and Pacific Islanders in the United States, 1995 to 1999. Cancer Epidemiol Biomarkers Prev 13:1215–1222
14. Qing SH, Rao KY, Jiang HY et al (2003) Racial differences in the anatomical distribution of colorectal cancer: a study of differences between American and Chinese patients. World J Gastroenterol 9:721–725
15. Kolonel LN, Wilkens LR (2006) Migrant studies. In: Schottenfeld D, Fraumeni JF (eds) Cancer epidemiology and prevention, 3rd edn. Oxford University Press, New York
16. Parkin DM, Khlat M (1996) Studies of cancer in migrants: rationale and methodology. Eur J Cancer 32A:761–771
17. Kolonel LN, Hinds MW, Hankin JH (1980) Cancer patterns among migrant and native-born Japanese in Hawaii in relation to smoking, drinking and dietary habits. In: Gelboin HV, Macmahon B, Matsushima T et al (eds) Genetics and environmental factors in experimental and human cancer. Japan Scientific Societies Press, Tokyo

18. King H, Locke FB (1980) Cancer mortality among Chinese in the United States. J Natl Cancer Inst 65:1141–1148
19. Thomas DB, Karagas MR (1987) Cancer in first and second generation Americans. Cancer Res 47:5771–5776
20. Flood DM, Weiss NS, Cook LS et al (2000) Colorectal cancer incidence in Asian migrants to the United States and their descendants. Cancer Causes Control 11:403–411
21. U.S. Department of Health and Human Services (2015) Percentage of adults who receive colorectal cancer screening as appropriate. https://healthmeasures.aspe.hhs.gov/measure/25. Accessed 15 Jun 2015
22. Liss DT, Baker DW (2014) Understanding current racial/ethnic disparities in colorectal cancer screening in the United States: the contribution of socioeconomic status and access to care. Am J Prev Med 46:228–236
23. Lee HY, Lundquist M, Ju E et al (2011) Colorectal cancer screening disparities in Asian Americans and Pacific Islanders: which groups are most vulnerable? Ethn Health 16:501–518
24. Thompson CA, Gomez SL, Chan A et al (2014) Patient and provider characteristics associated with colorectal, breast, and cervical cancer screening among Asian Americans. Cancer Epidemiol Biomarkers Prev 23:2208–2217
25. Wong ST, Gildengorin G, Nguyen T et al (2005) Disparities in colorectal cancer screening rates among Asian Americans and non-Latino Whites. Cancer 104:2940–2947
26. Honda K (2004) Factors associated with colorectal cancer screening among the US urban Japanese population. Am J Public Health 94:815–822
27. Kimura A, Sin MK, Spigner C et al (2014) Barriers and facilitators to colorectal cancer screening in Vietnamese Americans: a qualitative analysis. J Cancer Educ 29:728–734
28. Lee S, Chen L, Jung MY et al (2014) Acculturation and cancer screening among Asian Americans: role of health insurance and having a regular physician. J Community Health 39:201–212
29. Ma GX, Wang MQ, Toubbeh J et al (2012) Factors associated with colorectal cancer screening among Cambodians, Vietnamese, Koreans and Chinese living in the United States. N Am J Med Sci (Boston) 5:1–8
30. Maxwell AE, Danao LL, Crespi CM et al (2008) Disparities in the receipt of fecal occult blood test versus endoscopy among Filipino American immigrants. Cancer Epidemiol Biomarkers Prev 17:1963–1967
31. Menon U, Szalacha L, Prabhughate A et al (2014) Correlates of colorectal cancer screening among South Asian immigrants in the United States. Cancer Nurs 37:E19–E27
32. Oh KM, Jacobsen KH (2014) Colorectal cancer screening among Korean Americans: a systematic review. J Community Health 39:193–200
33. Ryu SY, Crespi CM, Maxwell AE (2014) Colorectal cancer among Koreans living in South Korea versus California: incidence, mortality, and screening rates. Ethn Health 19:406–423
34. Sentell TL, Tsoh JY, Davis T et al (2015) Low health literacy and cancer screening among Chinese Americans in California: a cross-sectional analysis. BMJ Open 5:e006104
35. Sun WY, Basch CE, Wolf RL et al (2004) Factors associated with colorectal cancer screening among Chinese-Americans. Prev Med 39:323–329
36. Carney PA, Lee-Lin F, Mongoue-Tchokote S et al (2014) Improving colorectal cancer screening in Asian Americans: results of a randomized intervention study. Cancer 120:1702–1712
37. Crawford J, Ahmad F, Beaton D et al (2016) Cancer screening behaviours among South Asian immigrants in the UK, US and Canada: a scoping study. Health Soc Care Community 24(2):123–153
38. Lee HY, Tran M, Jin SW et al (2014) Motivating underserved Vietnamese Americans to obtain colorectal cancer screening: evaluation of a culturally tailored DVD intervention. Asian Pac J Cancer Prev 15:1791–1796
39. Nguyen BH, Mcphee SJ, Stewart SL et al (2010) Effectiveness of a controlled trial to promote colorectal cancer screening in Vietnamese Americans. Am J Public Health 100:870–876

40. Nguyen-Truong CK, Lee-Lin F, Gedaly-Duff V (2013) Contributing factors to colorectal cancer and hepatitis B screening among Vietnamese Americans. Oncol Nurs Forum 40:238–251
41. Wang J, Burke A, Tsoh JY et al (2014) Engaging traditional medicine providers in colorectal cancer screening education in a Chinese American community: a pilot study. Prev Chronic Dis 11, E217
42. Wu TY, Kao JY, Hsieh HF et al (2010) Effective colorectal cancer education for Asian Americans: a Michigan program. J Cancer Educ 25:146–152
43. World Cancer Research Fund/American Institute for Cancer Research (2011) Continuous Update Project Report. Food, nutrition, physical activity, and the prevention of colorectal cancer. World Cancer Research Fund/American Institute for Cancer Research
44. Moghaddam AA, Woodward M, Huxley R (2007) Obesity and risk of colorectal cancer: a meta-analysis of 31 studies with 70,000 events. Cancer Epidemiol Biomarkers Prev 16:2533–2547
45. Deurenberg P, Deurenberg-Yap M, Guricci S (2002) Asians are different from Caucasians and from each other in their body mass index/body fat per cent relationship. Obes Rev 3:141–146
46. Goh LY, Goh KL (2013) Obesity: an epidemiological perspective from Asia and its relationship to gastrointestinal and liver cancers. J Gastroenterol Hepatol 28(Suppl 4):54–58
47. He Q, Horlick M, Thornton J et al (2002) Sex and race differences in fat distribution among Asian, African–American, and Caucasian prepubertal children. J Clin Endocrinol Metab 87:2164–2170
48. Lim U, Ernst T, Buchthal SD et al (2011) Asian women have greater abdominal and visceral adiposity than Caucasian women with similar body mass index. Nutr Diabetes 1:e6
49. Park YW, Allison DB, Heymsfield SB et al (2001) Larger amounts of visceral adipose tissue in Asian Americans. Obes Res 9:381–387
50. Chyou PH, Nomura AM, Stemmermann GN (1996) A prospective study of colon and rectal cancer among Hawaii Japanese men. Ann Epidemiol 6:276–282
51. Li H, Yang G, Xiang YB et al (2012) Body weight, fat distribution and colorectal cancer risk: a report from cohort studies of 134255 Chinese men and women. Int J Obes (Lond) 37(6):783–789
52. Jee SH, Yun JE, Park EJ et al (2008) Body mass index and cancer risk in Korean men and women. Int J Cancer 123:1892–1896
53. Song YM, Sung J, Ha M (2008) Obesity and risk of cancer in postmenopausal Korean women. J Clin Oncol 26:3395–3402
54. Matsuo K, Mizoue T, Tanaka K et al (2012) Association between body mass index and the colorectal cancer risk in Japan: pooled analysis of population-based cohort studies in Japan. Ann Oncol 23:479–490
55. Odegaard AO, Koh WP, Yu MC et al (2011) Body mass index and risk of colorectal cancer in Chinese Singaporeans: the Singapore Chinese Health Study. Cancer 117:3841–3849
56. Giovannucci E, Harlan DM, Archer MC et al (2010) Diabetes and cancer: a consensus report. Diabetes Care 33:1674–1685
57. Tsilidis KK, Allen NE, Appleby PN et al (2015) Diabetes mellitus and risk of prostate cancer in the European prospective investigation into cancer and nutrition. Int J Cancer 136: 372–381
58. Kolonel LN, Henderson BE, Hankin JH et al (2000) A multiethnic cohort in Hawaii and Los Angeles: baseline characteristics. Am J Epidemiol 151:346–357
59. He J, Stram DO, Kolonel LN et al (2010) The association of diabetes with colorectal cancer risk: the multiethnic cohort. Br J Cancer 103:120–126
60. Maskarinec G, Jacobs S, Morimoto Y et al (2015) Disparity in diabetes risk across native Hawaiians and different Asian groups: the multiethnic cohort. Asia Pac J Public Health 27:375–384
61. Jee SH, Ohrr H, Sull JW et al (2005) Fasting serum glucose level and cancer risk in Korean men and women. JAMA 293:194–202

62. International Agency for Research on Cancer (2012) Personal habits and indoor combustions. Volume 100 E. A review of human carcinogens. IARC Monogr Eval Carcinog Risks Hum 100:1–538
63. Cheng J, Chen Y, Wang X et al (2015) Meta-analysis of prospective cohort studies of cigarette smoking and the incidence of colon and rectal cancers. Eur J Cancer Prev 24:6–15
64. Tsoi KK, Pau CY, Wu WK et al (2009) Cigarette smoking and the risk of colorectal cancer: a meta-analysis of prospective cohort studies. Clin Gastroenterol Hepatol 7(682–688): e681–e685
65. Botteri E, Iodice S, Bagnardi V et al (2008) Smoking and colorectal cancer: a meta-analysis. JAMA 300:2765–2778
66. Walter V, Jansen L, Hoffmeister M et al (2014) Smoking and survival of colorectal cancer patients: systematic review and meta-analysis. Ann Oncol 25:1517–1525
67. Phipps AI, Baron J, Newcomb PA (2011) Prediagnostic smoking history, alcohol consumption, and colorectal cancer survival: the Seattle Colon Cancer Family Registry. Cancer 117:4948–4957
68. Luchtenborg M, White KK, Wilkens L et al (2007) Smoking and colorectal cancer: different effects by type of cigarettes? Cancer Epidemiol Biomarkers Prev 16:1341–1347
69. Nomura AM, Hankin JH, Henderson BE et al (2007) Dietary fiber and colorectal cancer risk: the multiethnic cohort study. Cancer Causes Control 18:753–764
70. Park SY, Wilkens LR, Kolonel LN, Henderson BE, Le Marchand L (2016) Inverse associations of dietary fiber and menopausal hormone therapy with colorectal cancer risk in the Multiethnic Cohort Study. Int J Cancer 139(6):1241–1250
71. Borugian MJ, Sheps SB, Whittemore AS et al (2002) Carbohydrates and colorectal cancer risk among Chinese in North America. Cancer Epidemiol Biomarkers Prev 11:187–193
72. Howarth NC, Murphy SP, Wilkens LR et al (2008) The association of glycemic load and carbohydrate intake with colorectal cancer risk in the multiethnic cohort study. Am J Clin Nutr 88:1074–1082
73. Aune D, Chan DS, Lau R et al (2012) Carbohydrates, glycemic index, glycemic load, and colorectal cancer risk: a systematic review and meta-analysis of cohort studies. Cancer Causes Control 23:521–535
74. Nomura AM, Wilkens LR, Murphy SP et al (2008) Association of vegetable, fruit, and grain intakes with colorectal cancer: the multiethnic cohort study. Am J Clin Nutr 88:730–737
75. Vogtmann E, Xiang YB, Li HL et al (2013) Fruit and vegetable intake and the risk of colorectal cancer: results from the Shanghai Men's Health Study. Cancer Causes Control 24: 1935–1945
76. Seow A, Yuan JM, Sun CL et al (2002) Dietary isothiocyanates, glutathione S-transferase polymorphisms and colorectal cancer risk in the Singapore Chinese Health Study. Carcinogenesis 23:2055–2061
77. Butler LM, Wang R, Koh WP et al (2008) Prospective study of dietary patterns and colorectal cancer among Singapore Chinese. Br J Cancer 99:1511–1516
78. Ollberding NJ, Wilkens LR, Henderson BE et al (2012) Meat consumption, heterocyclic amines and colorectal cancer risk: the multiethnic cohort study. Int J Cancer 131: E1125–E1133
79. Murff HJ, Shu XO, Li H et al (2009) A prospective study of dietary polyunsaturated fatty acids and colorectal cancer risk in Chinese women. Cancer Epidemiol Biomarkers Prev 18:2283–2291
80. Lee SA, Shu XO, Yang G et al (2009) Animal origin foods and colorectal cancer risk: a report from the Shanghai Women's Health Study. Nutr Cancer 61:194–205
81. Whittemore AS, Wu-Williams AH, Lee M et al (1990) Diet, physical activity, and colorectal cancer among Chinese in North America and China. J Natl Cancer Inst 82:915–926
82. Pham NM, Mizoue T, Tanaka K et al (2014) Meat consumption and colorectal cancer risk: an evaluation based on a systematic review of epidemiologic evidence among the Japanese population. Jpn J Clin Oncol 44:641–650

83. Pham NM, Mizoue T, Tanaka K et al (2013) Fish consumption and colorectal cancer risk: an evaluation based on a systematic review of epidemiologic evidence among the Japanese population. Jpn J Clin Oncol 43:935–941
84. Liu L, Zhuang W, Wang RQ et al (2011) Is dietary fat associated with the risk of colorectal cancer? A meta-analysis of 13 prospective cohort studies. Eur J Nutr 50:173–184
85. Stemmermann GN, Nomura AM, Heilbrun LK (1984) Dietary fat and the risk of colorectal cancer. Cancer Res 44:4633–4637
86. Tsushima M, Nomura AM, Lee J et al (2005) Prospective study of the association of serum triglyceride and glucose with colorectal cancer. Dig Dis Sci 50:499–505
87. Nomura AM, Stemmermann GN, Chyou PH (1991) Prospective study of serum cholesterol levels and large-bowel cancer. J Natl Cancer Inst 83:1403–1407
88. Yao X, Tian Z (2015) Dyslipidemia and colorectal cancer risk: a meta-analysis of prospective studies. Cancer Causes Control 26:257–268
89. Park SY, Murphy SP, Wilkens LR et al (2007) Calcium and vitamin D intake and risk of colorectal cancer: the multiethnic cohort study. Am J Epidemiol 165:784–793
90. Stemmermann GN, Nomura A, Chyou PH (1990) The influence of dairy and nondairy calcium on subsite large-bowel cancer risk. Dis Colon Rectum 33:190–194
91. Woolcott CG, Wilkens LR, Nomura AM et al (2010) Plasma 25-hydroxyvitamin D levels and the risk of colorectal cancer: the multiethnic cohort study. Cancer Epidemiol Biomarkers Prev 19:130–134
92. Le Marchand L, White KK, Nomura AM et al (2009) Plasma levels of B vitamins and colorectal cancer risk: the multiethnic cohort study. Cancer Epidemiol Biomarkers Prev 18:2195–2201
93. Takata Y, Shrubsole MJ, Li H et al (2014) Plasma folate concentrations and colorectal cancer risk: a case–control study nested within the Shanghai Men's Health Study. Int J Cancer 135:2191–2198
94. Shrubsole MJ, Yang G, Gao YT et al (2009) Dietary B vitamin and methionine intakes and plasma folate are not associated with colorectal cancer risk in Chinese women. Cancer Epidemiol Biomarkers Prev 18:1003–1006
95. Li Y, Yang H, Cao J (2011) Association between alcohol consumption and cancers in the Chinese population—a systematic review and meta-analysis. PLoS One 6:e18776
96. Fedirko V, Tramacere I, Bagnardi V et al (2011) Alcohol drinking and colorectal cancer risk: an overall and dose–response meta-analysis of published studies. Ann Oncol 22:1958–1972
97. Yang G, Zheng W, Xiang YB et al (2011) Green tea consumption and colorectal cancer risk: a report from the Shanghai Men's Health Study. Carcinogenesis 32:1684–1688
98. Yang G, Shu XO, Li H et al (2007) Prospective cohort study of green tea consumption and colorectal cancer risk in women. Cancer Epidemiol Biomarkers Prev 16:1219–1223
99. Sun CL, Yuan JM, Koh WP et al (2007) Green tea and black tea consumption in relation to colorectal cancer risk: the Singapore Chinese Health Study. Carcinogenesis 28:2143–2148
100. Peterson S, Yuan JM, Koh WP et al (2010) Coffee intake and risk of colorectal cancer among Chinese in Singapore: the Singapore Chinese Health Study. Nutr Cancer 62:21–29
101. Severson RK, Nomura AM, Grove JS et al (1989) A prospective analysis of physical activity and cancer. Am J Epidemiol 130:522–529
102. Lee KJ, Inoue M, Otani T et al (2007) Physical activity and risk of colorectal cancer in Japanese men and women: the Japan Public Health Center-based prospective study. Cancer Causes Control 18:199–209
103. Takahashi H, Kuriyama S, Tsubono Y et al (2007) Time spent walking and risk of colorectal cancer in Japan: the Miyagi Cohort study. Eur J Cancer Prev 16:403–408
104. Ollberding NJ, Nomura AM, Wilkens LR et al (2011) Racial/ethnic differences in colorectal cancer risk: the multiethnic cohort study. Int J Cancer 129:1899–1906
105. Rothwell PM, Wilson M, Elwin CE et al (2010) Long-term effect of aspirin on colorectal cancer incidence and mortality: 20-year follow-up of five randomised trials. Lancet 376: 1741–1750

106. Ranger GS (2014) Current concepts in colorectal cancer prevention with cyclooxygenase inhibitors. Anticancer Res 34:6277–6282
107. Stolfi C, De Simone V, Pallone F et al (2013) Mechanisms of action of non-steroidal anti-inflammatory drugs (NSAIDs) and mesalazine in the chemoprevention of colorectal cancer. Int J Mol Sci 14:17972–17985
108. Ye X, Fu J, Yang Y et al (2013) Dose-risk and duration-risk relationships between aspirin and colorectal cancer: a meta-analysis of published cohort studies. PLoS One 8:e57578
109. Flossmann E, Rothwell PM (2007) Effect of aspirin on long-term risk of colorectal cancer: consistent evidence from randomised and observational studies. Lancet 369:1603–1613
110. Goh CH, Leong WQ, Chew MH et al (2014) Post-operative aspirin use and colorectal cancer-specific survival in patients with stage I–III colorectal cancer. Anticancer Res 34: 7407–7414
111. Foster PA (2013) Oestrogen and colorectal cancer: mechanisms and controversies. Int J Colorectal Dis 28:737–749
112. Barnes EL, Long MD (2012) Colorectal cancer in women: hormone replacement therapy and chemoprevention. Climacteric 15:250–255
113. De La Chapelle A (2004) Genetic predisposition to colorectal cancer. Nat Rev Cancer 4:769–780
114. Tomlinson I (2012) Colorectal cancer genetics: from candidate genes to GWAS and back again. Mutagenesis 27:141–142
115. National Cancer Institute (2015) PDQ® Genetics of Colorectal Cancer. http://cancer.gov/cancertopics/pdq/genetics/colorectal/HealthProfessional. Accessed 15 Jun 2015
116. Chang CQ, Yesupriya A, Rowell JL et al (2014) A systematic review of cancer GWAS and candidate gene meta-analyses reveals limited overlap but similar effect sizes. Eur J Hum Genet 22:402–408
117. Esteban-Jurado C, Garre P, Vila M et al (2014) New genes emerging for colorectal cancer predisposition. World J Gastroenterol 20:1961–1971
118. Butterworth AS, Higgins JP, Pharoah P (2006) Relative and absolute risk of colorectal cancer for individuals with a family history: a meta-analysis. Eur J Cancer 42:216–227
119. Le Marchand L, Zhao LP, Quiaoit F et al (1996) Family history and risk of colorectal cancer in the multiethnic population of Hawaii. Am J Epidemiol 144:1122–1128
120. Ma X, Zhang B, Zheng W (2014) Genetic variants associated with colorectal cancer risk: comprehensive research synopsis, meta-analysis, and epidemiological evidence. Gut 63: 326–336
121. Yang Z, Zhang XF, Liu HX et al (2012) MTHFR C677T polymorphism and colorectal cancer risk in Asians, a meta-analysis of 21 studies. Asian Pac J Cancer Prev 13:1203–1208
122. Le Marchand L, Wilkens LR, Kolonel LN et al (2005) The MTHFR C677T polymorphism and colorectal cancer: the multiethnic cohort study. Cancer Epidemiol Biomarkers Prev 14:1198–1203
123. Andersen V, Holst R, Vogel U (2013) Systematic review: diet-gene interactions and the risk of colorectal cancer. Aliment Pharmacol Ther 37:383–391
124. Ferrari P, Mckay JD, Jenab M et al (2012) Alcohol dehydrogenase and aldehyde dehydrogenase gene polymorphisms, alcohol intake and the risk of colorectal cancer in the European Prospective Investigation into Cancer and Nutrition study. Eur J Clin Nutr 66:1303–1308
125. Andersen V, Vogel U (2015) Interactions between meat intake and genetic variation in relation to colorectal cancer. Genes Nutr 10:448
126. Kim J, Cho YA, Kim DH et al (2012) Dietary intake of folate and alcohol, MTHFR C677T polymorphism, and colorectal cancer risk in Korea. Am J Clin Nutr 95:405–412
127. Peng XE, Jiang YY, Shi XS et al (2013) NQO1 609C>T polymorphism interaction with tobacco smoking and alcohol drinking increases colorectal cancer risk in a Chinese population. Gene 521:105–110
128. Vogtmann E, Xiang YB, Li HL et al (2014) Cruciferous vegetables, glutathione S-transferase polymorphisms, and the risk of colorectal cancer among Chinese men. Ann Epidemiol 24:44–49

129. Lichtenstein P, Holm NV, Verkasalo PK et al (2000) Environmental and heritable factors in the causation of cancer—analyses of cohorts of twins from Sweden, Denmark, and Finland. N Engl J Med 343:78–85
130. Aaltonen L, Johns L, Jarvinen H et al (2007) Explaining the familial colorectal cancer risk associated with mismatch repair (MMR)-deficient and MMR-stable tumors. Clin Cancer Res 13:356–361
131. Zhang K, Civan J, Mukherjee S et al (2014) Genetic variations in colorectal cancer risk and clinical outcome. World J Gastroenterol 20:4167–4177
132. Jiao S, Peters U, Berndt S et al (2014) Estimating the heritability of colorectal cancer. Hum Mol Genet 23:3898–3905
133. Peters U, Hutter CM, Hsu L et al (2012) Meta-analysis of new genome-wide association studies of colorectal cancer risk. Hum Genet 131:217–234
134. Wang H, Burnett T, Kono S et al (2014) Trans-ethnic genome-wide association study of colorectal cancer identifies a new susceptibility locus in VTI1A. Nat Commun 5:4613
135. Jia WH, Zhang B, Matsuo K et al (2013) Genome-wide association analyses in East Asians identify new susceptibility loci for colorectal cancer. Nat Genet 45:191–196
136. Zhang B, Jia WH, Matsuo K et al (2014) Genome-wide association study identifies a new SMAD7 risk variant associated with colorectal cancer risk in East Asians. Int J Cancer 135:948–955
137. Zhang B, Jia WH, Matsuda K et al (2014) Large-scale genetic study in East Asians identifies six new loci associated with colorectal cancer risk. Nat Genet 46:533–542
138. Cui R, Okada Y, Jang SG et al (2011) Common variant in 6q26-q27 is associated with distal colon cancer in an Asian population. Gut 60:799–805
139. He J, Wilkens LR, Stram DO et al (2011) Generalizability and epidemiologic characterization of eleven colorectal cancer GWAS hits in multiple populations. Cancer Epidemiol Biomarkers Prev 20:70–81
140. Lim U, Wilkens LR, Monroe KR et al (2012) Susceptibility variants for obesity and colorectal cancer risk: the multiethnic cohort and PAGE studies. Int J Cancer 131:E1038–E1043
141. Cheng I, Caberto CP, Lum-Jones A et al (2011) Type 2 diabetes risk variants and colorectal cancer risk: the multiethnic cohort and PAGE studies. Gut 60:1703–1711
142. Qin Q, Liu L, Zhong R et al (2013) The genetic variant on chromosome 10p14 is associated with risk of colorectal cancer: results from a case–control study and a meta-analysis. PLoS One 8:e64310
143. Zou L, Zhong R, Lou J et al (2012) Replication study in Chinese population and meta-analysis supports association of the 11q23 locus with colorectal cancer. PLoS One 7:e45461
144. Li FX, Yang XX, He XQ et al (2012) Association of 10q23 with colorectal cancer in a Chinese population. Mol Biol Rep 39:9557–9562
145. Zheng X, Wang L, Zhu Y et al (2012) The SNP rs961253 in 20p12.3 is associated with colorectal cancer risk: a case–control study and a meta-analysis of the published literature. PLoS One 7:e34625
146. Zhu L, Du M, Gu D et al (2013) Genetic variant rs7758229 in 6q26-q27 is not associated with colorectal cancer risk in a Chinese population. PLoS One 8:e59256
147. Thean LF, Li HH, Teo YY et al (2012) Association of Caucasian-identified variants with colorectal cancer risk in Singapore Chinese. PLoS One 7:e42407
148. Matsuo K, Suzuki T, Ito H et al (2009) Association between an 8q24 locus and the risk of colorectal cancer in Japanese. BMC Cancer 9:379
149. Wang H, Haiman CA, Burnett T et al (2013) Fine-mapping of genome-wide association study-identified risk loci for colorectal cancer in African Americans. Hum Mol Genet 22:5048–5055

Prostate Cancer Among Asian Americans

Shannon M. Conroy, Song-Yi Park, Scarlett Lin Gomez, and Iona Cheng

Abstract Prostate cancer, the most commonly diagnosed cancers in men, is a clinically heterogeneous disease. Some tumors remain indolent with little impact on morbidity and survival, while others are aggressive and rapidly progress to advanced and lethal disease. Studies of prostate cancer incidence have shown considerably higher incidence rates among Asian-American men living in the United States (US) relative to Asian men living in Asian countries. Although differences in screening practices by prostate-specific antigen (PSA) testing likely account for some of the differences in incidence, the adoption of Western lifestyles with migration to the US may play a role and involve the interplay between genetic and environmental factors. Epidemiological studies have examined migration-related risk factors among Asian Americans, capitalizing on the unique heterogeneity of specific Asian populations by generational status and acculturation. Age, race/ethnicity, family history, and genetic susceptibility are established risk factors for prostate cancer. Additional risk factors that have been implicated include hormonal and infection/inflammatory factors, body mass index, diabetes, physical activity, smoking, and dietary intake of animal and polyunsaturated fat, soy products, and green tea. In this chapter, we summarize our current understanding of the epidemiology of prostate cancer in Asian-American populations.

Keywords Asian American • Prostate cancer • Risk factors • Epidemiology • Body mass index • Smoking • Isoflavones

S.M. Conroy • S.L. Gomez • I. Cheng (✉)
Cancer Prevention Institute of California,
2201 Walnut Avenue, Suite 300, Fremont, CA 94538, US
e-mail: iona.cheng@cpic.org

S.-Y. Park
Cancer Epidemiology Program, University of Hawaii Cancer Center,
701 Ilalo Street, Honolulu 96813, HI, US

A.H. Wu, D.O. Stram (eds.), *Cancer Epidemiology Among Asian Americans*,
DOI 10.1007/978-3-319-41118-7_7

Introduction

Prostate cancer develops in the prostate, a gland in male reproductive system that functions to produce seminal fluid to nourish and transport semen. It is one of the most common cancers in men, typically diagnosed in men ages 50 and older, who are often asymptomatic and identified by screening, with the majority of deaths due to prostate cancer occurring in men ages 75 and older. While many of the symptoms of prostate cancer are similar to benign prostate hyperplasia (BPH), the enlargement of the prostate, prostate cancer and BPH are distinct conditions. The presence of BPH may increase the detection of indolent prostate cancer through transurethral resection of the prostate (TURP) or prostate-specific antigen (PSA) testing; however, BPH is not a risk factor for disease. Prostate cancer is generally an indolent disease, yet some cases are aggressive and fast growing that rapidly progress to lethal prostate cancer. Autopsy studies have revealed an increase in prostate cancer prevalence with each decade of age, with an estimated prevalence of 59 % by age >79 years [1]. This indicates a high proportion of indolent tumors. It is clear that strategies are needed to distinguish between indolent and aggressive forms of the disease.

Incidence

In 2009–2013, the incidence rate of prostate cancer in Asian Americans/Pacific Islanders was 68.9 per 100,000 [2]. In comparison, incidence rates of prostate cancer among non-Hispanic Whites and African Americans were 1.8- and 3.0-fold higher, respectively [2]. In spite of the lower incidence rates of disease in Asian Americans, prostate cancer is the leading incident cancer site in Asian-American men. Notably, variation in the incidence rate of prostate cancer has been seen across specific Asian American populations, with four-fold variation in rates seen across groups [3]. For Asian Indian and Pakistani, Chinese, Filipino, and Japanese men in the US, prostate cancer was the most commonly diagnosed cancer from 1990 through 2008 [3]. From 1990 through 1993, Filipino men experienced a 19 % annual percent increase in prostate cancer rates and Japanese men demonstrated a similar sharp increase in incidence [3]. Asian Indian and Pakistani men in the US experienced a 2.2 % annual percent increase in prostate cancer incidence rates in the 1990s, followed by a sharp 3-year decline, and another significant increase from 2006 to 2008 [3]. Korean men also experienced an increase in incidence rates of prostate cancer at 2.9 % per year from 1990 through 2006, which subsequently decreased thereafter [3]. Prostate cancer rates were relatively stable in Chinese men during this period, while rates in Vietnamese and Laotians rose steadily. The trends in Filipino and Japanese largely followed the pattern seen in the US population; a rapid rise in the early 1990s that peaked in 1992 and a subsequent decline and stabilization after 1996 attributable to the introduction and adoption of PSA screening in the population [4]. The patterns in South Asians were similar with a delayed peak the early 2000s. Yet, the stable rates in Chinese and increasing rates in Koreans, Vietnamese, and Laotians may be related to differences in the adoption of PSA screening and changing health behaviors associated with US acculturation.

Mortality

The mortality rates of prostate cancer in Asian Americans/Pacific Islanders at 9.1 deaths per 100,000 in 2009–2013 were the lowest in comparison to the other major racial/ethnic groups in the US—Hispanics (17.1), non-Hispanic Whites (19.2), American Indians (15.0), and African Americans (44.2) [2]. Recent data from 2002 to 2011 displayed a stable mortality rate of prostate cancer among Asian Americans/ Pacific Islanders [5]. The racial/ethnic differences in cancer survival have been primarily attributed to underlying biological factors [6] and the receipt of quality cancer care [7]. In a national study comparing cancer-specific survival between Whites and Asian Americans, no differences in the prevalence of definitive treatment were seen for stage 1 prostate cancer, but significant differences were seen with stage 2 disease (range, 75.3 % among Filipinos to 81.9 % among South Asians) and stage 3 disease (range, 91.4 % among Filipinos and 99.2 % among South Asians) [8]. In a competing risk analysis among these men, accounting for known factors to affect survival outcomes, Japanese (relative risk (RR)=0.54; 95 % CI=0.38–0.78) and Filipinos (RR=0.63; 95 % CI=0.48–0.84) displayed significantly lower risk of prostate-cancer-specific mortality in comparison to Whites, while other groups such as Chinese, Korean, and Vietnamese had nonsignificant lower risks of mortality [8].

Prostate Cancer Heterogeneity

Prostate cancer has an extremely heterogeneous clinical behavior. Some tumors will remain indolent with little impact on morbidity and survival, while others are aggressive and progress rapidly in a potentially lethal manner. The adoption of PSA screening has led to a vast increase in the number of presumably indolent tumors that remain difficult to distinguish from aggressive disease. Asian-American men were reported to present with a greater proportion of advanced-stage [9–12] and high-grade disease [10, 12] than White men, which has significant implications for treatment and prognosis. In a large, multiethnic, population-based study that categorized prostate cancer patients into low-, intermediate-, and high-risk profiles based on clinical stage, Gleason score, and PSA levels at diagnosis, six Asian-American groups—US-born Chinese, foreign-born Chinese, US-born Japanese, foreign-born Japanese, foreign-born Filipino, and foreign-born Vietnamese—were found to have a more unfavorable clinical risk profile compared to non-Hispanic White men [13]. The odds ratios for high versus intermediate risk of disease ranged from 1.23 for

US-born Japanese men to 1.45 for Filipino men, and these associations appeared to be driven by higher grade and higher PSA values [13]. In a study of Asian-American prostate cancer patients, who were treated in an equal access health-care system, Asian Americans presented with a lower clinical stage but worse biopsy grade than other groups [11]. In addition, Asian Americans treated with radical prostatectomy or radiation therapy were more likely to have less prostate cancer progression and improved survival than other groups [11]. The observation that Asian-American men have a better prognosis in spite of their presentation with poorer prognostic features suggests that race/ethnicity may have an independent effect on prostate cancer progression.

Prostate Cancer Screening

Screening for prostate cancer by PSA testing was introduced in the US in the early 1990s and became widespread by the mid- to late-1990s [14], resulting in large increases in prostate cancer incidence rates across all racial/ethnic groups [2, 3]. Due to concerns for over-detection and -treatment of indolent disease and the results of clinical trials, documenting no or little reduction in mortality associated with PSA screening [15], the US Preventive Services Task Force (USPSTF) reversed the 2008 PSA screening guidelines. In 2008 the USPSTF recommended against screening for men aged 75 and older [14] and in 2012 recommended against PSA screening for all men regardless of age [16].

Data on PSA screening (never received a test, received a test 1 year or less, received a test more than 1 year ago) by Asian-American ethnicity are available from the 2009 California Health Interview Survey (CHIS), a population-based survey of California populations [17]. Strengths of CHIS data include over-sampled racial/ethnic minority groups and availability of the telephone survey in English, Spanish, Chinese (Mandarin and Cantonese), Korean, and Vietnamese. The proportion of Asian-American men in California aged 40–79 who have never received a PSA screening test ranged from 52.5 % among Japanese to 86.8 % among Vietnamese (Fig. 1), in comparison to 47.6 % among non-Hispanic Whites, 71.2 % among Latinos, and 63.6 % among African Americans. The proportion who received a test within the past year ranged from 8.5 % among Vietnamese to 27.8 % among Japanese and 27.5 % among South Asians. The generally higher rates of nonadherence to cancer screening guidelines among most Asian-American ethnic groups compared to non-Hispanic Whites has been attributed to cultural factors and stigmas related to disease prevention [18–22], but may also be due to provider factors [23, 24]. Prior research of factors associated with decreased prostate cancer screening (by PSA and other modalities) among Asian-American men suggests lack of awareness, not having regular health-care access, no recommendations from providers, being unmarried, being of lower SES, financial issues, time constraints, fear of a cancer diagnosis, and embarrassment [25–29].

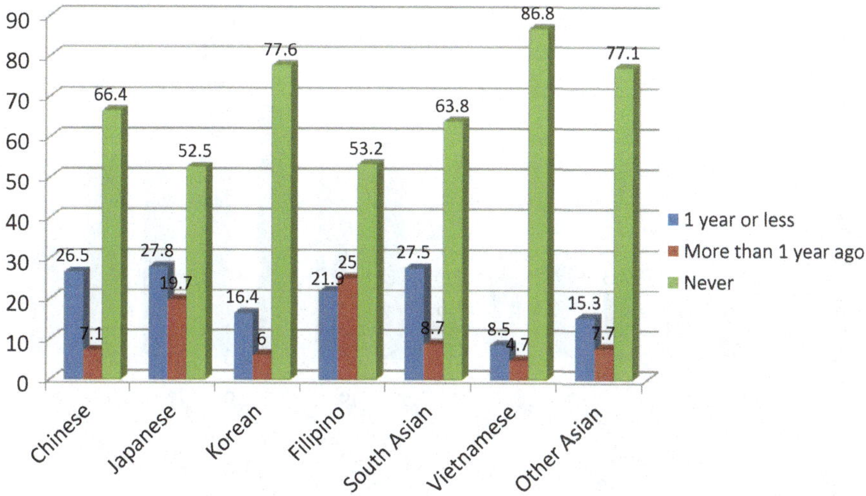

Fig. 1 Prostate-specific antigen screening for prostate cancer among men aged 40–79, California Health Interview Survey, 2009

Migrant Studies

Epidemiologic studies of risk of disease among persons or populations who migrate from one country to another lower- or higher-risk country can inform the relative contributions of environmental versus genetic risk factors and aid in the identification of putative risk factors [30–32]. International descriptive studies of prostate cancer incidence have shown considerably higher incidence rates among Asian-American men in the US relative to Asian men living in Asian countries [33]. In data from the International Association for Cancer Registries (IACR), prostate cancer incidence during the period 1998–2002 was about three times higher among Asian Americans than Asians living in Asia (Fig. 2) [34].

However, international differences in PSA screening has been cited as being a major driver of the incidence differences between Asians in the US and Asia [33], thus limiting interpretation of the incidence differentials, and the degree to which changes in prostate cancer incidence is due to changes in lifestyle and other exposures upon migration from Asia to the US. Moreover, to the extent that prostate cancer primarily impacts older men (e.g., 56.7 % of cases in the US are diagnosed among men aged 65 and older [2]) and incidence increases with increasing age, differences in life expectancy and competing causes of death across countries may also confound the interpretation of international descriptive statistics. Ito et al. compared the mortality/incidence rate ratio by Asian country and found considerably higher ratios among Asians in Asia than their counterparts in the US; for example, the mortality rate to incidence rate ratio was 0.42, 0.52, and 0.22 in China, the Philippines, and Japan, respectively, compared to 0.11, 0.14, and 0.15 among

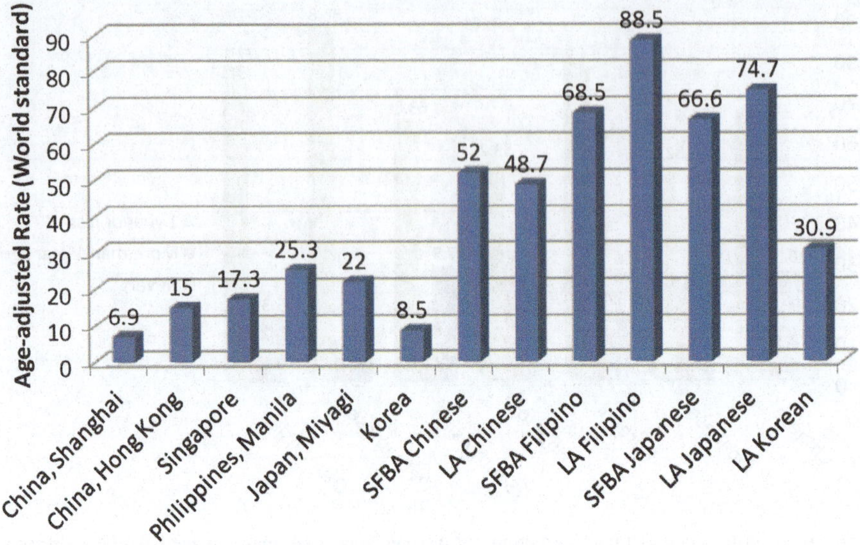

Fig. 2 Age-standardized incidence rates (1998–2002) by country and US Asian American ethnic group (data from Cancer Incidence in Five Continents, Vol. IX). Abbreviations: SFBA, San Francisco Bay Area, California; LA, Los Angeles County, California

California Chinese, Filipinos, and Japanese, respectively [33]. The lower ratios in the US Asian populations indicate a higher proportion of screen-detected cancers associated with lower mortality [33]. Indeed, the proportions of patients with metastatic disease are considerably higher in Asia, ranging from 26 % in a hospital-based cancer registry in Japan in 1998–2002 to 76.6 % in China in 2005–2007, compared to 3.1 % among Asian Americans in a hospital registry in Washington, DC, in 1989–2007 [33].

Risk Factors

Age, race/ethnicity, family history, and genetic susceptibility represent well-established risk factors for prostate cancer. Studies have investigated putative risk factors, including hormonal and infection/inflammatory factors, body mass index (BMI), diabetes, physical activity, smoking, and dietary intake. However, no definitive risk factor has emerged, particularly for incident prostate cancer. The lack of consistent associations with prostate cancer incidence likely reflects the heterogeneity in prostate cancer, specifically indolent screened cancers that likely have a different etiology than advanced cancers. Furthermore, the correlation between lifestyle factors with screening behavior may also confound these associations. In contrast, mortality and survival studies avoid screening-related biases and may highlight risk factors associated with aggressive and lethal disease phenotypes. The underlying etiology of prostate carcinogenesis likely involves the interaction of genetics and lifestyle factors, with differential effects by stage and disease characteristics.

Studies have examined migration-related risk factors among Asian-American populations, capitalizing on the unique heterogeneity in risk factor prevalence and disease risk with length of residency in the US. In particular, many studies have focused on the role of dietary factors that may differ by nativity and acculturation. Prominent cohorts have examined risk factors for prostate cancer in Asian Americans: (1) a cohort study among men of Japanese ancestry in Hawaii that were interviewed and examined as part of the Honolulu Heart Program from 1965 to 1968 [35] and (2) the Multiethnic Cohort (MEC), a population-based prospective study of African Americans, Native Hawaiians, Japanese Americans, Latinos, and Whites in Hawaii and Los Angeles that enrolled participants from 1993 to 1996 [36]. Another important study, a multicenter population-based case–control study in the US (Hawaii, Los Angeles, San Francisco) and Canada (Vancouver) used registry data to identify cases diagnosed between 1989 and 1991 of Black, White, Chinese American, or Japanese American race/ethnicities (with at least three grandparents all of same ethnicity) [37].

Age

Advancing age is an established risk factor for prostate cancer. Although prostate cancer incidence is extremely rare before the age of 40, the incidence rate increases exponentially up to the age 80 with advancing age [38, 39]. This rapid age-dependent rise in incidence is greater than any other cancer in Western countries; yet, this pattern is less evident in China and Japan [39, 40].

Race/Ethnicity

Race/ethnicity is an established risk factor for both prostate cancer incidence and mortality [2]. Asian Americans have lower incidence and mortality rates compared to other US racial/ethnic groups—African Americans, Hispanics, and Whites [33]. The key etiologic factors influencing racial/ethnic differences in prostate cancer epidemiology are complex. Genetic susceptibility may play an important role [41–43]; yet, the influence of other factors, such as racial/ethnic-specific differences in lifestyle, obesity, and diet, remains largely unknown. Further studies are needed to elucidate the underlying factors driving the lower risk among Asian Americans and thereby clarify the role of protective factors and potential interactions with genetic and environmental factors.

Family History

Family history is among the strongest epidemiologic risk factors for prostate cancer. Having one, two, or three affected first-degree relative(s) with prostate cancer has been found to increase the risk of prostate by 2.2-, 4.9-, and 10.9-fold, respectively [44]. While the prevalence of a father, brother, or son with prostate cancer has been reported to be lower in Asian Americans (4 %) in comparison to Whites (7 %) and Blacks (5 %), Asian Americans displayed a similar two- to threefold increased risk of prostate cancer associated with such a family history as other groups [45]. It has been estimated by a large study of twins that 42 % of the risk of prostate cancer is explained by inherited factors [46].

Genetic Susceptibility

Genome-wide association studies (GWAS) have successfully identified over 100 risk loci for prostate cancer to date. However, the majority of these studies have been conducted among men of European ancestry, with two studies conducted among Chinese [47] and Japanese [48] men in Asia and only one US study conducted among Japanese-American men in the MEC [49]. In a prostate cancer GWAS of 1033 Japanese-American prostate cancer cases and 1042 Japanese-American controls, no novel risk loci were discovered, and the majority (79 %) of established risk variants for prostate cancer at that time ($n = 56$) were positively associated with prostate cancer [49]. The cumulative effect of these variants were associated with a per allele odds ratio (OR) = 1.10; $P = 2.7 \times 10^{-25}$ [49]. In a study that examined 69 established prostate cancer risk variants, 64 variants were observed (frequency ≥ 0.01) in Japanese subjects (cases/controls = 2563/4391) with 84 % (54/64) positively associated with risk and 41 % (26/64) nominally statistically significant ($P < 0.05$) [43]. In addition, fine-mapping findings suggest that the 10q26 locus may be a Japanese-specific risk region as risk variants in this region are common across populations, yet strong associations with prostate cancer risk were only seen in Japanese and not in other racial/ethnic groups [43]. A separate study that included 288 Asian-American prostate cancer cases and 2938 controls examined 99 prostate cancer risk variants and found that 68 % (67/99) were in the same direction as previously reported [41]. Comparing the highest to lowest deciles of a risk score of these variants resulted in an OR = 3.38 (95 % CI, 1.91–5.97) for Asian Americans [41]. These findings indicate that the established risk variants for prostate cancer significantly contribute to risk in Asian Americans.

Androgens and Insulin-Like Growth Factors

The physiological development of the prostate is primarily regulated by testosterone and its most active metabolite, dihydrotestosterone (DHT), and androgens have long been hypothesized to play an etiologic role in prostate cancer [50, 51]. However, epidemiologic data on the relationship between endogenous androgens and prostate cancer have been inconclusive [52]. In a pooled analysis of 18 prospective studies consisting of 3886 men with incident prostate cancer and 6438 control subjects, no associations were found between risk of prostate cancer and pre-diagnostic serum androgens (total and free testosterone, DHT, and others) and estrogens (total and free estradiol), with no evidence of heterogeneity by length of time between blood collection and cancer diagnosis [52]. There was, however, a modest, inverse association between sex hormone-binding globulin (SHBG) and prostate cancer risk [52]. The lack of support of an androgen-prostate cancer risk link may reflect that these findings were based on androgen levels determined late in adult life. It may be that androgen levels in early adulthood may represent a more etiologically relevant period for the pathogenesis of prostate cancer. Population differences in testosterone levels of young men have been significantly associated with regional population disparities in the incidence of prostate cancer in older men [53]. There is limited evidence supporting racial/ethnic differences in testosterone or metabolites of testosterone in older men that correspond with respective population incidence rates [54, 55]. Similar levels of testosterone and 3α-androstanediol glucuronide have been found among middle-late-aged Singapore Chinese and Japanese American populations, whereas higher levels of testosterone or its metabolites have been found in middle-late-aged US Whites than Singapore Chinese [54], Japanese American [54, 55], Chinese American [55], and African American [55] men. Other growth factors, such as insulin-like growth factors (IGF) and their related binding proteins (IGFBP), may have an independent role in carcinogenesis as well as interact with the androgen signaling pathways [56].

The few studies conducted in Asian-American men observed null associations between androgens, SHBG, IGFs, and prostate cancer risk [57, 58]. In a case–control study (467 cases and 934 controls) nested in the MEC, pre-diagnostic serum levels of testosterone, DHT, SHBG, 3α-androstanediol glucuronide, IGF-I, IGF-II, IGFBP-1, and IGFBP-3 were not associated with risk of prostate cancer in all groups and in Japanese Americans [58]. In a prospective study (control arm of the multicenter case–control study in the US and Canada), null associations were observed for pre-diagnostic levels of IGF-I and IGFBP-3 with risk of developing prostate cancer in Asian Americans, yet the study was limited by the small number ($n=33$) of prostate cancer cases [57].

Infection/Inflammation

Inflammation has an etiological role in the pathogenesis of cancers [59], and prostatitis and sexually transmitted infections (STIs) may represent important risk factors for prostate cancer by inducing inflammation processes and chronic inflammation within the prostate [60]. Prostatitis is a common condition in men with an estimated prevalence ranging from 5 to 9 % [61] and includes acute and chronic bacterial infection of the prostate [62]. A meta-analysis of 20 case–control studies, primarily in Western countries, supports positive associations between prostatitis and prostate cancer with a stronger association in Chinese (meta-analysis OR=4.67; 95 % CI=3.08–7.07 based on two studies in China) than US (meta-analysis OR=1.50; 95 % CI=1.25–1.80) populations [63]. Additional meta-analyses, again relying primarily on case–control studies and studies conducted in Western countries, support modest associations of gonorrhea [64, 65] and any STI [65] with prostate cancer risk. The relationship between prostatitis, STIs, and prostate cancer risk was examined in the California Men's Health Study, representing an important study given the prospective study design of a large racial/ethnically diverse cohort of African American, Asian American, Latino, and White men from Northern and Southern California Kaiser Permanente [66]. After a median follow-up of 2 years (maximum 4 years), men reporting a history compared to those with no history of prostatitis had a significant 1.3-fold increased risk (95 % CI=1.10–1.54; 1658 cases) in the entire cohort and a nonsignificant positive association (RR=1.95; 95 % CI=0.89–4.24, 89 cases) in Asian Americans. Asian Americans experienced a significant positive association with history of syphilis (RR=3.72; 95 % CI=1.35–10.26) and chlamydia (RR=5.55; 95 % CI=1.70–18.09). Larger effects were observed among foreign-born versus US-born Asian Americans. For instance, among foreign-born Asian Americans, there was a significant 2.7-fold increased risk (95 % CI, 1.02–6.95; 38 cases) of prostate cancer associated with a history of prostatitis. Further cohort studies are needed to clarify the role of chronic inflammation and infectious agents in relation to prostate cancer susceptibility, especially among foreign-born Asian Americans.

Body Size and Obesity

Studies of the association between obesity and prostate incidence have been inconsistent [67, 68]. Studies of body size and obesity have examined BMI (kg/m^2) at various ages (pre-, early, middle, or late adulthood) [37, 69, 70], weight and weight change since early adulthood [71], waist circumference or waist-to-hip ratio as a measure of abdominal adiposity [37, 69], and various upper arm or skinfold thickness measurements [69, 70, 72]. A dose–response meta-analysis of 13 prospective studies (only one study from Japan) observed dual effects of obesity on risk of prostate cancer: a significant 6 % (RR=0.94; 95 % CI, 0.91–0.97) decreased risk for localized cancers but 9 % (RR=1.09; 95 % CI, 1.02–1.16) increased risk for advanced cancers per 5 kg/m^2 increase in BMI [68]. However, the prospective study in Japan showed nonsignificant increased risk with higher BMI at middle adulthood for both localized and advanced cancers [73]. A population-based case–control study in Shanghai, China, found a positive association with waist-to-hip ratio for both localized and advanced prostate cancers (quartile 4 versus 1, OR=4.20; 95 % CI=1.88–9.36 and OR=2.09; 95 % CI=1.18–3.70, respectively) yet no associations with adult BMI or BMI at various ages [69]. Detection bias may influence the ability to detect early-stage prostate cancers in obese men due to lower PSA values as observed in healthy US [74, 75] and Chinese men [76]. According to the World Cancer Research Fund/American Institute for Cancer Research (WCRF/AICR) 2014 report, there is strong evidence that being overweight or obese increases the risk of advanced (i.e., high-stage or grade) prostate cancers [67]. Obesity is also associated with 20 % (95 % CI 0.99–1.46) higher risk of prostate cancer-specific mortality per 5 kg/m^2 increase BMI [77]. Obesity-related biological, clinical, and lifestyle factors have been hypothesized as potential underlying mechanisms for the aggressive and lethal prostate cancer phenotype in obese men [78].

In Asian-American men, one case–control study [37] and three prospective cohorts [70–72, 79] examined obesity and prostate cancer risk with mixed results. In a multicenter population-based case–control study in the US and Canada, no consistent or convincing associations between BMI (at reference year or prior decades of life) and prostate cancer were observed in Chinese Americans (283 cases, 272 controls) or Japanese Americans (326 case, 329 controls) [37]. In contrast, a cohort study of Japanese-American men in Hawaii observed positive associations between obesity and prostate cancer risk with 20 years of follow-up ($n = 174$ cases identified 1965 through 1986) [72] and confirmed in a subsequent study ($n = 306$ cases identified 1965 through 1992) [79]. High BMI at baseline was associated with increased prostate cancer risk (BMI ≥ 26 versus <22 kg/m^2, RR = 1.21; 95 % CI = 0.87–1.68, p trend < 0.01) [79]. In a large, multiracial cohort of male subscribers to the Kaiser Permanente Medical Care Program, there was no evidence of an association between BMI at comprehensive medical examination (ages ranged from 18 to 84 years with 50 % of the men in their 30s or 40s) and prostate cancer risk among Asian Americans ($n = 53$ cases) or the other racial/ethnic groups ($n = 2026$ cases) after an average follow-up of 19.5 years [70]. The associations did not vary consistently by BMI at various ages or stage of prostate cancer at diagnosis [70]. In the MEC, an inverse association of borderline significance was observed between BMI at baseline and prostate cancer risk ($n = 1382$ cases in Japanese American men) after an average follow-up of 9.6 years (obese versus normal BMI, RR = 0.78; 95 % CI = 0.57–1.08; p trend 0.07) [71], but after an average 13.9 years of follow-up, no significant associations with baseline BMI were observed overall and across racial/ethnic groups [80]. It is uncertain whether length of follow-up affects the magnitude of association; however, the results from prospective studies appear mixed regardless of length of follow-up time [81]. Age (especially at early ages), duration of obesity, or significant weight gain may be etiologically relevant for prostate cancer development [82], and further studies are needed to clarify the association between obesity and prostate cancer in Asian Americans.

Diabetes

Diabetes is associated with increased risk for several cancers [83], yet evidence, primarily in White populations, suggests a significant decreased risk for prostate cancer [84]. A recent meta-analysis of 29 cohort and 16 case–control studies revealed an opposite pattern in Western versus Asian countries, with an inverse association between diabetes and prostate cancer risk in Western populations (meta-analysis RR=0.81; 95 % CI=0.76–0.85 for 37 studies in Western populations) and a positive association in Asian populations (meta-analysis RR=1.64; 95 % CI=1.0–2.28 for eight studies in Asian counties) [84]. The underlying mechanisms for the potential heterogeneity in the relationship between diabetes and prostate cancer risk in Western versus Asian populations are unknown.

In the MEC after a mean follow-up of 13.9 years, history of diabetes was significantly negatively associated with prostate cancer risk in multivariable models adjusted for BMI and smoking in all racial/ethnic groups combined (RR yes versus no diabetes=0.78; 95 % CI=0.72–0.85) and in Japanese Americans (RR yes versus no diabetes=0.85; 95 CI=0.72–0.85) [80] that confirmed earlier results from the MEC [85]. History of diabetes was related to a decrease risk of both localized and advanced tumors, and the inverse association persisted after adjustment for PSA screening history [80]. Proposed underlying mechanism of the lower prostate cancer risk associated with diabetes may involve low testosterone levels driven by insulin-related pathways. Although potential heterogeneity may exist early in the disease processes, hyperinsulinemia may drive a positive relationship; in contrast, with the progression of diabetes, hypoinsulinemia may result in an inverse relationship with prostate cancer [86].

Physical Activity

The WCRF/AICR 2014 report concluded that there was no convincing evidence to support the relationship between physical activity and prostate cancer risk [67]. Physical activity was not associated with prostate cancer risk in a cohort study of Japanese men in Hawaii [35] or in the MEC [80]. In the population-based case–control study, physical activity was not related to prostate cancer risk either in Asian American, White, or African American men [37].

Smoking

Cigarette smoke is a preventable risk factor for several cancers and contains known human carcinogens [87], yet the role of smoking in prostate cancer etiology appears inconsistent and may be relevant for prostate cancer mortality and more aggressive cancers. A recent systematic review and meta-analysis of prospective cohort studies showed a possible association between smoking and increased risk of prostate cancer in studies with case identification up to 1995 or earlier, representing the pre-PSA screening era (meta-analysis RR ever versus never smoking=1.06, 95 % CI=1.00–1.25, p heterogeneity=0.23), although studies completed afterwards or in the post-PSA screening era showed a null or inverse association (meta-analysis RR ever versus never smoking = 0.90, 95 % CI = 0.86–0.93, p heterogeneity < 0.001) [88]. Inverse [89, 90] or equivocal [91] associations were observed for studies in Japan, Korea, and Singapore. A recent large study in Europe (4623 cases) found current smoking was significantly negatively associated with risk of localized and low-grade prostate cancer, but nonsignificantly positively associated with advanced and high-grade prostate cancers [92]. The inverse smoking-prostate cancer association may reflect differences in screening behavior and health-care service availability among smokers versus nonsmokers [93]. More consistent associations have been documented between smoking and prostate cancer deaths in a meta-analysis of 21 studies conducted primarily in Western populations, with a modest increased (meta-analysis RR = 1.18; 95 % CI = 1.11–1.24) risk of mortality for ever versus never smokers and evidence of a dose–response with number of cigarettes smoked per day [88].

In a cohort study of Japanese-American men in Hawaii, although initially smoking was associated with a nonsignificant reduced risk of prostate cancer with 20 years of follow-up (n = 174 cases identified 1965 through 1986) [35], a subsequent study (249 cases identified 1971 through 1995) found a nonsignificant positive association between smoking and prostate cancer risk (OR current smokers versus nonsmokers = 1.3, 95 % CI = 0.8–2.0) [94]. In a recent study in the MEC, with an average follow-up of 13.9 years (through 2010), smoking (≥20 cigarettes per day) was inversely associated with prostate cancer risk in all racial/ethnic groups combined (RR current versus never smoker = 0.72; 95 % CI = 0.63–0.83; 7115 cases) and in Japanese Americans (RR current versus never smoker = 0.72; 95 % CI = 0.55–0.93; 2056 cases) that persisted after adjustment for PSA screening history [80]. These inverse associations were only observed for localized and not for advanced tumors [80]. Smoking is likely a weak risk factor for incident prostate cancer and subject to biases associated with PSA screening that make it difficult to unravel the complex relationships and heterogeneity by stage and disease characteristics.

Dietary Factors

Some dietary components have been implicated to increase prostate cancer risk (e.g., processed and red meats, milk and dairy products), whereas others are hypothesized to be protective (e.g., lycopene, selenium, legumes, alpha-tocopherol). However, according to the WCRF/AICR 2014 report that represents the most rigorous, systematic, global analysis of scientific research currently available on prostate cancer, there was no strong evidence to support the role of diet in prostate cancer risk including lycopene, vitamin D, and beta-carotene (either through food or supplements) [67]. Only a limited number of studies have examined the diet–prostate cancer relationship in Asian American populations as discussed further.

Fat

A traditional Asian diet is more plant-based and likely contains less fat, particularly animal fat, compared to the Western diet. Thus, dietary fat intake has been speculated to contribute to the lower risk of prostate cancer in Asian men compared to White men given its potential carcinogenic role [95]. The limited data of dietary fat intake and prostate cancer risk in Asian Americans have been inconclusive. In an ecological study of diet and cancer conducted in Hawaii during the 1970s, the ethnic-sex-specific fat intake of a representative sample of 4657 adults aged ≥45 years and corresponding population-based cancer incidence rates were compared across the five major ethnic groups [96, 97]. In general, fat intake was highest in Whites, followed by Hawaiians, lower in Japanese and Chinese, and lowest in Filipinos. Although total fat intakes in the five ethnic groups were not correlated with the corresponding incidence rates of prostate cancer [97], animal ($r=0.90$) and saturated ($r=0.87$) fat intakes were significantly positively correlated with prostate cancer incidence rates [96, 97]. In a subsequent population-based case–control study in the US and Canada, dietary fat, especially saturated fat, were associated with a higher risk of prostate cancer in Chinese Americans (quintile 5 versus 1, OR=1.5; 95 % CI=0.37–5.8; p trend<0.01) and Japanese Americans (OR=4.1; 95 % CI=1.4–11.8; p trend<0.01), while there was no association in African Americans and Whites [37]. In a cohort in Japan, intakes of some specific saturated fatty acids were related to an increased risk of prostate cancer; quartile 4 versus 1, RR=1.62; 95 % CI=1.15–2.29; p trend<0.01 for myristic acid and RR=1.53; 95 % CI=1.07–2.20; p trend=0.04 for palmitic acid [98]. However, a cohort study of Japanese-American men in Hawaii found no relationship between fat intake including saturated and unsaturated fat and prostate cancer risk [35]. In the MEC, no association was found with various types of dietary fat in Japanese men [99] or other racial/ethnic groups. However, circulating palmitic acid was associated with a higher risk of prostate cancer in Japanese men (tertile 3 versus 1, OR=3.21; 95 % CI=1.21–8.53; p trend<0.01) in a case–control study nested within the MEC [100]. The increased risk of prostate cancer with higher levels of palmitic acid in blood was also found in other prospective studies of men with European ancestry (Norway [101], European Prospective Investigation into Cancer and Nutrition (EPIC) study [102], Australia [103]).

Processed and Red Meat

Red meat intake has been examined in relation to cancer as it is a major source of cancer-promoting components including saturated fat, zinc, and heme iron. Also, heterocyclic amines, potent carcinogens, are formed when red meat is cooked and processed at high temperature. In a cohort study of Japanese American men in Hawaii, meat and processed meat intake were not related to prostate cancer risk [35]. In the MEC, no associations were found between various meat, including red meat, intakes and prostate cancer risk in Japanese men or in other ethnic groups

[99]. In a nested case–control study conducted within the MEC, well-done red meat consumption and *N*-acetyltransferase (*NAT*)*1* or *NAT2* genotypes, as modifiers of the carcinogenic effect of heterocyclic amines, were not related to prostate cancer risk [104].

Fruits/Vegetables

Fruits and vegetables contain various bioactive components with anticancer properties. In a case–control study of Chinese and Japanese men in the US and Canada, intake of carrots was related to a lower risk of prostate cancer in both Japanese (tertile 3 versus 1, OR=0.58; 95 % CI=0.38–0.87; *p* trend=0.01) and Chinese men (OR=0.49; 95 % CI=0.30–0.81; *p* trend=0.01) [105]. A decreased risk of prostate cancer was observed with a higher intake of yellow-orange vegetables in Japanese men (OR=0.61; 95 % CI=0.40–0.93; *p* trend=0.02) and with a higher intake of cruciferous vegetables in Chinese men (OR=0.68; 95 % CI=0.37–1.24; *p* trend=0.03) [105]. In contrast, in a cohort study of Japanese-American men in Hawaii, fruit intake was not associated with prostate cancer risk [35]. In the MEC, no associations were observed with intake of fruits and vegetables in Japanese Americans or in other racial/ethnic groups [106].

Soy

High intake of soy products or isoflavones has been hypothesized to contribute to the significantly lower incidence rate of prostate cancer among Asian compared to European/North American men [107]. The anticancer properties of isoflavones have been explored in animal and in vitro studies and support a potential beneficial role in the prevention of prostate cancer [108]. Meta-analyses of 15 studies suggested that soy food consumption is associated with a reduction in prostate cancer incidence and mortality, with a combined adjusted RR/OR of 0.74 (95 % CI=0.63–0.89) [109, 110]. Yet, the findings of individual studies were mixed, and the protection against prostate cancer may be dependent on the type and quantity of soy products consumed [110].

One case–control study and two cohort studies have examined soy intake in relation to prostate cancer risk in Asian Americans. In a case–control study in the US and Canada, soy food intake was not associated with prostate cancer risk in Japanese and Chinese men [105]. In a cohort study in Hawaii of Japanese-American men, there was an initial suggestive association between higher tofu consumption and decreased risk of prostate cancer with 20 years of follow-up (*n*=174 cases identified 1965 through 1986; 139,727 person-years) [35], but a subsequent study found tofu intake was not associated with prostate cancer risk (*n*=304 cases identified 1972 through 1995; 113,159 person-years) [111]. Furthermore, more recently in 25,052 Japanese-American men in the MEC, no association was found with intake of soy product, based on food frequency questionnaire, and prostate cancer risk

($n=1062$ cases) after an average follow-up of 8 years [112]. Similarly, in a case–control study nested in the MEC, no association was seen between isoflavone intake, based on urinary biomarkers, and prostate cancer risk in Japanese men ($n=70$ cases, $n=122$ controls matched on age, race/ethnicity, date/time specimen collection) [113].

Green Tea

It has been hypothesized that the lower incidence of prostate cancer in Asian men may be due to the consumption of green tea [114]. Green tea contains high concentrations of polyphenols with potential anticancer properties [115]. Although green tea appears to be effective in prostate cancer prevention in a recent review, most studies have been conducted in Asian countries [114]. Contrary to the hypothesis, green tea consumption (ever versus never) was associated with a nonsignificant increased risk of prostate cancer (HR = 1.47; 95 % CI = 0.99, 2.19; $n=174$ cases) in a cohort study of Japanese-American men in Hawaii followed for 20 years [35].

Micronutrients

An ecological study found no correlation between the ethnic-sex-specific intakes of vitamins A and C and corresponding prostate cancer incidence rates in the five major ethnic groups in Hawaii [96]. In the MEC, no association was observed with intakes of vitamins A, C, and E, carotenoids [106], vitamin D, and calcium [116] from foods and supplements in Japanese Americans. In addition to dietary intakes estimated by questionnaires, blood levels of micronutrients were examined in relation to prostate cancer risk. In a cohort of Japanese-American men in Hawaii, serum selenium was associated with a lower risk of prostate cancer [94], while no association was found for serum levels of vitamin D metabolites [117] and micronutrients including carotenoids, retinoids, and tocopherols [118]. In a nested case–control study within the MEC, serum zinc was positively associated with prostate cancer risk in Japanese Americans [119], while serum selenium, tocopherols, and carotenoids [120] and plasma 25-hydroxyvitamin D [121] were not associated with prostate cancer risk in Japanese-American men.

Others

According to the WCRF/AICR 2014 report, there is limited–suggestive evidence of an increased risk of prostate cancer associated with the intake of dairy products and no conclusion have been reached for alcohol drinks [67]. A dose–response meta-analysis of 32 studies showed a statistically significant 7 % increase per 400 grams of dairy products per day (meta-analysis RR = 1.07; 95 % CI = 1.02–1.12) [122]. Alcohol and milk consumptions were examined in a cohort study of

Japanese-American men in Hawaii and were not related to prostate cancer risk [35, 123]. In the MEC, milk and dairy product intakes were not associated with prostate cancer risk among Japanese-American men [116]. Serum uric acid, a potent antioxidant, was associated with a higher risk of prostate cancer in a cohort of Japanese-American men in Hawaii (quartile 4 versus 1, RR = 1.5; 95 % CI = 1.1–2.1; p trend = 0.04) [124].

Conclusion

Asian Americans are more likely to have advanced-stage, high-grade disease and overall a less favorable risk profile at diagnosis of prostate cancer than White men, with variation by Asian populations and nativity. This suggests that Asian-American men may be more susceptible to aggressive phenotypes, despite their low mortality rate of prostate cancer. Furthermore, variation in the incidence rates of prostate cancer has been seen across specific Asian-American populations. Yet, data on prostate cancer risk factors across Asian-American populations is limited as studies have focused primarily on Japanese and Chinese Americans. Additional studies are needed in other Asian-American populations as each Asian population has its own distinct culture, lifestyles, health behaviors, and prostate cancer risk profiles. Overall, studies in Asian-American men have found no consistent or convincing associations with BMI, dietary factors, including soy and green tea, or hormonal factors. Inverse associations of diabetes and smoking with prostate cancer have been observed that are consistent with associations observed in other US racial/ethnic groups. Infections of the prostate have emerged as important risk factors with potential higher risk among foreign-born Asian Americans. Inherited factors, including established risk variants for prostate cancer, are important risk factors for Asian Americans, similar to other US racial/ethnic groups. Further research is needed to better understand the interplay of genetic and environmental factors that influence prostate cancer risk, particularly in specific Asian populations by nativity and disease characteristics.

Acknowledgments Financial Disclosure: None.
Authors' declaration of personal interests: None declared.
Declaration of funding interests: None declared.

References

1. Bell KJ, Del Mar C, Wright G, Dickinson J, Glasziou P (2015) Prevalence of incidental prostate cancer: a systematic review of autopsy studies. Int J Cancer 137(7):1749–1757. doi:10.1002/ijc.29538
2. Howlader N, Noone AM, Krapcho M, Miller D, Bishop K, Altekruse SF, Kosary CL, Yu M, Ruhl J, Tatalovich Z, Mariotto A, Lewis DR, Chen HS, Feuer EJ, Cronin KA (eds) (2016)

SEER Cancer Statistics Review, 1975–2013, National Cancer Institute. Bethesda, MD. http://seer.cancer.gov/csr/1975_2013, based on November 2015 SEER data submission, posted to the SEER web site, April 2016
3. Gomez SL, Noone AM, Lichtensztajn DY, Scoppa S, Gibson JT, Liu L, Morris C, Kwong S, Fish K, Wilkens LR, Goodman MT, Deapen D, Miller BA (2013) Cancer incidence trends among Asian American populations in the United States, 1990–2008. J Natl Cancer Inst 105(15):1096–1110. doi:10.1093/jnci/djt157, djt157 [pii]
4. Welch HG, Albertsen PC (2009) Prostate cancer diagnosis and treatment after the introduction of prostate-specific antigen screening: 1986–2005. J Natl Cancer Inst 101(19):1325–1329. doi:10.1093/jnci/djp278, djp278 [pii]
5. Kohler BA, Sherman RL, Howlader N, Jemal A, Ryerson AB, Henry KA, Boscoe FP, Cronin KA, Lake A, Noone AM, Henley SJ, Eheman CR, Anderson RN, Penberthy L (2015) Annual Report to the Nation on the Status of Cancer, 1975–2011. Featuring incidence of breast cancer subtypes by race/ethnicity, poverty, and state. J Natl Cancer Inst 107(6):djv048. doi:10.1093/jnci/djv048, djv048 [pii]
6. Magi-Galluzzi C, Tsusuki T, Elson P, Simmerman K, LaFargue C, Esgueva R, Klein E, Rubin MA, Zhou M (2011) TMPRSS2-ERG gene fusion prevalence and class are significantly different in prostate cancer of Caucasian, African–American and Japanese patients. Prostate 71(5):489–497. doi:10.1002/pros.21265
7. Mahal BA, Aizer AA, Ziehr DR, Hyatt AS, Choueiri TK, Hu JC, Hoffman KE, Sweeney CJ, Beard CJ, D'Amico AV, Martin NE, Kim SP, Trinh QD, Nguyen PL (2014) Racial disparities in prostate cancer-specific mortality in men with low-risk prostate cancer. Clin Genitourin Cancer 12(5):e189–e195. doi:10.1016/j.clgc.2014.04.003, S1558-7673(14)00081-0 [pii]
8. Trinh QD, Nguyen PL, Leow JJ, Dalela D, Chao GF, Mahal BA, Nayak M, Schmid M, Choueiri TK, Aizer AA (2015) Cancer-specific mortality of Asian Americans diagnosed with cancer: a nationwide population-based assessment. J Natl Cancer Inst 107(6):djv054. doi:10.1093/jnci/djv054, djv054 [pii]
9. Fedewa SA, Etzioni R, Flanders WD, Jemal A, Ward EM (2010) Association of insurance and race/ethnicity with disease severity among men diagnosed with prostate cancer, National Cancer Database 2004–2006. Cancer Epidemiol Biomarkers Prev 19(10):2437–2444. doi:10.1158/1055-9965.EPI-10-0299, 1055-9965.EPI-10-0299 [pii]
10. Man A, Pickles T, Chi KN (2003) Asian race and impact on outcomes after radical radiotherapy for localized prostate cancer. J Urol 170(3):901–904. doi:10.1097/01.ju.0000081423.37043.b4, S0022-5347(05)63259-4 [pii]
11. Raymundo EM, Rice KR, Chen Y, Zhao J, Brassell SA (2011) Prostate cancer in Asian Americans: incidence, management and outcomes in an equal access healthcare system. BJU Int 107(8):1216–1222. doi:10.1111/j.1464-410X.2010.09685.x
12. Robbins AS, Koppie TM, Gomez SL, Parikh-Patel A, Mills PK (2007) Differences in prognostic factors and survival among white and Asian men with prostate cancer, California, 1995–2004. Cancer 110(6):1255–1263. doi:10.1002/cncr.22872
13. Lichtensztajn DY, Gomez SL, Sieh W, Chung BI, Cheng I, Brooks JD (2014) Prostate cancer risk profiles of Asian–American men: disentangling the effects of immigration status and race/ethnicity. J Urol 191(4):952–956. doi:10.1016/j.juro.2013.10.075, S0022-5347(13)05758-3 [pii]
14. U.S. Preventive Services Task Force (2008) Screening for prostate cancer: U.S. Preventive Services Task Force recommendation statement. Ann Intern Med 149(3):185–191, 149/3/185 [pii]
15. Djulbegovic M, Beyth RJ, Neuberger MM, Stoffs TL, Vieweg J, Djulbegovic B, Dahm P (2010) Screening for prostate cancer: systematic review and meta-analysis of randomised controlled trials. BMJ 14;341:c4543. doi:10.1136/bmj.c4543
16. Moyer VA (2012) Screening for prostate cancer: U.S. Preventive Services Task Force recommendation statement. Ann Intern Med 157(2):120–134. doi:10.7326/0003-4819-157-2-201207170-00459, 1216568 [pii]

17. UCLA Center for Health Policy Research. AskCHIS 2009. PSA Screening among adult males (California). http://ask.chis.ucla.edu. Accessed 4 Aug 2015
18. Lee SY (2015) Cultural factors associated with breast and cervical cancer screening in Korean American women in the US: an integrative literature review. Asian Nurs Res 9(2):81–90. doi:10.1016/j.anr.2015.05.003, S1976-1317(15)00036-5 [pii]
19. Lee-Lin F, Menon U, Pett M, Nail L, Lee S, Mooney K (2007) Breast cancer beliefs and mammography screening practices among Chinese American immigrants. J Obstet Gynecol Neonatal Nurs 36(3):212–221. doi:10.1111/j.1552-6909.2007.00141.x, JOGN141 [pii]
20. Poonawalla IB, Goyal S, Mehrotra N, Allicock M, Balasubramanian BA (2014) Attitudes of South Asian women to breast health and breast cancer screening: findings from a community based sample in the United States. Asian Pac J Cancer Prev 15(20):8719–8724
21. Wu TY, West B, Chen YW, Hergert C (2006) Health beliefs and practices related to breast cancer screening in Filipino, Chinese and Asian–Indian women. Cancer Detect Prev 30(1):58–66. doi:10.1016/j.cdp.2005.06.013, S0361-090X(05)00095-4 [pii]
22. Harmon BE, Little MA, Woekel ED, Ettienne R, Long CR, Wilkens LR, Le Marchand L, Henderson BE, Kolonel LN, Maskarinec G (2014) Ethnic differences and predictors of colonoscopy, prostate-specific antigen, and mammography screening participation in the multiethnic cohort. Cancer Epidemiol 38(2):162–167. doi:10.1016/j.canep.2014.02.007, S1877-7821(14)00029-0 [pii]
23. May FP, Almario CV, Ponce N, Spiegel BM (2015) Racial minorities are more likely than whites to report lack of provider recommendation for colon cancer screening. Am J Gastroenterol 110(10):1388–1394. doi:10.1038/ajg.2015.138, ajg2015138 [pii]
24. Thompson CA, Gomez SL, Chan A, Chan JK, McClellan SR, Chung S, Olson C, Nimbal V, Palaniappan LP (2014) Patient and provider characteristics associated with colorectal, breast, and cervical cancer screening among Asian Americans. Cancer Epidemiol Biomarkers Prev 23(11):2208–2217. doi:10.1158/1055-9965.EPI-14-0487, 23/11/2208 [pii]
25. Bao Y, Fox SA, Escarce JJ (2007) Socioeconomic and racial/ethnic differences in the discussion of cancer screening: "between-" versus "within-" physician differences. Health Serv Res 42(3 Pt 1):950–970. doi:10.1111/j.1475-6773.2006.00638.x, HESR638 [pii]
26. Conde FA, Landier W, Ishida D, Bell R, Cuaresma CF, Misola J (2011) Barriers and facilitators of prostate cancer screening among Filipino men in Hawaii. Oncol Nurs Forum 38(2):227–233. doi:10.1188/11.ONF.227-233, JG51R3X46013V673 [pii]
27. Glenn BA, Bastani R, Maxwell AE, Mojica CM, Herrmann AK, Gallardo NV, Swanson KA, Chang LC (2012) Prostate cancer screening among ethnically diverse first-degree relatives of prostate cancer cases. Health Psychol 31(5):562–570. doi:10.1037/a0028626, 2012-16094-001 [pii]
28. Lee HY, Jung Y (2013) Older Korean American men's prostate cancer screening behavior: the prime role of culture. J Immigr Minor Health 15(6):1030–1037. doi:10.1007/s10903-013-9804-x
29. Seo HS, Lee NK (2010) Predictors of PSA screening among men over 40 years of age who had ever heard about PSA. Korean J Urol 51(6):391–397. doi:10.4111/kju.2010.51.6.391
30. Kolonel LN, Wilkens LR (2006) Migrant studies. In: Schottenfeld D, Fraumeni JF Jr (eds) Cancer epidemiology and prevention, 3rd edn. Oxford University Press, New York
31. Parkin DM, Khlat M (1996) Studies of cancer in migrants: rationale and methodology. Eur J Cancer 32A(5):761–771
32. Thomas DB, Karagas MR (1996) Migrant studies. In: Schottenfeld D, Fraumeni JF Jr (eds) Cancer epidemiology and prevention, 2nd edn. Oxford University Press, Oxford
33. Ito K (2014) Prostate cancer in Asian men. Nat Rev Urol 11(4):197–212. doi:10.1038/nrurol.2014.42, nrurol.2014.42 [pii]
34. Curado MP, Edwards B, Shin HR, Storm H, Ferlay J, M. Heanue, Boyle P (eds). (2007) Cancer Incidence in Five Continents Volume IX. International Agency for Research on Cancer. Lyon, France, http://www.iarc.fr/en/publications/pdfs-online/epi/sp160/. Accessed Aug 2015
35. Severson RK, Nomura AM, Grove JS, Stemmermann GN (1989) A prospective study of demographics, diet, and prostate cancer among men of Japanese ancestry in Hawaii. Cancer Res 49(7):1857–1860

36. Kolonel LN, Henderson BE, Hankin JH, Nomura AM, Wilkens LR, Pike MC, Stram DO, Monroe KR, Earle ME, Nagamine FS (2000) A multiethnic cohort in Hawaii and Los Angeles: baseline characteristics. Am J Epidemiol 151(4):346–357
37. Whittemore AS, Kolonel LN, Wu AH, John EM, Gallagher RP, Howe GR, Burch JD, Hankin J, Dreon DM, West DW et al (1995) Prostate cancer in relation to diet, physical activity, and body size in Blacks, Whites, and Asians in the United States and Canada. J Natl Cancer Inst 87(9):652–661
38. Cook PJ, Doll R, Fellingham SA (1969) A mathematical model for the age distribution of cancer in man. Int J Cancer 4(1):93–112
39. Hsing AW, Tsao L, Devesa SS (2000) International trends and patterns of prostate cancer incidence and mortality. Int J Cancer 85(1):60–67. doi:10.1002/(SICI)1097-0215(20000101)85:1<60::AID-IJC11>3.0.CO;2-B [pii]
40. Brawley OW, Knopf K, Thompson I (1998) The epidemiology of prostate cancer part II: the risk factors. Semin Urol Oncol 16(4):193–201
41. Hoffmann TJ, Van Den Eeden SK, Sakoda LC, Jorgenson E, Habel LA, Graff RE, Passarelli MN, Cario CL, Emami NC, Chao CR, Ghai NR, Shan J, Ranatunga DK, Quesenberry CP, Aaronson D, Presti J, Wang Z, Berndt SI, Chanock SJ, McDonnell SK, French AJ, Schaid DJ, Thibodeau SN, Li Q, Freedman ML, Penney KL, Mucci LA, Haiman CA, Henderson BE, Seminara D, Kvale MN, Kwok PY, Schaefer C, Risch N, Witte JS (2015) A large multiethnic genome-wide association study of prostate cancer identifies novel risk variants and substantial ethnic differences. Cancer Discov 5(8):878–891. doi:10.1158/2159-8290.CD-15-0315, 2159-8290.CD-15-0315 [pii]
42. Liu JH, Li HW, Tong M, Li M, Na YQ (2004) Genetic risk factors of prostate cancer in Han nationality population in Northern China and a preliminary study of the reason of racial difference in prevalence of prostate cancer. Zhonghua Yi Xue Za Zhi 84(5):364–368
43. Han Y, Hazelett DJ, Wiklund F, Schumacher FR, Stram DO, Berndt SI, Wang Z, Rand KA, Hoover RN, Machiela MJ, Yeager M, Burdette L, Chung CC, Hutchinson A, Yu K, Xu J, Travis RC, Key TJ, Siddiq A, Canzian F, Takahashi A, Kubo M, Stanford JL, Kolb S, Gapstur SM, Diver WR, Stevens VL, Strom SS, Pettaway CA, Al Olama AA, Kote-Jarai Z, Eeles RA, Yeboah ED, Tettey Y, Biritwum RB, Adjei AA, Tay E, Truelove A, Niwa S, Chokkalingam AP, Isaacs WB, Chen C, Lindstrom S, Le Marchand L, Giovannucci EL, Pomerantz M, Long H, Li F, Ma J, Stampfer M, John EM, Ingles SA, Kittles RA, Murphy AB, Blot WJ, Signorello LB, Zheng W, Albanes D, Virtamo J, Weinstein S, Nemesure B, Carpten J, Leske MC, Wu SY, Hennis AJ, Rybicki BA, Neslund-Dudas C, Hsing AW, Chu L, Goodman PJ, Klein EA, Zheng SL, Witte JS, Casey G, Riboli E, Li Q, Freedman ML, Hunter DJ, Gronberg H, Cook MB, Nakagawa H, Kraft P, Chanock SJ, Easton DF, Henderson BE, Coetzee GA, Conti DV, Haiman CA (2015) Integration of multiethnic fine-mapping and genomic annotation to prioritize candidate functional SNPs at prostate cancer susceptibility regions. Hum Mol Genet 24(19):5603–5618. doi:10.1093/hmg/ddv269, ddv269 [pii]
44. Steinberg GD, Carter BS, Beaty TH, Childs B, Walsh PC (1990) Family history and the risk of prostate cancer. Prostate 17(4):337–347
45. Whittemore AS, Wu AH, Kolonel LN, John EM, Gallagher RP, Howe GR, West DW, Teh CZ, Stamey T (1995) Family history and prostate cancer risk in Black, White, and Asian men in the United States and Canada. Am J Epidemiol 141(8):732–740
46. Lichtenstein P, Holm NV, Verkasalo PK, Iliadou A, Kaprio J, Koskenvuo M, Pukkala E, Skytthe A, Hemminki K (2000) Environmental and heritable factors in the causation of cancer—analyses of cohorts of twins from Sweden, Denmark, and Finland. N Engl J Med 343(2):78–85. doi:10.1056/NEJM200007133430201
47. Xu J, Mo Z, Ye D, Wang M, Liu F, Jin G, Xu C, Wang X, Shao Q, Chen Z, Tao Z, Qi J, Zhou F, Wang Z, Fu Y, He D, Wei Q, Guo J, Wu D, Gao X, Yuan J, Wang G, Xu Y, Yao H, Dong P, Jiao Y, Shen M, Yang J, Ou-Yang J, Jiang H, Zhu Y, Ren S, Zhang Z, Yin C, Dai B, Hu Z, Yang Y, Wu Q, Chen H, Peng P, Zheng Y, Zheng X, Xiang Y, Long J, Gong J, Na R, Lin X, Yu H, Tao S, Feng J, Sun J, Liu W, Hsing A, Rao J, Ding Q, Wiklund F, Gronberg H, Shu XO, Zheng

W, Shen H, Jin L, Shi R, Lu D, Zhang X, Zheng SL, Sun Y (2012) Genome-wide association study in Chinese men identifies two new prostate cancer risk loci at 9q31.2 and 19q13.4. Nat Genet 44(11):1231–1235. doi:10.1038/ng.2424, ng.2424 [pii]

48. Takata R, Akamatsu S, Kubo M, Takahashi A, Hosono N, Kawaguchi T, Tsunoda T, Inazawa J, Kamatani N, Ogawa O, Fujioka T, Nakamura Y, Nakagawa H (2010) Genome-wide association study identifies five new susceptibility loci for prostate cancer in the Japanese population. Nat Genet 42(9):751–754. doi:10.1038/ng.635, ng.635 [pii]
49. Cheng I, Chen GK, Nakagawa H, He J, Wan P, Laurie CC, Shen J, Sheng X, Pooler LC, Crenshaw AT, Mirel DB, Takahashi A, Kubo M, Nakamura Y, Al Olama AA, Benlloch S, Donovan JL, Guy M, Hamdy FC, Kote-Jarai Z, Neal DE, Wilkens LR, Monroe KR, Stram DO, Muir K, Eeles RA, Easton DF, Kolonel LN, Henderson BE, Le Marchand L, Haiman CA (2012) Evaluating genetic risk for prostate cancer among Japanese and Latinos. Cancer Epidemiol Biomarkers Prev 21(11):2048–2058. doi:10.1158/1055-9965.EPI-12-0598, 1055-9965.EPI-12-0598 [pii]
50. Platz EA, Giovannucci E (2004) The epidemiology of sex steroid hormones and their signaling and metabolic pathways in the etiology of prostate cancer. J Steroid Biochem Mol Biol 92(4):237–253. doi:10.1016/j.jsbmb.2004.10.002, S0960-0760(04)00364-4 [pii]
51. Hsing AW (2001) Hormones and prostate cancer: what's next? Epidemiol Rev 23(1):42–58
52. Roddam AW, Allen NE, Appleby P, Key TJ (2008) Endogenous sex hormones and prostate cancer: a collaborative analysis of 18 prospective studies. J Natl Cancer Inst 100(3):170–183. doi:10.1093/jnci/djm323, djm323 [pii]
53. Calistro Alvarado L (2010) Population differences in the testosterone levels of young men are associated with prostate cancer disparities in older men. Am J Hum Biol 22(4):449–455. doi:10.1002/ajhb.21016
54. Cheng I, Yu MC, Koh WP, Pike MC, Kolonel LN, Henderson BE, Stram DO (2005) Comparison of prostate-specific antigen and hormone levels among men in Singapore and the United States. Cancer Epidemiol Biomarkers Prev 14(7):1692–1696. doi:10.1158/1055-9965.EPI-04-0864, 14/7/1692 [pii]
55. Wu AH, Whittemore AS, Kolonel LN, Stanczyk FZ, John EM, Gallagher RP, West DW (2001) Lifestyle determinants of 5alpha-reductase metabolites in older African–American, White, and Asian–American men. Cancer Epidemiol Biomarkers Prev 10(5):533–538
56. Heidegger I, Massoner P, Sampson N, Klocker H (2015) The insulin-like growth factor (IGF) axis as an anticancer target in prostate cancer. Cancer Lett 367(2):113–121. doi:10.1016/j.canlet.2015.07.026, S0304-3835(15)00481-4 [pii]
57. Borugian MJ, Spinelli JJ, Sun Z, Kolonel LN, Oakley-Girvan I, Pollak MD, Whittemore AS, Wu AH, Gallagher RP (2008) Prostate cancer risk in relation to insulin-like growth factor (IGF)-I and IGF-binding protein-3: a prospective multiethnic study. Cancer Epidemiol Biomarkers Prev 17(1):252–254. doi:10.1158/1055-9965.EPI-07-2694, 17/1/252 [pii]
58. Gill JK, Wilkens LR, Pollak MN, Stanczyk FZ, Kolonel LN (2010) Androgens, growth factors, and risk of prostate cancer: the multiethnic cohort. Prostate 70(8):906–915. doi:10.1002/pros.21125
59. Hanahan D, Weinberg RA (2011) Hallmarks of cancer: the next generation. Cell 144(5):646–674. doi:10.1016/j.cell.2011.02.013, S0092-8674(11)00127-9 [pii]
60. Sutcliffe S (2010) Sexually transmitted infections and risk of prostate cancer: review of historical and emerging hypotheses. Future Oncol 6(8):1289–1311. doi:10.2217/fon.10.95
61. Krieger JN, Lee SW, Jeon J, Cheah PY, Liong ML, Riley DE (2008) Epidemiology of prostatitis. Int J Antimicrob Agents 31(Suppl 1):S85–S90. doi:10.1016/j.ijantimicag.2007.08.028, S0924-8579(07)00552-3 [pii]
62. Krieger JN, Nyberg L Jr, Nickel JC (1999) NIH consensus definition and classification of prostatitis. JAMA 282(3):236–237, doi:jlt0721 [pii]
63. Jiang J, Li J, Yunxia Z, Zhu H, Liu J, Pumill C (2013) The role of prostatitis in prostate cancer: meta-analysis. PLoS One 8(12):e85179. doi:10.1371/journal.pone.0085179, PONE-D-13-36344 [pii]

64. Lian WQ, Luo F, Song XL, Lu YJ, Zhao SC (2015) Gonorrhea and prostate cancer incidence: an updated meta-analysis of 21 epidemiologic studies. Med Sci Monit 21:1902–1910. doi:10.12659/MSM.893579, 893579 [pii]
65. Caini S, Gandini S, Dudas M, Bremer V, Severi E, Gherasim A (2014) Sexually transmitted infections and prostate cancer risk: a systematic review and meta-analysis. Cancer Epidemiol 38(4):329–338. doi:10.1016/j.canep.2014.06.002, S1877-7821(14)00105-2 [pii]
66. Cheng I, Witte JS, Jacobsen SJ, Haque R, Quinn VP, Quesenberry CP, Caan BJ, Van Den Eeden SK (2010) Prostatitis, sexually transmitted diseases, and prostate cancer: the California Men's Health Study. PLoS One 5(1):e8736. doi:10.1371/journal.pone.0008736
67. World Cancer Research Fund International (2014) Continuous Update Project Report. Diet, nutrition, physical activity, and prostate cancer. World Cancer Research Fund International/American Institute for Cancer Research, London
68. Discacciati A, Orsini N, Wolk A (2012) Body mass index and incidence of localized and advanced prostate cancer—a dose–response meta-analysis of prospective studies. Ann Oncol 23(7):1665–1671. doi:10.1093/annonc/mdr603, mdr603 [pii]
69. Hsing AW, Deng J, Sesterhenn IA, Mostofi FK, Stanczyk FZ, Benichou J, Xie T, Gao YT (2000) Body size and prostate cancer: a population-based case–control study in China. Cancer Epidemiol Biomarkers Prev 9(12):1335–1341
70. Habel LA, Van Den Eeden SK, Friedman GD (2000) Body size, age at shaving initiation, and prostate cancer in a large, multiracial cohort. Prostate 43(2):136–143. doi:10.1002/(SICI)1097-0045(20000501)43:2<136::AID-PROS8>3.0.CO;2-L [pii]
71. Hernandez BY, Park SY, Wilkens LR, Henderson BE, Kolonel LN (2009) Relationship of body mass, height, and weight gain to prostate cancer risk in the multiethnic cohort. Cancer Epidemiol Biomarkers Prev 18(9):2413–2421. doi:10.1158/1055-9965.EPI-09-0293, 1055-9965.EPI-09-0293 [pii]
72. Severson RK, Grove JS, Nomura AM, Stemmermann GN (1988) Body mass and prostatic cancer: a prospective study. BMJ 297(6650):713–715
73. Kurahashi N, Iwasaki M, Sasazuki S, Otani T, Inoue M, Tsugane S (2006) Association of body mass index and height with risk of prostate cancer among middle-aged Japanese men. Br J Cancer 94(5):740–742. doi:10.1038/sj.bjc.6602983, 6602983 [pii]
74. Baillargeon J, Pollock BH, Kristal AR, Bradshaw P, Hernandez J, Basler J, Higgins B, Lynch S, Rozanski T, Troyer D, Thompson I (2005) The association of body mass index and prostate-specific antigen in a population-based study. Cancer 103(5):1092–1095. doi:10.1002/cncr.20856
75. Grubb RL 3rd, Black A, Izmirlian G, Hickey TP, Pinsky PF, Mabie JE, Riley TL, Ragard LR, Prorok PC, Berg CD, Crawford ED, Church TR, Andriole GL Jr (2009) Serum prostate-specific antigen hemodilution among obese men undergoing screening in the prostate, lung, colorectal, and ovarian cancer screening trial. Cancer Epidemiol Biomarkers Prev 18(3):748–751. doi:10.1158/1055-9965.EPI-08-0938, 1055-9965.EPI-08-0938 [pii]
76. Zhang J, Sheng B, Ma M, Nan X (2015) An inverse association of body mass index and prostate-specific antigen in northwest men of China: a population-based analysis. Int J Clin Exp Med 8(3):4557–4562
77. Cao Y, Ma J (2011) Body mass index, prostate cancer-specific mortality, and biochemical recurrence: a systematic review and meta-analysis. Cancer Prev Res (Phila) 4(4):486–501. doi:10.1158/1940-6207.CAPR-10-0229, 1940-6207.CAPR-10-0229 [pii]
78. Buschemeyer WC 3rd, Freedland SJ (2007) Obesity and prostate cancer: epidemiology and clinical implications. Eur Urol 52(2):331–343. doi:10.1016/j.eururo.2007.04.069, S0302-2838(07)00664-1 [pii]
79. Chyou PH, Nomura AM, Stemmermann GN (1994) A prospective study of weight, body mass index and other anthropometric measurements in relation to site-specific cancers. Int J Cancer 57(3):313–317
80. Park SY, Haiman CA, Cheng I, Park SL, Wilkens LR, Kolonel LN, Le Marchand L, Henderson BE (2015) Racial/ethnic differences in lifestyle-related factors and prostate cancer risk: the

multiethnic cohort study. Cancer Causes Control 26(10):1507–1515. doi:10.1007/s10552-015-0644-y [pii]
81. Golabek T, Bukowczan J, Chlosta P, Powroznik J, Dobruch J, Borowka A (2014) Obesity and prostate cancer incidence and mortality: a systematic review of prospective cohort studies. Urol Int 92(1):7–14. doi:10.1159/000351325, 000351325 [pii]
82. Moyad MA (2002) Is obesity a risk factor for prostate cancer, and does it even matter? A hypothesis and different perspective. Urology 59(4 Suppl 1):41–50, doi:S009042950101175X [pii]
83. Giovannucci E, Harlan DM, Archer MC, Bergenstal RM, Gapstur SM, Habel LA, Pollak M, Regensteiner JG, Yee D (2010) Diabetes and cancer: a consensus report. CA Cancer J Clin 60(4):207–221. doi:10.3322/caac.20078, caac.20078 [pii]
84. Bansal D, Bhansali A, Kapil G, Undela K, Tiwari P (2013) Type 2 diabetes and risk of prostate cancer: a meta-analysis of observational studies. Prostate Cancer Prostatic Dis 16(2):151–158. doi:10.1038/pcan.2012.40, S151pcan201240 [pii]
85. Waters KM, Henderson BE, Stram DO, Wan P, Kolonel LN, Haiman CA (2009) Association of diabetes with prostate cancer risk in the multiethnic cohort. Am J Epidemiol 169(8):937–945. doi:10.1093/aje/kwp003, kwp003 [pii]
86. Rastmanesh R, Hejazi J, Marotta F, Hara N (2014) Type 2 diabetes: a protective factor for prostate cancer? An overview of proposed mechanisms. Clin Genitourin Cancer 12(3):143–148. doi:10.1016/j.clgc.2014.01.001, S1558-7673(14)00002-0 [pii]
87. Cogliano VJ, Baan R, Straif K, Grosse Y, Lauby-Secretan B, El Ghissassi F, Bouvard V, Benbrahim-Tallaa L, Guha N, Freeman C, Galichet L, Wild CP (2011) Preventable exposures associated with human cancers. J Natl Cancer Inst 103(24):1827–1839. doi:10.1093/jnci/djr483, djr483 [pii]
88. Islami F, Moreira DM, Boffetta P, Freedland SJ (2014) A systematic review and meta-analysis of tobacco use and prostate cancer mortality and incidence in prospective cohort studies. Eur Urol 66(6):1054–1064. doi:10.1016/j.eururo.2014.08.059, S0302-2838(14)00812-4 [pii]
89. Bae JM, Li ZM, Shin MH, Kim DH, Lee MS, Ahn YO (2013) Cigarette smoking and prostate cancer risk: negative results of the Seoul Male Cancer Cohort Study. Asian Pac J Cancer Prev 14(8):4667–4669
90. Sawada N, Inoue M, Iwasaki M, Sasazuki S, Yamaji T, Shimazu T, Tsugane S (2014) Alcohol and smoking and subsequent risk of prostate cancer in Japanese men: the Japan Public Health Center-based prospective study. Int J Cancer 134(4):971–978. doi:10.1002/ijc.28423
91. Butler LM, Wang R, Wong AS, Koh WP, Yu MC (2009) Cigarette smoking and risk of prostate cancer among Singapore Chinese. Cancer Causes Control 20(10):1967–1974. doi:10.1007/s10552-009-9391-2
92. Rohrmann S, Linseisen J, Allen N, Bueno-de-Mesquita HB, Johnsen NF, Tjonneland A, Overvad K, Kaaks R, Teucher B, Boeing H, Pischon T, Lagiou P, Trichopoulou A, Trichopoulos D, Palli D, Krogh V, Tumino R, Ricceri F, Arguelles Suarez MV, Agudo A, Sanchez MJ, Chirlaque MD, Barricarte A, Larranaga N, Boshuizen H, van Kranen HJ, Stattin P, Johansson M, Bjartell A, Ulmert D, Khaw KT, Wareham NJ, Ferrari P, Romieux I, Gunter MJ, Riboli E, Key TJ (2013) Smoking and the risk of prostate cancer in the European Prospective Investigation into cancer and nutrition. Br J Cancer 108(3):708–714. doi:10.1038/bjc.2012.520, bjc2012520 [pii]
93. Rolison JJ, Hanoch Y, Miron-Shatz T (2012) Smokers: at risk for prostate cancer but unlikely to screen. Addict Behav 37(6):736–738. doi:10.1016/j.addbeh.2012.02.006, S0306-4603(12)00059-7 [pii]
94. Nomura AM, Lee J, Stemmermann GN, Combs GF Jr (2000) Serum selenium and subsequent risk of prostate cancer. Cancer Epidemiol Biomarkers Prev 9(9):883–887
95. Huang M, Narita S, Numakura K, Tsuruta H, Saito M, Inoue T, Horikawa Y, Tsuchiya N, Habuchi T (2012) A high-fat diet enhances proliferation of prostate cancer cells and activates MCP-1/CCR2 signaling. Prostate 72(16):1779–1788. doi:10.1002/pros.22531
96. Kolonel LN, Hankin JH, Lee J, Chu SY, Nomura AM, Hinds MW (1981) Nutrient intakes in relation to cancer incidence in Hawaii. Br J Cancer 44(3):332–339

97. Kolonel LN, Hankin JH, Nomura AM, Chu SY (1981) Dietary fat intake and cancer incidence among five ethnic groups in Hawaii. Cancer Res 41(9 Pt 2):3727–3728
98. Kurahashi N, Inoue M, Iwasaki M, Sasazuki S, Tsugane AS (2008) Dairy product, saturated fatty acid, and calcium intake and prostate cancer in a prospective cohort of Japanese men. Cancer Epidemiol Biomarkers Prev 17(4):930–937. doi:10.1158/1055-9965.EPI-07-2681, 17/4/930 [pii]
99. Park SY, Murphy SP, Wilkens LR, Henderson BE, Kolonel LN (2007) Fat and meat intake and prostate cancer risk: the multiethnic cohort study. Int J Cancer 121(6):1339–1345. doi:10.1002/ijc.22805
100. Park SY, Wilkens LR, Henning SM, Le Marchand L, Gao K, Goodman MT, Murphy SP, Henderson BE, Kolonel LN (2009) Circulating fatty acids and prostate cancer risk in a nested case–control study: the multiethnic cohort. Cancer Causes Control 20(2):211–223. doi:10.1007/s10552-008-9236-4
101. Harvei S, Bjerve KS, Tretli S, Jellum E, Robsahm TE, Vatten L (1997) Prediagnostic level of fatty acids in serum phospholipids: omega-3 and omega-6 fatty acids and the risk of prostate cancer. Int J Cancer 71(4):545–551. doi:10.1002/(SICI)1097-0215(19970516)71:4<545::AID-IJC7>3.0.CO;2-U [pii]
102. Crowe FL, Allen NE, Appleby PN, Overvad K, Aardestrup IV, Johnsen NF, Tjonneland A, Linseisen J, Kaaks R, Boeing H, Kroger J, Trichopoulou A, Zavitsanou A, Trichopoulos D, Sacerdote C, Palli D, Tumino R, Agnoli C, Kiemeney LA, Bueno-de-Mesquita HB, Chirlaque MD, Ardanaz E, Larranaga N, Quiros JR, Sanchez MJ, Gonzalez CA, Stattin P, Hallmans G, Bingham S, Khaw KT, Rinaldi S, Slimani N, Jenab M, Riboli E, Key TJ (2008) Fatty acid composition of plasma phospholipids and risk of prostate cancer in a case–control analysis nested within the European Prospective Investigation into Cancer and Nutrition. Am J Clin Nutr 88(5):1353–1363, doi:88/5/1353 [pii]
103. Bassett JK, Severi G, Hodge AM, MacInnis RJ, Gibson RA, Hopper JL, English DR, Giles GG (2013) Plasma phospholipid fatty acids, dietary fatty acids and prostate cancer risk. Int J Cancer 133(8):1882–1891. doi:10.1002/ijc.28203
104. Sharma S, Cao X, Wilkens LR, Yamamoto J, Lum-Jones A, Henderson BE, Kolonel LN, Le Marchand L (2010) Well-done meat consumption, NAT1 and NAT2 acetylator genotypes and prostate cancer risk: the multiethnic cohort study. Cancer Epidemiol Biomarkers Prev 19(7):1866–1870. doi:10.1158/1055-9965.EPI-10-0231, 1055-9965.EPI-10-0231 [pii]
105. Kolonel LN, Hankin JH, Whittemore AS, Wu AH, Gallagher RP, Wilkens LR, John EM, Howe GR, Dreon DM, West DW, Paffenbarger RS Jr (2000) Vegetables, fruits, legumes and prostate cancer: a multiethnic case–control study. Cancer Epidemiol Biomarkers Prev 9(8):795–804
106. Stram DO, Hankin JH, Wilkens LR, Park S, Henderson BE, Nomura AM, Pike MC, Kolonel LN (2006) Prostate cancer incidence and intake of fruits, vegetables and related micronutrients: the multiethnic cohort study* (United States). Cancer Causes Control 17(9):1193–1207. doi:10.1007/s10552-006-0064-0
107. Akaza H (2012) Prostate cancer chemoprevention by soy isoflavones: role of intestinal bacteria as the "second human genome". Cancer Sci 103(6):969–975. doi:10.1111/j.1349-7006.2012.02257.x
108. Mahmoud AM, Yang W, Bosland MC (2014) Soy isoflavones and prostate cancer: a review of molecular mechanisms. J Steroid Biochem Mol Biol 140:116–132. doi:10.1016/j.jsbmb.2013.12.010, S0960-0760(13)00283-5 [pii]
109. Yan L, Spitznagel EL (2005) Meta-analysis of soy food and risk of prostate cancer in men. Int J Cancer 117(4):667–669. doi:10.1002/ijc.21266
110. Yan L, Spitznagel EL (2009) Soy consumption and prostate cancer risk in men: a revisit of a meta-analysis. Am J Clin Nutr 89(4):1155–1163. doi:10.3945/ajcn.2008.27029, ajcn.2008.27029 [pii]
111. Nomura AM, Hankin JH, Lee J, Stemmermann GN (2004) Cohort study of tofu intake and prostate cancer: no apparent association. Cancer Epidemiol Biomarkers Prev 13(12):2277–2279, doi:13/12/2277 [pii]

112. Park SY, Murphy SP, Wilkens LR, Henderson BE, Kolonel LN (2008) Legume and isoflavone intake and prostate cancer risk: the multiethnic cohort study. Int J Cancer 123(4):927–932. doi:10.1002/ijc.23594
113. Park SY, Wilkens LR, Franke AA, Le Marchand L, Kakazu KK, Goodman MT, Murphy SP, Henderson BE, Kolonel LN (2009) Urinary phytoestrogen excretion and prostate cancer risk: a nested case–control study in the multiethnic cohort. Br J Cancer 101(1):185–191. doi:10.1038/sj.bjc.6605137, 6605137 [pii]
114. Mandair D, Rossi RE, Pericleous M, Whyand T, Caplin ME (2014) Prostate cancer and the influence of dietary factors and supplements: a systematic review. Nutr Metab (Lond) 11:30. doi:10.1186/1743-7075-11-30, 1743-7075-11-30 [pii]
115. Yang CS, Wang X, Lu G, Picinich SC (2009) Cancer prevention by tea: animal studies, molecular mechanisms and human relevance. Nat Rev Cancer 9(6):429–439. doi:10.1038/nrc2641
116. Park SY, Murphy SP, Wilkens LR, Stram DO, Henderson BE, Kolonel LN (2007) Calcium, vitamin D, and dairy product intake and prostate cancer risk: the multiethnic cohort study. Am J Epidemiol 166(11):1259–1269. doi:10.1093/aje/kwm269, kwm269 [pii]
117. Nomura AM, Stemmermann GN, Lee J, Kolonel LN, Chen TC, Turner A, Holick MF (1998) Serum vitamin D metabolite levels and the subsequent development of prostate cancer (Hawaii, United States). Cancer Causes Control 9(4):425–432
118. Nomura AM, Stemmermann GN, Lee J, Craft NE (1997) Serum micronutrients and prostate cancer in Japanese Americans in Hawaii. Cancer Epidemiol Biomarkers Prev 6(7):487–491
119. Park SY, Wilkens LR, Morris JS, Henderson BE, Kolonel LN (2013) Serum zinc and prostate cancer risk in a nested case–control study: the multiethnic cohort. Prostate 73(3):261–266. doi:10.1002/pros.22565
120. Gill JK, Franke AA, Steven Morris J, Cooney RV, Wilkens LR, Le Marchand L, Goodman MT, Henderson BE, Kolonel LN (2009) Association of selenium, tocopherols, carotenoids, retinol, and 15-isoprostane F(2t) in serum or urine with prostate cancer risk: the multiethnic cohort. Cancer Causes Control 20(7):1161–1171. doi:10.1007/s10552-009-9304-4
121. Park SY, Cooney RV, Wilkens LR, Murphy SP, Henderson BE, Kolonel LN (2010) Plasma 25-hydroxyvitamin D and prostate cancer risk: the multiethnic cohort. Eur J Cancer 46(5):932–936. doi:10.1016/j.ejca.2009.12.030, S0959-8049(09)00961-7 [pii]
122. Aune D, Navarro Rosenblatt DA, Chan DS, Vieira AR, Vieira R, Greenwood DC, Vatten LJ, Norat T (2015) Dairy products, calcium, and prostate cancer risk: a systematic review and meta-analysis of cohort studies. Am J Clin Nutr 101(1):87–117. doi:10.3945/ajcn.113.067157, ajcn.113.067157 [pii]
123. Pollack ES, Nomura AM, Heilbrun LK, Stemmermann GN, Green SB (1984) Prospective study of alcohol consumption and cancer. N Engl J Med 310(10):617–621. doi:10.1056/NEJM198403083101003
124. Kolonel LN, Yoshizawa C, Nomura AM, Stemmermann GN (1994) Relationship of serum uric acid to cancer occurrence in a prospective male cohort. Cancer Epidemiol Biomarkers Prev 3(3):225–228

Breast Cancer Among Asian Americans

Anna H. Wu, Eunjung Lee, and Daniel O. Stram

Abstract Breast cancer is the most commonly diagnosed cancer in women. Studies of breast cancer incidence have shown consistently two to threefold higher incidence rates among Asian-American women living in the United States (USA) relative to Asian women living in Asia. For example, breast cancer incidence in Japanese Americans is now approaching rates in Non-Hispanic (NH) Whites after two or three generations living in the USA. Epidemiologic data from studies conducted in Asian Americans, NH Whites, and in Asia reviewed in this chapter show that differences between incidence rates in NH Whites and US-born Asians are explained, in part, by menstrual and reproductive factors, body size, and use of hormonal replacement therapy. Changing prevalence of risk factors likely have had a major role in explaining the rise in breast cancer incidence with migration while the magnitude of risk associations for most of the risk factors are comparable to those of NH Whites. We review etiological risk factors that may explain the continued differences in rates between Asian Americans, Asians, and NH White women.

Keywords Asian Americans • Menstrual and reproductive factors • Exogenous and endogenous hormones • Body size • Alcohol • Diet • Mammographic density • Genetics

Incidence Rates and Secular Trends

Breast cancer is the most common cancer in Asian Americans as it is in other racial/ethnic groups in the USA. In 2007–2011, breast cancer incidence among Asian Americans/Pacific Islanders (AAPI) was 86.0 per 100,000 women, about 33 % lower than the incidence in NH Whites (127.6) [1]. However, the incidence of breast

A.H. Wu (✉) • E. Lee • D.O. Stram
Department of Preventive Medicine, Keck School of Medicine of USC, University of Southern California, Los Angeles, CA, USA
e-mail: anna.wu@med.usc.edu

A.H. Wu, D.O. Stram (eds.), *Cancer Epidemiology Among Asian Americans*,
DOI 10.1007/978-3-319-41118-7_8

Table 1 Breast cancer incidence in different Asian ethnic groups in the United States and in Asia compared to rates in Non-Hispanic Whites

	In the United States[a]			In Asia[b]	
	1990–1994	1998–2002	2004–2008	1990	2013
Asian Indian/Pakistani	56.1	76.2	88.3	40.8[c]	62.4[c]
Chinese	66.1	75.5	78.8	33.2[d]	55.0[d]
Filipino	85.8	99.2	103.7	42.4	87.5
Japanese	98.8	120.1	104.9	29.7	45.4
Kampuchean (Cambodian)	19.6	35.3	43.4	24.3	54.9
Korean	34.9	53.9	69.5	23.2	33.3
Laotian	22.5	34.4	41.3	22.4	48.2
Vietnamese	52.3	54.0	63.0	26.7	21.4
Non-Hispanic Whites	140.5	148.9	135.3		

[a]Data from Gomez et al. [2]

[b]Data from Global Burden of Disease Cancer Prevention (2015) [216]

[c]Based on average of rates in India (22.4 in 1990 and 31.4 in 2013) and Pakistan (59.1 in 1990 and 93.4 in 2013)

[d]Based on average of rates in China (21.6 in 1990 and 32.8 in 2013), Singapore (50.1 in 1990 and 61.3 in 2013) and Taiwan (27.5 in 1990 and 71.0 in 2013)

cancer varied more than twofold across different Asian ethnic groups. Data from 13 Surveillance, Epidemiology, and End Results (SEER) registries for 2004–2008 showed that breast cancer incidence was highest in Japanese (104.9) and Filipinas (103.7), intermediate among Asian Indians/Pakistani (88.3) and Chinese (78.8), lower in Koreans (69.5) and Vietnamese (63.0), and lowest in Laotians (41.3) and Kampucheans (Cambodians) (43.4) [2] (Table 1).

Steady increases in incidence were observed in nearly all Asian ethnic groups between 1990 through 2008 (Table 1). The annual percent increases ranged from 1.2 % in both Chinese and Vietnamese to 4.7 % in Koreans and there was no indication of a leveling in breast cancer incidence across these groups [2]. Japanese Americans displayed an incidence pattern that was most similar to that of NH Whites with rates increased steadily between the early 1990s and 2000s and appeared to be on a downward trend since the early 2000s [2].

Age at Diagnosis

Asian Americans present at a younger mean age at diagnosis of breast cancer than NH Whites [3, 4]. Data from the California Cancer Registry (CCR) (2000–2011) showed that the mean age at diagnosis was 56.4 years in Asian Americans and 62.4 years in NH Whites. Among Asian-American ethnic groups, mean age at diagnosis was youngest in Koreans (54.2), intermediate in Chinese (56.3) and Filipina (56.9), and oldest in Japanese (61.9) [3]. Age of breast cancer diagnosis also tended to be younger in Asia than in the West [5–7]. However, a recent study that included invasive breast cancer data (1988–2009) from five cancer registries in Asia, and made longitudinal extrapolations adjusting for calendar-period changes and conditioned upon birth cohort suggested that the age distributions of breast cancer are becoming more similar between Asian and Western women than previously recognized [8].

Stage and Tumor Characteristics

Asian Americans had slightly later stage at diagnosis than NH Whites but this varied by Asian ethnic groups [3, 4, 9]. Results from SEER (2000–2006) showed that the respective prevalences of stage III and IV cancers were less common among Chinese (7.8 and 2.9 %) and Japanese (6.2 and 2.7 %) but these later stages were more common among Filipina (10 and 4.4 %) and Asian Indian/ Pakistani women (11.2 and 5.2 %) than NH Whites (8.9 and 4.2 %) [9]. Similar patterns in Asian-American subgroups were found in other SEER-based studies [4, 10]. Differences in the distribution of tumor stage by Asian ethnicity may be attributable to differences in the prevalence of breast cancer screening and access to medical care, but may also reflect differences in tumor biology and tumor aggressiveness.

Breast cancer is a heterogeneous cancer consisting of a number of subtypes that are now recognized to have distinct risk factors, molecular characteristics, response to treatment, and prognosis [11]. Hormone receptor (HR) (estrogen receptor (ER) and progesterone receptor (PR)) and human epidermal growth factor receptor 2 (HER2) are classified in SEER database as positive, negative, borderline, not tested, not recorded, or unknown [12, 13]. In a review of over 220,000 invasive breast cancers among women ages 40–79 years, Asian Americans as a group had a lower proportion of breast cancers classified as ER + PR+ (66.2 %) than NH Whites (68.4 %), and were more likely to have ER-PR- tumors (21.1 % in Asian Americans and 18.6 % in NH Whites; OR 1.2, 95 % CI 1.2–1.3). Except for Japanese Americans who had a lower proportion of ER-PR- tumors (14.4 %), a higher proportion of breast cancers in Korean (26.1 %), Vietnamese (25.6 %), Asian Indian/Pakistani (25.6 %), Filipina (22.8 %), and Chinese (20.4 %) were ER-PR- compared to NH Whites [9]. In a CCR-based study of breast cancers (2000–2006) that also considered HER2 status, the diagnosis of HER2+ breast cancer was more common in Asian Americans (28 %) than NH Whites (19 %), particularly among Koreans (36 %) and Filipina (31 %). The proportion of triple negative tumors was similar between Asian Americans (12 %) and NH Whites (12 %) [12]. A subsequent study using CCR data from 2000 to 2011 classified breast cancer into eight subtypes based on ER, PR, and HER2 status. This larger study confirmed that HER2+ tumors were more common in Asian Americans (25 %) than in NH Whites (18 %), showing an excess of both ER + PR+ HER2+ (11.6 % vs. 8.8 %) and ER-PR- HER2+ (9.4 % vs. 5.6 %) tumors; this was most apparent among Korean and Filipina-Americans [3].

There is also tremendous interest to classify breast cancer into intrinsic subtypes using ER, PR, HER2, and ki-67 status (or tumor grade) or by gene expression profiling. However, to date, these studies tended to include few Asian Americans and the results were presented for Asian Americans as a group [14] or the sample size was too sparse to conduct meaningful analysis by Asian ethnicity [15]. In one study that classified breast cancer subtypes into four intrinsic subtypes, compared to NH Whites ($n=14{,}268$), Asian Americans ($n=533$) showed similar distributions of luminal A-like (48.0 % vs. 47.4 %) and triple negatives (15.3 % vs. 15.9 %), but were less likely to have luminal B-like (25.8 % vs. 29.8 %) and more likely to have HER2-type tumors (10.9 % vs. 7.9 %) [14]. In a study of gene expression profiling (e.g., PAM50) to classify breast cancer subtypes ($n=1319$ women, 72.6 % NH Whites, 9.2 % Asian Americans), the proportion of luminal A tumors were the same in Asian Americans (55.2 %) and NH Whites (55.2 %) but basal-like tumors was less common in Asian Americans (5.0 %) than in NH Whites (8.2 %) [16, 17]. Further studies by specific Asian-American subgroups will be needed to characterize the distribution of breast cancer intrinsic subtypes and to investigate risk factors by breast cancer subtypes.

Survival

In a study of invasive breast cancer diagnosed between 1988 and 2008 from 17 registries in SEER, the 5-year overall survival rate was better in Asian Americans (85.5 %) than NH Whites (79.8 %). Asian Americans also had better breast cancer-specific survival rate than NH Whites after adjusting for ER, PR, tumor grade, disease stage, radiation therapy, year of diagnosis, and age at diagnosis (HR=0.92, 95 % CI 0.89–0.95) [4]. The more favorable breast cancer-specific survival rates was clearest among Japanese (HR=0.63), Korean (HR=0.92) and Chinese (HR=0.98) but this was not found in Filipina (HR=1.06), Asian Indians/Pakistani (HR=1.14), and Vietnamese Americans (HR=1.14) [4, 9]. Receipt of definitive treatment by stage [18] and guideline concordant treatment for specific breast cancer subtypes [10] was high in Asian-American patients and was comparable to that reported in NH Whites. Reasons for the more favorable outcome in Japanese Americans are not known. The California Breast Cancer Survivorship Consortium (CBCSC) harmonized and pooled lifestyle information on 12,210 patients, including 1505 Asian Americans, to explore reasons for these outcome differences. Results from the CBCSC showed that breast cancer-specific mortality was significantly better in Asian Americans than NH Whites (HR=0.60, 95 % CI 0.37–0.97) after adjustment for tumor and lifestyle characteristics (e.g., smoking, alcohol) [19]. Although high waist–hip ratio [20] and a history of comorbidities including previous cancer, diabetes, and myocardial infarction [21] were associated with increased breast cancer-specific mortality in Asian Americans, high body mass index (BMI), physical inactivity, and neighborhood characteristics were not associated with outcome and did not explain the lower breast cancer-specific mortality in Asian

Americans [20, 22–24]. A limitation of this analysis was that the sample size of Asian Americans was modest and did not allow analysis separately by specific Asian ethnic subgroups. Thus, further investigation is needed to better understand the more favorable outcome in some Asian-American breast cancer patients.

Breast Cancer Risk Factors

Despite the numerous epidemiologic studies of breast cancer, only a handful of studies have included enough Asian Americans to be able to report statistically meaningful findings for this population. The Multiethnic Cohort (MEC) conducted in Hawaii and Los Angeles County is an ongoing prospective cohort study of over 200,000 men and women, ages 45–79 years, that has included 45,000 Japanese American women, who were recruited between 1993 and 1996 [25, 26]. In addition, three case–control studies have reported on findings on breast cancer in Asian Americans: (1) a case–control of 183 Japanese breast cancer cases and corresponding controls, ages 45–74, from Hawaii (1975–1980) [27, 28]; (2) a case–control study of 597 Chinese, Japanese, and Filipina breast cancer cases and 966 controls (aged 20–55 years) from Hawaii, the San Francisco Bay Area, and Los Angeles County (1983–1987) (referred to hereafter as CA-HW study); and (3) a case–control study of 2303 breast cancer cases (929 Chinese, 547 Japanese, 827 Filipino) and 2035 controls (923 Chinese, 518 Japanese, 594 Filipino), ages 30–79 years old, from Los Angeles County (1995–2006) (referred to hereafter as LAC study) [29]. Thus, our coverage of breast cancer risk factors in Asian Americans will be based on results of Japanese Americans from the MEC, and those of Chinese, Japanese, and Filipina women from the CA-HW and LAC case–control studies that were conducted 10–15 years apart. Results of Japanese Americans in the MEC represent mainly data on postmenopausal women and allowed comparison to those of NH Whites in the MEC. The CA-HW focused on primarily premenopausal or perimenopausal women, and had higher proportion of US-born Asians (46 % of cases and 42 % of controls), mainly from Hawaii and the San Francisco Bay Area. In contrast, the LAC study included both pre- and postmenopausal women, was based on a single geographic area, and consisted of mostly migrants (79 % of cases and 73 % of controls were non-US born) but this differed for the three Asian ethnic groups (95 % of Filipina, 86 % of Chinese, and 26 % of Japanese control women were foreign born) [30].

Menstrual and Reproductive Factors

Age at Menarche

Early age at menarche is a well-established risk factor that is attributed to extended exposure to estrogens and possibly progesterone [31]. In some studies, the earlier onset of menstrual cycles was related to more intensive exposure to estrogen and a persistent effect of age at menarche on estrogen concentration [32]. The most comprehensive international evaluation showed that breast cancer risk increased by a factor of 1.05 (95 % CI = 1.044–1.057) for every year of younger age at menarche; results were similar in pre- and postmenopausal women [33]. In the CA-HW study, there was a trend of lower risk associated with later age at menarche, the risk reduction for each year that menarche was delayed was 0.94 (95 % CI 0.86–1.03) [34]. In the LAC study, there was also a significant trend of lower risk with later age at menarche, but this was only observed in premenopausal Asian-American women (*P* trend = 0.03) and not in postmenopausal women (*P* trend = 0.67) [35]. The mean age of menarche of LAC Asian-American control women (12.9) was similar to that of Whites and African Americans in the Women's Contraceptive and Reproductive Experiences (CARE) case–control study (12.5) [36] but considerably younger than that reported for the Japan Public Health Center (JPHC) (14.4) or Miyagi (14.4) cohorts [33]. Although results were not statistically significant in some studies, the strength of the overall evidence implies that the steady decline in age at menarche among Asian Americans [34] and in Asia [37, 38] will continue to have an important impact on their breast cancer risk [39].

Parity, Age at First Birth, Breastfeeding

With westernization and urbanization, there have been striking changes in reproductive patterns in Asia and in Asian Americans, including increases in age at first birth and nulliparity and decreases in number of births and breastfeeding. Most of the established reproductive variables related to breast cancer risk are observed in Asians and Asian Americans. In some cases, changes in the reproductive patterns in the countries of origin (e.g., China's one child policy) [40] have been as dramatic as those in migrant groups to the USA. Thus, reproductive variables may underlie both secular increases in risk and some risk difference between Asians in the USA and in Asia.

Studies conducted in Asian Americans show a strong increased risk associated with nulliparity [34], similar to the findings in western populations [26, 36]. In both CA-HW and LAC studies, parous Chinese, Japanese, and Filipina American women displayed a significant trend of decreasing risk with increasing number of births [34, 35]. The respective ORs for 0, 1, 2, 3, 4+ births were 1.0, 0.94, 0.72, 0.58, 0.33 (*P* trend <0.001); the risk pattern was similar in pre- and postmenopausal Asian Americans [35]. A significant increase in risk per 5 year delay in first birth was observed in the CA-HW study (OR = 1.22, 95 % CI 1.05–1.42) [34] and also the LAC study although the effect in the latter study was weaker [51]. Nulliparity and later age at first birth were statistically significant risk factors for Japanese Americans, as well as NH Whites in the MEC [26]. The prevalence of nulliparity among Asian Americans in LAC (16.8 %) [30] and Japanese Americans in the MEC (12.9 %) was similar to that of NH Whites in the MEC (15.5 %) [41] but considerably higher than that in Japan (5–6 %) [42, 43] and Shanghai China (3–4 %) [44]. A striking change was in the age at first birth; few Asian Americans had a first birth before age 21 (5.4 % of LAC Asian Americans, 10.9 % of Japanese Americans in the MEC and 30.8 % of NH Whites in the MEC) and many had delayed their first birth to after age 30 (26 % of LAC Asian Americans, 10.2 % of Japanese Americans in the MEC and 7.2 % of NH Whites in the MEC) [30, 41]. Delay in first birth to age 30 or later was also common in Shanghai, China (23 %) [44], but less frequent in Japanese cohorts (5–8 %) that were conducted during the same time periods [42, 45].

An international pooled analysis of 47 studies showed a significant 4.3 % (95 % CI 2.9–5.8 %) reduction in breast cancer risk for every 12 months of breastfeeding [46]. In studies conducted in the early 1970s and 1980s, long duration of breastfeeding (i.e., >3 years) had a profound protective effect on breast cancer risk in urban China [47–49]. However, the breastfeeding-breast cancer association was weak in Asian-American women [34], and recent studies in Japan [42, 45, 50] and Shanghai, China [44]. While approximately 80 % of Asian women have breastfed in recent studies conducted in Asia [42, 44, 45], the duration of breastfeeding was short. For example, the highest category of breastfeeding (18 months or more) was reported by 23 % of Chinese control women in Shanghai in the 1990s [44] whereas 41 % reported 3 or more years of breastfeeding in Shanghai in the mid-1980s [48]. Also, the prevalence of breastfeeding was lower (48 %) among Asian Americans in LAC and only 18 % had breastfed for 1 year or longer [51]. The interrelated changes in number of births, age at first birth, and breastfeeding [52] have likely played a very important role in contributing to changes in breast cancer incidence in both Asian women in the USA and in Asia.

Menopause

The timing of natural menopause is an important risk factor for breast cancer. Women who experience later natural menopause have higher rates of breast cancer than do women with earlier natural menopause. In an international pooled analysis, breast cancer risk increased by a factor of 1.029 (95 % CI 1.025–1.032) for every year older at menopause [33]. Late age at natural menopause was associated with an increased risk of breast cancer in LAC Asian Americans but the effect was weaker (RR per 5 year delay in natural menopause was 1.02, 95 % CI 0.99–1.04, $P=0.17$) [51]. Although age at menopause did not differ between NH Whites, Japanese, and Chinese Americans in the Study of Women's Health Across the Nation (SWAN) study [53], age at natural menopause was later in Japanese than NH Whites in the MEC, after accounting for age at menarche, parity, body mass index, and smoking [54]. Among women who had a natural menopause in the MEC, 42.7 % of Japanese Americans vs. 33.7 % of NH Whites experienced menopause at or after age 55 [54]; this proportion of Japanese with a late menopause was considerably higher than women (5–8 %) in the Miyagi and JACC cohorts [43, 45]. Better understanding of the lifestyle determinants of age at natural menopause in Asian Americans and Asians is needed.

Use of Exogenous Hormones

Oral Contraceptives

In an international pooled analysis of mostly studies in western women, risk of breast cancer increased in relation to any oral contraceptives (OC) use (OR = 1.10, 95 % CI 1.02–1.19) and recent use within 5 years (OR = 1.20, 95 % CI 1.1–1.20) [46]. In the CA-HW study, OC use increased with time since migration and was reported by 49.6 % of Asian women born in the USA compared to 15.0 % of Asia-born women who had lived in the USA for less than 8 years. OC use was inversely associated with risk; relative to Asian-American women who were nonusers, those who used OCs for 1–12, 13–60, 60+ months showed ORs of 1.20, 0.81, and 0.71, respectively (*P* trend = 0.03). The pattern of risk reduction was found in all three Asian ethnic groups [55] and also in the recent LAC study [51]. OC use was not approved in Japan until 1999 and usage is still low. There is little evidence of an increased risk between OC use and breast cancer risk in recent studies conducted in Japan [45, 56], Shanghai, China [57], or elsewhere in Asia (see review [55]). However, duration of OC use was typically short among users in Asia and the factors associated with use may differ between Asian and NH White women. Pharmacokinetic differences in metabolism of OCs between Asians and Whites have been suggested [58, 59]. Nevertheless, while OC use has increased among Asian Americans, there is little suggestion that OC use is positively associated with breast cancer risk in Asian Americans or in Asia and thus OC use cannot explain the elevated risk observed in Asian women who migrated to the USA.

Hormone Replacement Therapy

Results from the Women's Health Initiative (WHI) trial with <2 % of Asian-American women support findings from previous observational studies that current or recent use of estrogen–progestin therapy (EPT) use is associated with an increase in breast cancer risk [60]. Use of hormone therapy (HT) has been uncommon in Asia and Asian Americans until recently, but has become more prevalent especially among Japanese Americans. In the MEC, reported use of estrogen alone therapy (ET) and EPT were similar between Japanese Americans and NH Whites at baseline. Among Japanese Americans, 25.2 % were current EPT users, 18.5 % were current ET users, 9.6 % were past EPT users, and 13.0 % were past ET users; the corresponding percentages in NH Whites were 25.3, 20.1, 14.4, and 16.4 %. For Japanese Americans, the hazard ratios per 5 years of current EPT and current ET use were 1.33 (95 % CI 1.24–1.43) and 1.18 (95 % CI 1.08–1.30), respectively; similar to the risk estimates observed in NH Whites [61]. Results from LAC showed that HT use was highest in US-born Asians (69 %), intermediate (55 %) in migrants who have lived in the USA for 21+ years, and lowest (31 %) in recent migrants who have lived in the USA for less than 21 years. In LAC Chinese, Japanese, and Filipina American women, the risk of breast cancer per 5 years of current EPT use was 1.26

(95 % CI 1.04–1.52) but there was no increased risk associated with current ET use 0.99 (95 % CI 0.83–1.19) [35]. Studies on HT use and breast cancer risk in Asia generally show no statistically significant associations but these studies had low statistical power as use of HT was uncommon (<5 %) and duration of use was rarely considered in the analyses [42, 44, 45]. Thus the increase in HT, particularly EPT use among Asian Americans can explain, in part, the elevated risk observed in postmenopausal women.

Anthropometric Measures

There is extensive evidence that body size measures from birth, young adult life, to late adult life have profound effects on risk of breast cancer although these associations are more consistent and better understood in relation to risk in postmenopausal than premenopausal women. Adult height may serve as an indicator of childhood or adolescent nutrition and energy balance in that shorter women may have been energy restricted during childhood and adolescence. The predominant hypothesis is that after menopause, adipose tissues becomes the primary site of estrogen production through the aromatization of androgens, and that the higher concentrations of circulating estrogens are associated with increases in breast cancer risk [62].

Adult Body Size Measures and Risk in Premenopausal Women

Most studies conducted in western populations found that height was weakly positively associated with breast cancer risk in premenopausal women [63]. Height was significantly associated with breast cancer risk in premenopausal Asian Americans in the CA-HW study (RR 1.9, 95 % CI 1.1–3.6 for ≥167.6 vs. ≤149.9 cm; *P* trend = 0.03) but this was not observed in the LAC study (*P* trend = 0.63). In a meta-analysis of six studies that included Asians and Asian Americans, the RR per 10 cm increase in height was 1.02 (95 % CI 1.00–1.03); the corresponding RR in Whites was 1.03 (95 % CI 1.02–1.05) [64].

Results on BMI before diagnosis and risk of breast cancer in premenopausal Asian-American women have not been consistent. In the CA-HW study, higher risk was seen with higher BMI (90th vs. 10th percentile = 1.60, 95 % CI 0.87–2.94) [65] but in the LAC study, risk was lower with higher BMI (RR for Q4 vs. Q1 = 0.67, 95 % CI 0.48–0.98, *P* trend = 0.07) [35]. In a meta-analysis of studies in Asians (nine in Asia and one among Asian Americans; eight case–control, two cohort), the RR was 1.05 (95 % 1.01–1.09) per 5 kg/m^2 increase in BMI [64]; this is in contrast to a RR of 0.93 (95 % CI = 0.91–0.95) in premenopausal white women from 16 studies (nine case–control, seven cohort) [64]. Thus while high BMI is inversely associated with breast cancer risk in premenopausal Whites, the evidence in Asians suggests a positive association [64]. Interestingly, despite the Asian-white difference in the BMI-risk association in premenopausal women, high waist/hip ratio (WHR) appeared to be a risk factor for premenopausal breast cancer in both Whites and Asian women. In a meta-analysis of six studies in Whites and four studies in Asians that had information on both WHR and BMI, in Asians, the respective RR per 0.1 increase in WHR was 1.05 (95 % CI = 1.01–1.08) and per 5 kg/m^2 in BMI was 1.19 (95 % CI = 1.15–1.24); the corresponding RRs in Whites were 1.05 (95 % CI = 1.01–1.09) and 0.90 (95 % CI 0.86–0.94) [64]. Better understanding is needed of the differing roles of general adiposity, measured by BMI, and the comparable roles of central obesity, measured by WHR, in the etiology of premenopausal breast cancer in Asia as well as among Asians and Whites in the USA.

Adult Body Size Measures and Risk in Postmenopausal Women

Height, current BMI, weight changes, and WHR are all significantly positively associated with breast cancer risk in postmenopausal Asian Americans as in western populations [66, 67]. In the MEC, the RRs associated with height (per 10 cm), current BMI (per 5 kg/m^2), and weight gain (per 5 kg since age 21) were 1.21 (95 % CI 1.07–1.36), 1.25 (95 % CI 1.1–1.36), and 1.16 (95 % CI 1.12–1.21), respectively, among Japanese Americans; the corresponding RRs among NH Whites were 1.09 (95 % CI 0.98–1.21), 1.06 (95 % CI 1.00–1.14), and 1.06 (95 % CI 1.03–1.09) [41]. High BMI at age 21 was inversely associated with breast cancer risk in postmenopausal Japanese and NH Whites; the respective ORs per 5 kg/m^2 increase was 0.85 (95 % CI 0.74–0.98) and 0.82 (95 % CI 0.72–0.95). Results from the LAC study showed that high BMI and weight gain increased the risk of postmenopausal breast cancer in Chinese, Japanese, and Filipina in a manner similar to the results observed in the MEC. In addition, high WHR was a significant risk factor for postmenopausal breast cancer among Asian Americans; RR was 1.48 (95 % CI 1.02–2.15) for highest vs. lowest category of WHR [35] which is similar to the meta-analysis findings of 1.33 (95 % CI 1.19–1.48) [66]. In a pooled analysis of eight cohort studies in Japan, the risk among postmenopausal women was 1.06 ($P<0.001$) per 1 kg/m^2 increase in BMI [68]. Although BMI at age 20 years was unrelated to breast cancer risk in postmenopausal women in Japan [69] and Shanghai, China [70], weight gain between age 20 years and current weight appeared to be significantly associated with risk in Japan [69–71].

Birth Weight

In utero exposure to elevated concentrations of estrogens has been hypothesized to adversely affect risk of breast cancer [72]. Findings from meta-analyses of studies conducted mainly in western populations show a significant positive association between breast cancer risk and body size, measured by birth weight, birth length, or head circumference [73, 74] although the confounding effect of adult height may exist [75]. Results from the few studies on birth weight and breast cancer risk in Asian Americans and Asians are mixed. Nonsignificantly reduced risk of breast cancer in association with higher birth weight was found in a small study conducted among Asians and Whites in Hawaii [76] and in Shanghai, China [77]. However, among Chinese, Japanese, and Filipina women in the LAC study, women in the highest birth weight category (≥4000 g) compared to those in the lowest (<2500 g) category had a doubling of risk after adjustment for age at menarche, adult BMI, and other potential confounding factors. Risk increased (RR = 1.08, 95 % CI 0.99–1.19) per 500 g increase in birth weight [30]. With the current trends of increasing birth weight in Asians and Asian Americans [78, 79], further investigation of the influence of birth weight is warranted since birth weight has been found to influence age at menarche [80, 81] and mammographic density [82, 83].

Physical Activity

Numerous studies have investigated the role of physical activity in relation to breast cancer risk based on the hypothesis that regular activity may beneficially influence the profile of endogenous hormones and growth factors, and lessen inflammation [84, 85]. A meta-analysis of 31 prospective studies (including three studies from Asia) found lower breast cancer risk (RR = 0.87, 95 % CI 0.83–0.91) in association with highest vs. lowest category of physical activity in multivariable models with adjustment for BMI; 0.77 (95 % CI 0.65–0.81) in premenopausal and 0.87 (95 % CI 0.83–1.05) in postmenopausal women [86]. The combined effect associated with high vs. low activity was similar (RR 0.82, 95 % CI 0.87–1.08) for the three cohort studies from Asia which investigated risk in relation to leisure-time physical activity including walking [87, 88] and occupational physical activity [89]. In the LAC study, Asian-American women showed a trend of decreasing risk with increasing years of physical activity (0–4, 5–9, 10–19, 20+ years); the respective ORs were 0.94, 0.77, and 0.57 (*P* trend <0.01) [35].

Diabetes

Diabetes has been implicated as a breast cancer risk factor; the postulated mechanisms are activation of insulin and insulin-like growth factor pathways and regulation of endogenous sex hormones [90]. In a meta-analysis of observational studies (15 case–control, three cross-sectional, 22 prospective) conducted in mostly western populations, prediagnostic diabetes was associated with breast cancer risk (RR = 1.27, 95 % CI 1.16–1.39) [91]. In LAC, Asian Americans who had a history of diabetes had a higher risk of breast cancer (RR = 1.71, 95 % CI 1.15–2.54) after adjustment for BMI, WHR, and other covariates, this was statistically significant in postmenopausal but not in premenopausal women [92]. Although diabetes was unrelated to breast cancer risk in a pooled analysis of six cohort studies from Japan (RR = 1.03, 95 % CI 0.69–1.56) [93], diabetes was a significant risk factor for breast cancer in a prospective cohort from Korea [94]. Given the secular increase in diabetes in Asia and in Asian Americans, even a small increase in breast cancer risk among diabetics will have substantial public health implications.

Dietary Factors

The role of diet in the causation of breast cancer continues to be controversial. According to the 2014 updated report from the World Cancer Research Fund/American Institute for Cancer Research (WCRF/AICR), alcohol intake is the only dietary factor that shows consistent positive associations with risk of breast cancer. The role of specific nutrients and foods (dietary fat, specific fats, red meat, fruits, and vegetables) remains unclear with reports of significant results in some prospective studies but contradictory results in others (see below). There are suggestions that specific dietary patterns and intake of soy may be associated with breast cancer risk. The traditional Asian diet is rich in plant foods and low in animal protein and fat with soy as a staple. These dietary patterns may underlie risk differences and have been investigated in numerous studies in the past two decades.

Alcohol

Alcohol consumption is a well-established risk factor for breast cancer; the association is thought to be largely hormonally driven. A meta-analysis of 98 studies reported a 10 % increase in breast cancer risk per 10 g of alcohol (~one 12 oz bottle or can of beer, one 4 oz glass of wine, or a 1.5 oz drink or shot of liquor) per day [95]. Although alcohol intake was unrelated to breast cancer risk in Asian Americans in the CA-HW study [96], results from the larger LAC study that allowed analysis by Asian ethnicity showed that alcohol intake was associated with breast cancer risk among Japanese Americans (per 5 g/day RR=1.17, 95 % CI 0.99–1.39, P=0.073) but not among Chinese and Filipina Americans. Regular alcohol intake was less common among Chinese (14 %) and Filipina (14 %) compared to Japanese Americans (27 %) in the LAC study [29]. Intake of alcohol was lower among Japanese American (17.0 % consumed <10 g/day and 3.7 % consumed ≥10 g/day) than NH Whites in the MEC (34.3 % consumed <10 g/day and 24.3 % consumed ≥10 g/day). However, the RR per 10 g/day was 1.08 (95 % CI 1.01–1.15) in Japanese Americans, similar to the risk estimate for NH Whites (RR=1.04, 95 % CI 1.02–1.07) [97]. Alcohol intake also emerged as a breast cancer risk factor in Japan. In the JACC cohort, the RR for current drinkers was 1.27 (95 % CI 0.87–1.84) compared to nondrinkers and risk was significantly increased for women who consumed ≥15 g/day of alcohol (RR=2.93, 95 % CI 1.55–5.54) [98]. In the JPHC, consumption of 10 g ethanol/day was associated with a 6 % (95 % CI 1–13 %) (P trend=0.047) increase in the risk of breast cancer [99]. These results in Asian Americans and in Japan are important given that alcohol intake is one of the few modifiable risk factors for breast cancer.

Dietary Fat

Dietary fat has been the major focus in the search for dietary causes of breast cancer for decades, and despite compelling results from ecologic and animal studies, findings from analytic epidemiologic studies have been inconsistent. In the large MEC study, breast cancer risk in postmenopausal women was unrelated to intake of total fat and by type of fat. These null results were found in Japanese Americans as well as the other racial/ethnic groups in the MEC and remain unchanged when body mass index and age at menarche were removed as adjustment factors to avoid adjusting for intermediate variables in the pathway from dietary fat and breast cancer risk [100].

The generally null findings in the MEC are consistent with pooled analyses of cohort studies that have found no association between dietary fat and breast cancer risk [101], although a positive association with total fat was suggested in a meta-analysis of 31 case–control and 14 cohort studies [102]. In addition, findings from the WHI dietary trial showed that after 10 years of intervention, those in the low-fat arm with a goal of consuming 20 % of energy from fat showed a small reduction in risk (HR 0.91, 95 % CI 0.83–1.01) [103] although the risk reduction was no longer evident with additional years of follow-up [104]. Recent results from the NIH-AARP [105], the EPIC [106], and VITAL [107] cohorts suggest that risk of breast cancer, and particularly certain subtypes of breast cancer in postmenopausal women, may be positively associated with intake of total fat, saturated fat, and specific fatty acids. A meta-analysis of 21 cohort studies found that high intake of marine *n*-3 polyunsaturated fatty acids (PUFA) was inversely associated with breast cancer risk (RR = 0.86, 95 % CI 0.78–0.94); this effect was stronger (RR = 0.69, 95 % CI 0.56–0.86) [108] in the subset of studies conducted in Asia [109–111]. Meta-analysis of another six prospective nested case–control studies and five cohort studies found a significantly 6–10 % lower breast cancer risk in association with high dietary or serum ratio of *n*-3/*n*-6 PUFA [112]. Results from the JPHC cohort suggests that the effects of total fish (the major dietary source of *n*-3 PUFAs in this population), *n*-3 PUFA and *n*-6 PUFA on breast cancer risk may vary by ER/PR status. A significant positive association was reported between intake of *n*-6 PUFA and risk of ER + PR+ breast cancer [113].

Meat, Red Meat, and Processed Meat Intake

Results from prospective cohort studies have found no consistent associations between breast cancer risk and meat intake [114, 115]. However, an updated meta-analysis of 14 prospective studies (one from China, 13 from western populations) reported elevated summary RRs for the highest vs. the lowest categories for red meat (RR = 1.10, 95 % CI 1.02–1.19) and processed meat (RR = 1.08; 95 % CI 1.01–1.15) [116]. Results from the LAC study showed elevated risk of breast cancer in Asian Americans with increasing intake of meat (RR per 23 g/1000 kcal=1.12, 95 % CI 1.02–1.22) [117]. Breast cancer risk was also positively associated with intake of total meat and red meat in case–control studies conducted in Shanghai, China [118, 119]; there was a significant trend of increasing risk with increasing intake of all meats (Q5 vs. Q1 RR = 2.18, 95 % CI 1.82–2.61), and red meat (Q5 vs. Q1 RR = 1.45, 95 % CI 1.22–1.72) [119]. The association with red meat intake may be due to a combination of nutritionally related factors, such as content of fat, protein, iron [120, 121] and/or meat preparation methods including the presence of carcinogenic compounds such as the heterocyclic amines and polycyclic aromatic hydrocarbons by-products that are produced in the process of high-temperature cooking of red meats [122].

Plant Foods—Fruit and Vegetable Intake

Fruits and vegetables are rich sources of carotenoids, flavonoids, and glucosinolates, and have been hypothesized to reduce the risk of breast cancer. Results from the Pooling Project of Prospective Studies of Diet and Cancer that included 20 cohort studies (including the JPHC cohort) found no overall association between breast cancer risk and intake of fruits (*P* trend = 0.36), vegetables (*P* trend = 0.77), or fruits and vegetables combined (*P* trend = 0.30) [123]. In subgroup analysis by hormone receptor status, the pooled RR comparing the highest vs. lowest quintile of total vegetable intake was 0.83 (95 % CI 0.74–0.90) for ER- but not for ER+ breast cancer [123]. In the LAC study, risk of breast cancer in Asian Americans decreased in association with intake of vegetables (RR per 89 g/1000 kcal = 0.90 (95 % CI 0.82–0.99), fruits and nuts (RR per 109 g/1000 kcal = 0.95, 95 % CI 0.86–1.04), and legumes (RR per 30 g/1000 kcal = 0.87, 95 % CI: 0.79–0.95) after adjustment for relevant covariates [117]. Although breast cancer risk was unrelated to intake of both fruits and vegetables, or specific types of vegetables in the JPHC cohort [124], intake of vegetables (RR per 200 g/day = 0.77, 95 % CI: 0.47–1.24), but not fruits (RR per 200 g/day = 1.04, 95 % CI 0.88–1.25) was inversely associated with risk in the Singapore Chinese Health Study [125]. Intake of total vegetables (particularly allium vegetables and fresh legumes) but not fruits was significantly inversely related to breast cancer risk in Shanghai, China [119]. A meta-analysis of eight studies, including three studies from China found that high intake of cruciferous vegetables was significantly associated with reduced risk (RR = 0.85, 95 % CI 0.77–0.94) [126]. In a pooled analysis of eight prospective studies (including the MEC) that used prediagnostic blood samples, statistically significant inverse associations with breast cancer were observed for total and specific carotenoids; associations appeared to be stronger for ER- breast cancers [127].

Soy Products

Soybeans are a rich source of isoflavones, which are hypothesized to be natural estrogen receptor modulators that possess both estrogen-like and anti-estrogenic like properties. In the CA-HW study, high intake of tofu was significantly inversely associated with breast cancer risk in Asian Americans [128]. In the LAC study that included a more complete assessment of soy intake among Chinese, Japanese, and Filipinas, there was a significant trend of decreasing risk with increasing intake of isoflavones. Specifically, Asian Americans who were high consumers during adolescence and adult life, derived the strongest benefit [129]. In a 2008 meta-analysis of mostly case–control studies, a dose–response relationship was observed with a statistically significant trend of decreasing risk with increasing soy food intake. Compared to the lowest level of soy food intake (≤5 mg isoflavones per day), risk was intermediate (OR=0.88, 95 % CI 0.78–0.98) among those with modest (~10 mg isoflavones per day) intake, and lowest (OR=0.71, 95 % CI 0.60–0.85) among those with high intake (≥20 mg isoflavones per day). This inverse association was observed in pre- and postmenopausal women [130]. However, there is concern the effect of soy may be due to residual confounding by correlated foods and other factors associated with traditional Asian lifestyle. In the MEC, self-reported soy food intake based on food frequency questionnaire did not show a statistically significant inverse association in all postmenopausal women but the association was borderline statistically significant in Japanese Americans (upper vs. lower quartile RR=0.86, 95 % CI 0.70,1.05, *P* trend=0.06) [131]. In addition, in a case–control study nested within the MEC, a significantly lower breast cancer risk was observed in postmenopausal women with higher urinary prediagnostic isoflavone excretion levels, especially among Japanese American women (upper vs. lower quartile RR=0.53, 95 % CI 0.24, 1.16, *P* trend=0.005) [132]. A meta-analysis of mainly prospective studies [133] as well as a systematic review of studies from Japan are supportive of a role of soy food in the etiology of breast cancer [134].

Dietary Patterns

Studies of the role of diet and breast cancer have expanded to include investigation of dietary patterns which can accommodate the complex interplay of foods within a diet. These studies aim to reduce a large amount of original data (food items/groups and portion sizes) into indices or factors that might reflect the composite dietary habits. In the LAC study, breast cancer risk in Chinese, Japanese, and Filipina American women decreased significantly with increasing intake of a vegetable-soy pattern (*P* for trend=0.013) [117]. In the prospective Singapore Chinese Health Study [125] and case–control studies conducted in Japan [135], Korea [136], and southern China [137], breast cancer risk was inversely associated with higher consumption of a dietary pattern comprising fruit, vegetables, soy, and soy-bean products. However, in a case–control study in Shanghai, China, breast cancer risk was not associated with intake of a "vegetable and soy" pattern [138]. Identification of the key factors within the Asian fruit-vegetable-soy dietary pattern that are responsible for observed inverse relationships with breast cancer is needed.

Green and Black Tea

Green tea is rich in tea catechins and have many cancer chemopreventive attributes including anti-oxidation, anti-inflammatory, anti-proliferative, and anti-angiogenic effects [139]. Asian-American women who were regular green tea drinkers had a significantly lower risk of breast cancer in the LAC study [140]. Supportive results also were found in case–control studies in China [141, 142]. The combined OR from these case–control studies was 0.70 (95 % CI 0.61–0.79) for women who drank green tea regularly compared to non-green tea drinkers [143]. However, cohort studies from Japan [144–146], Singapore [147, 148], and Shanghai, China [149], showed no association between breast cancer risk and green tea intake (combined OR = 1.06, 95 % CI 0.93–1.20). In a meta-analysis, black tea intake was not associated with breast cancer risk [150].

Active Smoking, Passive smoking

Experimental studies have shown that compounds found in tobacco smoke, such as polycyclic hydrocarbons, aromatic amines, and N-nitrosamines, may induce mammary tumors [151, 152]. Although smoking has been suggested to have antiestrogenic effects [153], recent results have found higher concentrations of androstenedione, testosterone, and estrogen concentrations in postmenopausal women who were current smokers than nonsmokers [154, 155].

While many epidemiological studies conducted in western populations have found no association or at most a weak positive association with active smoking (see review [156]), recent cohort studies [157–159] including the MEC [160] have reported elevated risk of breast cancer among smokers. A 2013 meta-analysis of prospective studies estimated a combined risk of 1.12 (95 % CI 1.08–1.16) for current smokers and 1.09 (95 % CI = 1.04–1.15) for former smokers. Risk was also elevated among those who started smoking at a young age and smoking before first birth suggesting that a long duration of smoking may have a deleterious effect [159]. With few exceptions [161], active smoking was not significantly associated with breast cancer risk in studies conducted in Japan [162, 163]. Prevalence of active smoking is generally low in Japan and lifetime history of smoking was often not ascertained in studies of breast cancer.

The evidence on passive smoking and risk of breast cancer is also controversial. A meta-analysis of case–control studies in China reported a significant positive association between passive smoking and breast cancer risk (RR = 1.67, 95 % CI 1.27–2.21) [164] but null results (RR = 1.01, 95 % CI 0.96–1.06) were found in a meta-analysis of ten prospective studies; the RR was 0.82 (95 % CI 0.54–1.23) for the four studies conducted in Asia [165]. Breast cancer risk was unrelated to passive smoking in most studies in Japan [161, 163, 166] but results from the Takayama cohort differed [167]. Results from the EPIC study found that breast cancer risk increased significantly by 10–16 % in association with passive and active smoking

[158]. With the large numbers of active smokers in China and elsewhere in Asia, the potential effects of passive smoking on breast cancer risk requires continued monitoring but differences in active smoking and passive smoking are unlikely to explain the increase of breast cancer in Asian Americans.

In summary, results described in the above sections show clear effects of menstrual and reproductive factors, body mass index (postmenopausally), use of hormone therapy, and intake of alcohol and soy, but less clear effects of other specific dietary factors as explanations of the rising incidence of breast cancer among Asian Americans. Besides the above factors, there are three other factors, genetics, endogenous hormones, and mammographic density, that could underlie racial/ethnic differences in risk and substantial new information on Asians and Asian Americans have become available in studies conducted in the past two decades.

Family History

Studies conducted in Western populations have consistently reported a two to threefold increased risk of breast cancer in association with a family history of breast cancer among mothers or sisters [168]. Family history of breast cancer is a significant risk factor in Asian Americans [27, 28, 35] and in the LAC study, in both premenopausal (RR = 2.44, 95 % CI 1.55–3.87) and postmenopausal Asian Americans (RR = 1.64, 95 % CI 1.12–2.41) [35]. The prevalence of family history of breast cancer among LAC Asian Americans was 9–11 %, similar to that of Japanese Americans in the MEC (10 %) [41], but higher than prevalences of 1–5 % reported in Singapore, China, or Japan [42, 45, 169, 170].

Examination of the familial risk as above implies that close relatives have similar risk profiles. These shared risk profiles may be environmental or behavioral but may be also indicative of an important role for genetic variation as underlying risk of this disease. The relative importance of genetic variation, compared to modifiable causes, and how much they explain the risk patterns seen in Asian Americans must be judged in light of the experience of migration. The fact that risk increases dramatically with migration to the USA (especially for ER+ postmenopausal disease) indicates the complexity of the disease, and implies an interplay of genetics, environment, and behavior causes.

Genetic Susceptibility

Familial breast cancer accounts for 5–10 % of all breast cancers and are due to genetic predisposition caused by germline mutations; the most commonly tested genes are *BRCA1/BRCA2.* Among Asian Americans with a strong family history of breast cancer, mutation prevalence was 11.5 % for *BRCA1* and 13.2 % for *BRCA2*, the corresponding estimate in Whites was 25–40 % for *BRCA1* and 6–15 % for *BRCA2* [171, 172]. However, among Asian Americans and in Asia, the prevalence of *BRCA1/BRCA2* mutations (BRCA1: 0.5–4.1 %; BRCA2: 1.1–4.4 %) was comparable to Western populations (1.8–3.6 %) [173]. In a comprehensive analysis of the frequency and mutation spectrum from 11 Asian countries, the overall prevalence of *BRCA1/BRCA2* in Asians was comparable to that in other ethnic groups [173].

In addition, genome-wide association studies (GWAS) have identified approximately 100 genetic loci associated with breast cancer risk [174–176]. Approximately ten of these loci were initially identified in GWAS conducted in East Asian descendants [177]. In a consortium analysis that included 23,637 breast cancer cases and 25,579 controls of East Asian ancestry and tested 70 SNPs previously associated with breast cancer mostly in studies of European descendants, 31 loci was associated with breast cancer risk at $P<0.05$ in a direction consistent with previous reports [178]; 21 of them remained statistically significant at a Bonferroni-corrected significance level. These common genetic variants explain a lower fraction of excess familial risk of breast cancer in Asian (~10 %) than in European-ancestry populations (~14 %) [178]; this is expected since most known common genetic variants were identified in GWAS conducted in European-ancestry populations, and they tended to show a stronger association in European than Asian-ancestry populations. In addition to these SNPs reported from the collaborative analysis, two GWAS of East Asian women identified four additional susceptibility loci (1q32.1, 5q14.3 and 15q26.1 [177] and 2q34 [179]). When three of these four SNPs were tested in women of European ancestry, all three SNPs showed associations in the same direction ($P<0.05$), but the magnitude of association was weaker than in women of East Asian ancestry [177].

Lee et al. [170] created a genetic risk score based on 51 genetic variants identified in previous GWAS and tested this in a nested case–control study of 411 breast cancer cases and 1212 controls within the Singapore Chinese Health Study. They found that the genetic risk score was an independent predictor of breast cancer risk, and improved the classification of 6.2 % of women for their absolute risk of breast cancer in the next 5 years. These findings indicate that the established risk variants for breast cancer also contribute to risk in Asian women.

Endogenous Hormones

Many of the breast cancer risk factors, particularly, those related to menstrual and reproductive factors and some lifestyle factors (e.g., body weight) can be understood as measures of the cumulative exposure of the breast to estrogen, and perhaps progesterone. A compelling body of epidemiologic and experimental data implicates endogenous estrogens in the etiology of breast cancer [180–182].

Prospective studies have provided convincing evidence. An international pooled analysis of nine prospective studies found that prediagnostic estrogenic (including estrone, estradiol) and androgenic (including testosterone, androstenedione) steroid sex hormones were significantly positively associated with increased breast cancer risk in postmenopausal women, and that sex hormone binding globulin (SHBG) was significantly inversely associated with risk even after adjustment for BMI and other factors [62, 183]. However, this evidence was based primarily in White women; only 23 cases and 45 controls were from Japan. Results from a nested case–control study conducted in the MEC further strengthened the evidence that high endogenous estrogen levels confer a similar or slightly higher risk of breast cancer in Japanese Americans relative to NH Whites and other race/ethnicities. The risks associated with a doubling of estradiol levels was 2.88 (95 % CI 1.63–5.10) in Japanese Americans and 1.87 (95 % CI 1.17–2.99) in the other racial/ethnic groups combined. A significant twofold increased risk in association with a doubling of estrone, estrone sulfate, free estradiol levels were observed in postmenopausal Japanese Americans [184].

The evidence on circulating sex hormones and breast cancer risk in premenopausal women is less consistent but points to a role of androgens in nested case–control studies that were conducted in EPIC [185] and the NHS [186] studies. We are not aware of such prospective studies conducted among premenopausal Asian Americans or in Asia.

While findings from earlier cross-sectional studies of mostly convenience samples tended to show lower urinary or blood estrogen levels among women in Asia, and Asian Americans compared to Whites in the USA, body weight and other potential confounders were usually not adjusted for (see review [187, 188]). In fact, postmenopausal Japanese American in the MEC study ($n=96$) had similar levels of estrone, estradiol, bioavailable estradiol, and other hormones to that of NH Whites ($n=91$) in age-adjusted analyses, but showed 15 % higher estradiol ($P=0.036$) and 18 % higher bioavailable estradiol ($P=0.024$) levels than NH Whites after adjustment for BMI and age at menarche [155]. There is little evidence in contemporaneous cross-sectional studies that reproductive hormones are lower in Asian Americans than in NH Whites [189] or lower in non-US-born Asian Americans than US-born Asian Americans [190, 191].

Mammographic Density and Screening

Mammographic density reflect the distribution of fat, connective tissue, and epithelium in the breast. Boyd and colleagues hypothesized that the relative amount of epithelium and connective tissues or the mammographic densities represent the cumulative exposure to factors that stimulate growth of breast cells since puberty and would influence the risk of breast cancer development [192, 193]. Numerous studies conducted in North America and Europe have shown that women with densities greater than 75 % of the breast have a 4–6 times higher breast cancer risk than women of the same age with no densities [192, 194].

A few studies have investigated mammographic density and risk of breast cancer in Asian Americans. In a study of Chinese, Japanese, and Filipina Americans in LAC (143 cases, 67 controls), which also included NH Whites (280 cases, 227 controls) for comparison, the OR per 10 % increase in percent density was 1.30 (95 %

CI 1.05–1.61) in Asian Americans, and 1.15 (95 % CI 1.04–1.27) in NH Whites. Per 10 % increase in percent density, breast cancer risk increased 10 % (95 % CI 0.84–1.45) in the younger (<50 year-old) and 59 % (95 % CI 1.09–2.32) in the older (≥50 year-old) Asian Americans. The risk associations in NH Whites were 1.10 (95 % CI 0.96–1.26) and 1.24 (95 % CI 1.05–1.34), respectively [195]. Results were similar in the MEC; the OR per 10 % increase in percent density was 1.15 (95 % CI 1.04–1.27) in Japanese Americans, and 1.33 (95 % CI 1.18–1.51) in NH Whites [196]. Among Chinese in Singapore, after multivariable adjustment, the 76–100 % density category had an OR of 5.54 (95 % CI 2.38–12.9) compared with 0–10 % [197]. Thus there is general consistency that mammographic density is an equally strong breast cancer risk factor for Asian women in the USA as in NH Whites [195–197].

In cross-sectional studies that use a quantitative method to compare mammographic densities in Asian Americans and NH Whites [198–200], women of Asian ethnicities tended to have lower absolute density but higher percent densities than NH Whites because of their relatively small breast size. These differences in percent densities tended to attenuate after adjustment for BMI, parity, and other factors [199–201]. In a study that compared breast densities of Japanese Americans in Hawaii to those in Japan, absolute breast density was higher among Japanese Americans in Hawaii than among women in Japan reflecting the higher breast cancer risk of Japanese in Hawaii [202, 203], although the specific factors responsible for the high densities are not clear. However, percent densities do not differ consistently between US-born and non-US-born Asian Americans [200] or by measures of acculturation [200, 204]. Results from these studies suggest that absolute but not percent mammographic density reflects the lower breast cancer incidence rates of Asian Americans in relation to those of NH Whites [199].

Data from twin and family studies suggest that genetic factors explain 30–60 % of the variation in mammographic density, when adjusted for age, BMI, and other covariates [205–207]. However, only a few genetic loci (*ZNF365, LSP1*, and *RAD51L1*) have been associated with mammographic density, mainly in European Whites [208–210]. In one of the larger studies involving Asian women, a candidate gene approach was used and identified SNPS in *PPARγ* and *TGFB1* to be associated with mammographic density in Singapore Chinese women [211, 212]. A recent study that investigated 36 SNPs, mostly GWAS-identified, found that 6q25.1 region near *ESR1* was associated with mammographic density in Malaysian Chinese women [213]. However, the previously reported PPARγ-density association in Singapore Chinese was not replicated and the *TGFB1* SNP was not evaluated (i.e., did not pass genotyping quality control).

Data on mammography screening by Asian-American ethnicity are reviewed in detail (see Chap. 4). Briefly, data from the 2011 to 2012 California Health Interview Survey of women ages 40 and over showed that 72 % of Asian Americans reported a recent mammogram in the past 2 years compared to 83 % of African Americans, 81 % of Whites, and 77 % of Latinas [214]. In analysis by specific Asian ethnicity, screening rates were lowest in Koreans (52 %), intermediate in Filipina (78 %), Vietnamese (76 %), Chinese (73 %), and other South Asians (69 %), and highest in Japanese Americans (84 %). These differences remained after adjustment for acculturation, sociodemographic characteristics, access to health care, and breast cancer risk factors. In addition to Korean ethnicity, low screening rates were found among women with low level of acculturation, lack of health insurance, and low level of education [215]. Thus, continued efforts to promote utilization of screening services need to be emphasized in Asian Americans.

Conclusion

The adoption of a westernized lifestyle with migration to the USA, characterized by early age at menarche, few children, delayed age at first birth, less breastfeeding, and a sedentary lifestyle have contributed to the risk of breast cancer in Asian-American women. Diabetes, increase in body weight, and use of menopausal hormones are additional risk factors for breast cancer in postmenopausal Asian-American women. High alcohol intake, a dietary pattern that is low in vegetables and soy, and high in meat are contributing factors as well. The pattern of dietary differences remains highly suggestive of a contributing role, especially between breast cancer between Asians and the USA. Failure to identify dietary factors in analytic studies could be due to measurement errors, correlation between dietary components, and assessment of dietary patterns during adult life when diet during earlier life (e.g., before puberty) may be more relevant.

Three other factors, genetics, endogenous hormones, and mammographic density, are also significant risk factors for breast cancer in Asian-American women. Thus, the available data suggest that it is unlikely that risk factors for breast cancer in Asian Americans differ markedly from those in other racial/ethnic groups. While we now have excellent data on Japanese Americans from the MEC, information on other Asian ethnic groups is still sparse. Most studies typically present results for Asian Americans combined and not separately for Asian ethnic subgroup. It is quite likely that changes in various lifestyle exposures are not identical across different Asian race/ethnicities such that the relative importance of each individual risk factor will depend on the changing prevalence of these risk factors.

Financial Disclosures This work was in part supported by the National Cancer Institute grants P30 CA014089 and 2P30 EW007048021.

1. Authors' declaration of personal interests: None declared.
2. Declaration of funding interests: None declared.

References

1. Siegel RL, Miller KD, Jemal A (2015) Cancer statistics, 2015. CA Cancer J Clin 65:5–29
2. Gomez SL, Noone AM, Lichtensztajn DY, Scoppa S, Gibson JT, Liu L et al (2013) Cancer incidence trends among Asian American populations in the United States, 1990–2008. J Natl Cancer Inst 105:1096–1110

3. Parise C, Caggiano V (2014) Disparities in the risk of the ER/PR/HER2 breast cancer subtypes among Asian Americans in California. Cancer Epidemiol 38:556–562
4. Yi M, Liu P, Li X, Mittendorf EA, He J, Ren Y et al (2012) Comparative analysis of clinicopathologic features, treatment, and survival of Asian women with a breast cancer diagnosis residing in the United States. Cancer 118:4117–4125
5. Fan L, Strasser-Weippl K, Li JJ, St Louis J, Finkelstein DM, Yu KD et al (2014) Breast cancer in China. Lancet Oncol 15:e279–e289
6. Toi M, Ohashi Y, Seow A, Moriya T, Tse G, Sasano H et al (2010) The Breast Cancer Working Group presentation was divided into three sections: the epidemiology, pathology and treatment of breast cancer. Jpn J Clin Oncol 40(Suppl 1):i13–i18
7. Matsuno RK, Anderson WF, Yamamoto S, Tsukuma H, Pfeiffer RM, Kobayashi K et al (2007) Early- and late-onset breast cancer types among women in the United States and Japan. Cancer Epidemiol Biomarkers Prev 16:1437–1442
8. Sung H, Rosenberg PS, Chen WQ, Hartman M, Lim WY, Chia KS et al (2015) Female breast cancer incidence among Asian and Western populations: more similar than expected. J Natl Cancer Inst 107:djv107
9. Ooi SL, Martinez ME, Li CI (2011) Disparities in breast cancer characteristics and outcomes by race/ethnicity. Breast Cancer Res Treat 127:729–738
10. Chen L, Li CI (2015) Racial disparities in breast cancer diagnosis and treatment by hormone receptor and HER2 status. Cancer Epidemiol Biomarkers Prev 24:1666–1672
11. Perou CM, Sorlie T, Eisen MB, van de Rijn M, Jeffrey SS, Rees CA et al (2000) Molecular portraits of human breast tumours. Nature 406:747–752
12. Telli ML, Chang ET, Kurian AW, Keegan TH, McClure LA, Lichtensztajn D et al (2010) Asian ethnicity and breast cancer subtypes: a study from the California Cancer Registry. Breast Cancer Res Treat 127:471–478
13. Clarke CA, Keegan TH, Yang J, Press DJ, Kurian AW, Patel AH et al (2012) Age-specific incidence of breast cancer subtypes: understanding the black–white crossover. J Natl Cancer Inst 104:1094–1101
14. Warner ET, Tamimi RM, Hughes ME, Ottesen RA, Wong YN, Edge SB et al (2015) Racial and ethnic differences in breast cancer survival: mediating effect of tumor characteristics and sociodemographic and treatment factors. J Clin Oncol 33:2254–2261
15. Chuang E, Paul C, Flam A, McCarville K, Forst M, Shin S et al (2012) Breast cancer subtypes in Asian–Americans differ according to Asian ethnic group. J Immigr Minor Health 14:754–758
16. Carey LA, Perou CM, Livasy CA, Dressler LG, Cowan D, Conway K et al (2006) Race, breast cancer subtypes, and survival in the Carolina Breast Cancer Study. JAMA 295:2492–2502
17. Sorlie T, Perou CM, Tibshirani R, Aas T, Geisler S, Johnsen H et al (2001) Gene expression patterns of breast carcinomas distinguish tumor subclasses with clinical implications. Proc Natl Acad Sci U S A 98:10869–10874
18. Trinh QD, Nguyen PL, Leow JJ, Dalela D, Chao GF, Mahal BA et al (2015) Cancer-specific mortality of Asian Americans diagnosed with cancer: a nationwide population-based assessment. J Natl Cancer Inst 107:djv054
19. Wu AH, Gomez SL, Vigen C, Kwan ML, Keegan TH, Lu Y et al (2013) The California Breast Cancer Survivorship Consortium (CBCSC): prognostic factors associated with racial/ethnic differences in breast cancer survival. Cancer Causes Control 24:1821–1836
20. Kwan ML, John EM, Caan BJ, Lee VS, Bernstein L, Cheng I et al (2014) Obesity and mortality after breast cancer by race/ethnicity: the California Breast Cancer Survivorship Consortium. Am J Epidemiol 179:95–111
21. Wu AH, Kurian AW, Kwan ML, John EM, Lu Y, Keegan TH et al (2015) Diabetes and other comorbidities in breast cancer survival by race/ethnicity: the California Breast Cancer Survivorship Consortium (CBCSC). Cancer Epidemiol Biomarkers Prev 24:361–368
22. Lu Y, John EM, Sullivan-Halley J, Vigen C, Gomez SL, Kwan ML et al (2015) History of recreational physical activity and survival after breast cancer: the California Breast Cancer Survivorship Consortium. Am J Epidemiol 181:944–955

23. Cheng I, Shariff-Marco S, Koo J, Monroe KR, Yang J, John EM et al (2015) Contribution of the neighborhood environment and obesity to breast cancer survival: the California Breast Cancer Survivorship Consortium. Cancer Epidemiol Biomarkers Prev 24:1282–1290
24. Shariff-Marco S, Yang J, John EM, Kurian AW, Cheng I, Leung R et al (2015) Intersection of race/ethnicity and socioeconomic status in mortality after breast cancer. J Community Health 40:1287–1299
25. Kolonel LN, Henderson BE, Hankin JH, Nomura AM, Wilkens LR, Pike MC et al (2000) A multiethnic cohort in Hawaii and Los Angeles: baseline characteristics. Am J Epidemiol 151:346–357
26. Pike MC, Kolonel LN, Henderson BE, Wilkens LR, Hankin JH, Feigelson HS et al (2002) Breast cancer in a multiethnic cohort in Hawaii and Los Angeles: risk factor-adjusted incidence in Japanese equals and in Hawaiians exceeds that in whites. Cancer Epidemiol Biomarkers Prev 11:795–800
27. Nomura AM, Hirohata T, Kolonel LN, Hankin JH, Lee J, Stemmermann G (1985) Breast cancer in Caucasian and Japanese women in Hawaii. Natl Cancer Inst Monogr 69:191–196
28. Hirohata T, Nomura AM, Hankin JH, Kolonel LN, Lee J (1987) An epidemiologic study on the association between diet and breast cancer. J Natl Cancer Inst 78:595–600
29. Wu AH, Vigen C, Razavi P, Tseng CC, Stancyzk FZ (2012) Alcohol and breast cancer risk among Asian-American women in Los Angeles County. Breast Cancer Res 14:R151
30. Wu AH, McKean-Cowdin R, Tseng CC (2011) Birth weight and other prenatal factors and risk of breast cancer in Asian-Americans. Breast Cancer Res Treat 130:917–925
31. Henderson BE, Pike MC, Casagrande JT (1981) Breast cancer and the oestrogen window hypothesis. Lancet 2:363–364
32. Apter D, Reinila M, Vihko R (1989) Some endocrine characteristics of early menarche, a risk factor for breast cancer, are preserved into adulthood. Int J Cancer 44:783–787
33. Collaborative Group on Hormonal Factors in Breast C (2012) Menarche, menopause, and breast cancer risk: individual participant meta-analysis, including 118 964 women with breast cancer from 117 epidemiological studies. Lancet Oncol 13:1141–1151
34. Wu AH, Ziegler RG, Pike MC, Nomura AM, West DW, Kolonel LN et al (1996) Menstrual and reproductive factors and risk of breast cancer in Asian-Americans. Br J Cancer 73:680–686
35. Wu AH, Yu MC, Tseng CC, Pike MC (2007) Body size, hormone therapy and risk of breast cancer in Asian-American women. Int J Cancer 120:844–852
36. Ursin G, Bernstein L, Wang Y, Lord SJ, Deapen D, Liff JM et al (2004) Reproductive factors and risk of breast carcinoma in a study of white and African–American women. Cancer 101:353–362
37. Hosokawa M, Imazeki S, Mizunuma H, Kubota T, Hayashi K (2012) Secular trends in age at menarche and time to establish regular menstrual cycling in Japanese women born between 1930 and 1985. BMC Womens Health 12:19
38. Cho GJ, Park HT, Shin JH, Hur JY, Kim YT, Kim SH et al (2010) Age at menarche in a Korean population: secular trends and influencing factors. Eur J Pediatr 169:89–94
39. Hoel DG, Wakabayashi T, Pike MC (1983) Secular trends in the distributions of the breast cancer risk factors—menarche, first birth, menopause, and weight—in Hiroshima and Nagasaki, Japan. Am J Epidemiol 118:78–89
40. Linos E, Spanos D, Rosner BA, Linos K, Hesketh T, Qu JD et al (2008) Effects of reproductive and demographic changes on breast cancer incidence in China: a modeling analysis. J Natl Cancer Inst 100:1352–1360
41. White KK, Park SY, Kolonel LN, Henderson BE, Wilkens LR (2012) Body size and breast cancer risk: the multiethnic cohort. Int J Cancer 131:E705–E716
42. Iwasaki M, Otani T, Inoue M, Sasazuki S, Tsugane S, Japan Public Health Center-based Prospective Study Group (2007) Role and impact of menstrual and reproductive factors on breast cancer risk in Japan. Eur J Cancer Prev 16:116–123
43. Tamakoshi K, Yatsuya H, Wakai K, Suzuki S, Nishio K, Lin Y et al (2005) Impact of menstrual and reproductive factors on breast cancer risk in Japan: results of the JACC Study. Cancer Sci 96:57–62

44. Bao PP, Shu XO, Gao YT, Zheng Y, Cai H, Deming SL et al (2011) Association of hormone-related characteristics and breast cancer risk by estrogen receptor/progesterone receptor status in the Shanghai Breast Cancer Study. Am J Epidemiol 174:661–671
45. Kawai M, Minami Y, Kuriyama S, Kakizaki M, Kakugawa Y, Nishino Y et al (2010) Reproductive factors, exogenous female hormone use and breast cancer risk in Japanese: the Miyagi Cohort Study. Cancer Causes Control 21:135–145
46. Collaborative Group on Hormonal Factors in Breast C (2002) Breast cancer and breastfeeding: collaborative reanalysis of individual data from 47 epidemiological studies in 30 countries, including 50302 women with breast cancer and 96973 women without the disease. Lancet 360:187–195
47. Tao SC, Yu MC, Ross RK, Xiu KW (1988) Risk factors for breast cancer in Chinese women of Beijing. Int J Cancer 42:495–498
48. Yuan JM, Yu MC, Ross RK, Gao YT, Henderson BE (1988) Risk factors for breast cancer in Chinese women in Shanghai. Cancer Res 48:1949–1953
49. Wang QS, Ross RK, Yu MC, Ning JP, Henderson BE, Kimm HT (1992) A case–control study of breast cancer in Tianjin, China. Cancer Epidemiol Biomarkers Prev 1:435–439
50. Nagata C, Mizoue T, Tanaka K, Tsuji I, Tamakoshi A, Wakai K et al (2012) Breastfeeding and breast cancer risk: an evaluation based on a systematic review of epidemiologic evidence among the Japanese population. Jpn J Clin Oncol 42:124–130
51. Wu AH, Vigen C, Lee, E, Tseng CC, Bulter LM (2016) Traditional breast cancer risk factors in Filipino Americans compared to Chinese and Japanese Americans in Los Angeles County. Cancer Epidemiol Biomarkers Prev. Aug 22 [Epub ahead of print]
52. Maskarinec G, Zhang Y, Takata Y, Pagano I, Shumay DM, Goodman MT et al (2006) Trends of breast cancer incidence and risk factor prevalence over 25 years. Breast Cancer Res Treat 98:45–55
53. Gold EB, Crawford SL, Avis NE, Crandall CJ, Matthews KA, Waetjen LE et al (2013) Factors related to age at natural menopause: longitudinal analyses from SWAN. Am J Epidemiol 178:70–83
54. Henderson KD, Bernstein L, Henderson B, Kolonel L, Pike MC (2008) Predictors of the timing of natural menopause in the Multiethnic Cohort Study. Am J Epidemiol 167:1287–1294
55. Ursin G, Wu AH, Hoover RN, West DW, Nomura AM, Kolonel LN et al (1999) Breast cancer and oral contraceptive use in Asian-American women. Am J Epidemiol 150:561–567
56. Ichida M, Kataoka A, Tsushima R, Taguchi T (2015) No increase in breast cancer risk in Japanese women taking oral contraceptives: a case–control study investigating reproductive, menstrual and familial risk factors for breast cancer. Asian Pac J Cancer Prev 16:3685–3690
57. Xu WH, Shu XO, Long J, Lu W, Cai Q, Zheng Y et al (2011) Relation of FGFR2 genetic polymorphisms to the association between oral contraceptive use and the risk of breast cancer in Chinese women. Am J Epidemiol 173:923–931
58. de Visser SJ, Uchida N, van Vliet-Daskalopoulou E, Fukazawa I, van Doorn MB, van den Heuvel MW et al (2003) Pharmacokinetic differences between Caucasian and Japanese subjects after single and multiple doses of a potential combined oral contraceptive (Org 30659 and EE). Contraception 68:195–202
59. Blode H, Kowal K, Roth K, Reif S (2012) Pharmacokinetics of drospirenone and ethinylestradiol in Caucasian and Japanese women. Eur J Contracept Reprod Health Care 17:284–297
60. Rossouw JE, Anderson GL, Prentice RL, LaCroix AZ, Kooperberg C, Stefanick ML et al (2002) Risks and benefits of estrogen plus progestin in healthy postmenopausal women: principal results from the Women's Health Initiative randomized controlled trial. JAMA 288:321–333
61. Lee S, Kolonel L, Wilkens L, Wan P, Henderson B, Pike M (2006) Postmenopausal hormone therapy and breast cancer risk: the multiethnic cohort. Int J Cancer 118:1285–1291
62. Key TJ, Appleby PN, Reeves GK, Roddam A, Dorgan JF, Longcope C et al (2003) Body mass index, serum sex hormones, and breast cancer risk in postmenopausal women. J Natl Cancer Inst 95:1218–1226

63. Van Den Brandt PA, Spiegelman D, Yaun SS, Adami HO, Beeson L, Folsom AR et al (2000) Pooled analysis of prospective cohort studies on height, weight, and breast cancer risk. Am J Epidemiol 152:514–527
64. Amadou A, Ferrari P, Muwonge R, Moskal A, Biessy C, Romieu I et al (2013) Overweight, obesity and risk of premenopausal breast cancer according to ethnicity: a systematic review and dose–response meta-analysis. Obes Rev 14:665–678
65. Ziegler RG, Hoover RN, Nomura AM, West DW, Wu AH, Pike MC et al (1996) Relative weight, weight change, height, and breast cancer risk in Asian-American women. J Natl Cancer Inst 88:650–660
66. Amadou A, Hainaut P, Romieu I (2013) Role of obesity in the risk of breast cancer: lessons from anthropometry. J Oncol 2013:906495
67. Renehan AG, Tyson M, Egger M, Heller RF, Zwahlen M (2008) Body-mass index and incidence of cancer: a systematic review and meta-analysis of prospective observational studies. Lancet 371:569–578
68. Wada K, Nagata C, Tamakoshi A, Matsuo K, Oze I, Wakai K et al (2014) Body mass index and breast cancer risk in Japan: a pooled analysis of eight population-based cohort studies. Ann Oncol 25:519–524
69. Suzuki R, Iwasaki M, Inoue M, Sasazuki S, Sawada N, Yamaji T et al (2011) Body weight at age 20 years, subsequent weight change and breast cancer risk defined by estrogen and progesterone receptor status—the Japan public health center-based prospective study. Int J Cancer 129:1214–1224
70. Shu XO, Jin F, Dai Q, Shi JR, Potter JD, Brinton LA et al (2001) Association of body size and fat distribution with risk of breast cancer among Chinese women. Int J Cancer 94:449–455
71. Suzuki S, Kojima M, Tokudome S, Mori M, Sakauchi F, Wakai K et al (2013) Obesity/weight gain and breast cancer risk: findings from the Japan collaborative cohort study for the evaluation of cancer risk. J Epidemiol 23:139–145
72. Trichopoulos D (1990) Hypothesis: does breast cancer originate in utero? Lancet 335:939–940
73. Xue F, Michels KB (2007) Intrauterine factors and risk of breast cancer: a systematic review and meta-analysis of current evidence. Lancet Oncol 8:1088–1100
74. dos Santos SI, de Stavola B, McCormack V, Collaborative Group on Pre-Natal Risk Factors and Subsequent Risk of Breast Cancer (2008) Birth size and breast cancer risk: re-analysis of individual participant data from 32 studies. PLoS Med 5:e193
75. Yang TO, Reeves GK, Green J, Beral V, Cairns BJ, Million Women Study C et al (2014) Birth weight and adult cancer incidence: large prospective study and meta-analysis. Ann Oncol 25:1836–1843
76. Le Marchand L, Kolonel LN, Myers BC, Mi MP (1988) Birth characteristics of premenopausal women with breast cancer. Br J Cancer 57:437–439
77. Sanderson M, Shu XO, Jin F, Dai Q, Ruan Z, Gao YT et al (2002) Weight at birth and adolescence and premenopausal breast cancer risk in a low-risk population. Br J Cancer 86:84–88
78. Kramer MS, Morin I, Yang H, Platt RW, Usher R, McNamara H et al (2002) Why are babies getting bigger? Temporal trends in fetal growth and its determinants. J Pediatr 141:538–542
79. Yu Z, Sun JQ, Haas JD, Gu Y, Li Z, Lin X (2008) Macrosomia is associated with high weight-for-height in children aged 1–3 years in Shanghai, China. Int J Obes (Lond) 32:55–60
80. Adair LS (2001) Size at birth predicts age at menarche. Pediatrics 107:E59
81. Morris DH, Jones ME, Schoemaker MJ, Ashworth A, Swerdlow AJ (2010) Determinants of age at menarche in the UK: analyses from the Breakthrough Generations Study. Br J Cancer 103(11):1760–1764
82. Tamimi RM, Eriksson L, Lagiou P, Czene K, Ekbom A, Hsieh CC et al (2010) Birth weight and mammographic density among postmenopausal women in Sweden. Int J Cancer 126:985–991
83. Cerhan JR, Sellers TA, Janney CA, Pankratz VS, Brandt KR, Vachon CM (2005) Prenatal and perinatal correlates of adult mammographic breast density. Cancer Epidemiol Biomarkers Prev 14:1502–1508

84. Bernstein L, Ross RK, Lobo RA, Hanisch R, Krailo MD, Henderson BE (1987) The effects of moderate physical activity on menstrual cycle patterns in adolescence: implications for breast cancer prevention. Br J Cancer 55:681–685
85. Frisch RE, Wyshak G, Albright NL, Albright TE, Schiff I, Jones KP et al (1985) Lower prevalence of breast cancer and cancers of the reproductive system among former college athletes compared to non-athletes. Br J Cancer 52:885–891
86. Wu Y, Zhang D, Kang S (2013) Physical activity and risk of breast cancer: a meta-analysis of prospective studies. Breast Cancer Res Treat 137:869–882
87. Suzuki S, Kojima M, Tokudome S, Mori M, Sakauchi F, Fujino Y et al (2008) Effect of physical activity on breast cancer risk: findings of the Japan Collaborative Cohort Study. Cancer Epidemiol Biomarkers Prev 17:3396–3401
88. Suzuki R, Iwasaki M, Yamamoto S, Inoue M, Sasazuki S, Sawada N et al (2011) Leisure-time physical activity and breast cancer risk defined by estrogen and progesterone receptor status—the Japan Public Health Center-Based Prospective Study. Prev Med 52:227–233
89. Pronk A, Ji BT, Shu XO, Chow WH, Xue S, Yang G et al (2011) Physical activity and breast cancer risk in Chinese women. Br J Cancer 105:1443–1450
90. Wolf I, Sadetzki S, Catane R, Karasik A, Kaufman B (2005) Diabetes mellitus and breast cancer. Lancet Oncol 6:103–111
91. Boyle P, Boniol M, Koechlin A, Robertson C, Valentini F, Coppens K et al (2012) Diabetes and breast cancer risk: a meta-analysis. Br J Cancer 107:1608–1617
92. Wu AH, Yu MC, Tseng CC, Stanczyk FZ, Pike MC (2007) Diabetes and risk of breast cancer in Asian-American women. Carcinogenesis 28:1561–1566
93. Sasazuki S, Charvat H, Hara A, Wakai K, Nagata C, Nakamura K et al (2013) Diabetes mellitus and cancer risk: pooled analysis of eight cohort studies in Japan. Cancer Sci 104:1499–1507
94. Jee SH, Ohrr H, Sull JW, Yun JE, Ji M, Samet JM (2005) Fasting serum glucose level and cancer risk in Korean men and women. JAMA 293:194–202
95. Key J, Hodgson S, Omar RZ, Jensen TK, Thompson SG, Boobis AR et al (2006) Meta-analysis of studies of alcohol and breast cancer with consideration of the methodological issues. Cancer Causes Control 17:759–770
96. Brown LM, Gridley G, Wu AH, Falk RT, Hauptmann M, Kolonel LN et al (2010) Low level alcohol intake, cigarette smoking and risk of breast cancer in Asian-American women. Breast Cancer Res Treat 120:203–210
97. Park SY, Kolonel LN, Lim U, White KK, Henderson BE, Wilkens LR (2014) Alcohol consumption and breast cancer risk among women from five ethnic groups with light to moderate intakes: the Multiethnic Cohort Study. Int J Cancer 134:1504–1510
98. Lin Y, Kikuchi S, Tamakoshi A, Wakai K, Kawamura T, Iso H et al (2005) Alcohol consumption and mortality among middle-aged and elderly Japanese men and women. Ann Epidemiol 15:590–597
99. Suzuki R, Orsini N, Mignone L, Saji S, Wolk A (2008) Alcohol intake and risk of breast cancer defined by estrogen and progesterone receptor status—a meta-analysis of epidemiological studies. Int J Cancer 122:1832–1841
100. Park SY, Kolonel LN, Henderson BE, Wilkens LR (2012) Dietary fat and breast cancer in postmenopausal women according to ethnicity and hormone receptor status: the Multiethnic Cohort Study. Cancer Prev Res (Phila) 5:216–228
101. Hunter DJ, Spiegelman D, Adami HO, Beeson L, van den Brandt PA, Folsom AR et al (1996) Cohort studies of fat intake and the risk of breast cancer—a pooled analysis. N Engl J Med 334:356–361
102. Boyd NF, Stone J, Vogt KN, Connelly BS, Martin LJ, Minkin S (2003) Dietary fat and breast cancer risk revisited: a meta-analysis of the published literature. Br J Cancer 89:1672–1685
103. Prentice RL, Caan B, Chlebowski RT, Patterson R, Kuller LH, Ockene JK et al (2006) Low-fat dietary pattern and risk of invasive breast cancer: the women's health initiative randomized controlled dietary modification trial. JAMA 295:629–642

104. Thomson CA, Van Horn L, Caan BJ, Aragaki AK, Chlebowski RT, Manson JE et al (2014) Cancer incidence and mortality during the intervention and postintervention periods of the women's health initiative dietary modification trial. Cancer Epidemiol Biomarkers Prev 23:2924–2935
105. Thiebaut AC, Kipnis V, Chang SC, Subar AF, Thompson FE, Rosenberg PS et al (2007) Dietary fat and postmenopausal invasive breast cancer in the National Institutes of Health-AARP Diet and Health Study Cohort. J Natl Cancer Inst 99:451–462
106. Sieri S, Chiodini P, Agnoli C, Pala V, Berrino F, Trichopoulou A et al (2014) Dietary fat intake and development of specific breast cancer subtypes. J Natl Cancer Inst 106:dju068
107. Sczaniecka AK, Brasky TM, Lampe JW, Patterson RE, White E (2012) Dietary intake of specific fatty acids and breast cancer risk among postmenopausal women in the VITAL cohort. Nutr Cancer 64:1131–1142
108. Zheng JS, Hu XJ, Zhao YM, Yang J, Li D (2013) Intake of fish and marine n-3 polyunsaturated fatty acids and risk of breast cancer: meta-analysis of data from 21 independent prospective cohort studies. BMJ 346:f3706
109. Gago-Dominguez M, Yuan JM, Sun CL, Lee HP, Yu MC (2003) Opposing effects of dietary n-3 and n-6 fatty acids on mammary carcinogenesis: the Singapore Chinese Health Study. Br J Cancer 89:1686–1692
110. Murff HJ, Shu XO, Li H, Yang G, Wu X, Cai H et al (2011) Dietary polyunsaturated fatty acids and breast cancer risk in Chinese women: a prospective cohort study. Int J Cancer 128:1434–1441
111. Wakai K, Tamakoshi K, Date C, Fukui M, Suzuki S, Lin Y et al (2005) Dietary intakes of fat and fatty acids and risk of breast cancer: a prospective study in Japan. Cancer Sci 96:590–599
112. Yang B, Ren XL, Fu YQ, Gao JL, Li D (2014) Ratio of n-3/n-6 PUFAs and risk of breast cancer: a meta-analysis of 274135 adult females from 11 independent prospective studies. BMC Cancer 14:105
113. Kiyabu GY, Inoue M, Saito E, Abe SK, Sawada N, Ishihara J et al (2015) Fish, n-3 polyunsaturated fatty acids and n-6 polyunsaturated fatty acids intake and breast cancer risk: the Japan Public Health Center-Based Prospective Study. Int J Cancer 137:2915–2926
114. Alexander DD, Morimoto LM, Mink PJ, Cushing CA (2010) A review and meta-analysis of red and processed meat consumption and breast cancer. Nutr Res Rev 23:349–365
115. Missmer SA, Smith-Warner SA, Spiegelman D, Yaun SS, Adami HO, Beeson WL et al (2002) Meat and dairy food consumption and breast cancer: a pooled analysis of cohort studies. Int J Epidemiol 31:78–85
116. Guo J, Wei W, Zhan L (2015) Red and processed meat intake and risk of breast cancer: a meta-analysis of prospective studies. Breast Cancer Res Treat 151:191–198
117. Wu AH, Yu MC, Tseng CC, Stanczyk FZ, Pike MC (2009) Dietary patterns and breast cancer risk in Asian American women. Am J Clin Nutr 89:1145–1154
118. Dai Q, Shu XO, Jin F, Gao YT, Ruan ZX, Zheng W (2002) Consumption of animal foods, cooking methods, and risk of breast cancer. Cancer Epidemiol Biomarkers Prev 11:801–808
119. Bao PP, Shu XO, Zheng Y, Cai H, Ruan ZX, Gu K et al (2012) Fruit, vegetable, and animal food intake and breast cancer risk by hormone receptor status. Nutr Cancer 64:806–819
120. Kallianpur AR, Lee SA, Gao YT, Lu W, Zheng Y, Ruan ZX et al (2008) Dietary animal-derived iron and fat intake and breast cancer risk in the Shanghai Breast Cancer Study. Breast Cancer Res Treat 107:123–132
121. Inoue-Choi M, Sinha R, Gierach GL, Ward MH (2015) Red and processed meat, nitrite, and heme iron intakes and postmenopausal breast cancer risk in the NIH-AARP Diet and Health Study. Int J Cancer 138(7):1609–1618
122. Sinha R (2002) An epidemiologic approach to studying heterocyclic amines. Mutat Res 506–507:197–204
123. Jung S, Spiegelman D, Baglietto L, Bernstein L, Boggs DA, van den Brandt PA et al (2013) Fruit and vegetable intake and risk of breast cancer by hormone receptor status. J Natl Cancer Inst 105:219–236

124. Suzuki R, Iwasaki M, Hara A, Inoue M, Sasazuki S, Sawada N et al (2013) Fruit and vegetable intake and breast cancer risk defined by estrogen and progesterone receptor status: the Japan Public Health Center-Based Prospective Study. Cancer Causes Control 24:2117–2128
125. Butler LM, Wu AH, Wang R, Koh WP, Yuan JM, Yu MC (2010) A vegetable-fruit-soy dietary pattern protects against breast cancer among postmenopausal Singapore Chinese women. Am J Clin Nutr 91(4):1013–1019
126. Liu X, Lv K (2013) Cruciferous vegetables intake is inversely associated with risk of breast cancer: a meta-analysis. Breast 22:309–313
127. Eliassen AH, Hendrickson SJ, Brinton LA, Buring JE, Campos H, Dai Q et al (2012) Circulating carotenoids and risk of breast cancer: pooled analysis of eight prospective studies. J Natl Cancer Inst 104:1905–1916
128. Wu AH, Ziegler RG, Horn-Ross PL, Nomura AM, West DW, Kolonel LN et al (1996) Tofu and risk of breast cancer in Asian-Americans. Cancer Epidemiol Biomarkers Prev 5:901–906
129. Wu AH, Wan P, Hankin J, Tseng CC, Yu MC, Pike MC (2002) Adolescent and adult soy intake and risk of breast cancer in Asian-Americans. Carcinogenesis 23:1491–1496
130. Wu AH, Yu MC, Tseng CC, Pike MC (2008) Epidemiology of soy exposures and breast cancer risk. Br J Cancer 98:9–14
131. Morimoto Y, Maskarinec G, Park SY, Ettienne R, Matsuno RK, Long C et al (2014) Dietary isoflavone intake is not statistically significantly associated with breast cancer risk in the multiethnic cohort. Br J Nutr 112:976–983
132. Goodman MT, Shvetsov YB, Wilkens LR, Franke AA, Le Marchand L, Kakazu KK et al (2009) Urinary phytoestrogen excretion and postmenopausal breast cancer risk: the Multiethnic Cohort Study. Cancer Prev Res (Phila) 2:887–894
133. Dong JY, Qin LQ (2011) Soy isoflavones consumption and risk of breast cancer incidence or recurrence: a meta-analysis of prospective studies. Breast Cancer Res Treat 125:315–323
134. Nagata C, Mizoue T, Tanaka K, Tsuji I, Tamakoshi A, Matsuo K et al (2014) Soy intake and breast cancer risk: an evaluation based on a systematic review of epidemiologic evidence among the Japanese population. Jpn J Clin Oncol 44:282–295
135. Hirose K, Matsuo K, Iwata H, Tajima K (2007) Dietary patterns and the risk of breast cancer in Japanese women. Cancer Sci 98:1431–1438
136. Cho YA, Kim J, Shin A, Park KS, Ro J (2010) Dietary patterns and breast cancer risk in Korean women. Nutr Cancer 62:1161–1169
137. Zhang CX, Ho SC, Fu JH, Cheng SZ, Chen YM, Lin FY (2011) Dietary patterns and breast cancer risk among Chinese women. Cancer Causes Control 22:115–124
138. Cui X, Dai Q, Tseng M, Shu XO, Gao YT, Zheng W (2007) Dietary patterns and breast cancer risk in the Shanghai Breast Cancer Study. Cancer Epidemiol Biomarkers Prev 16:1443–1448
139. Yang CS, Wang X, Lu G, Picinich SC (2009) Cancer prevention by tea: animal studies, molecular mechanisms and human relevance. Nat Rev Cancer 9:429–439
140. Wu AH, Yu MC, Tseng CC, Hankin J, Pike MC (2003) Green tea and risk of breast cancer in Asian Americans. Int J Cancer 106:574–579
141. Shrubsole MJ, Lu W, Chen Z, Shu XO, Zheng Y, Dai Q et al (2009) Drinking green tea modestly reduces breast cancer risk. J Nutr 139:310–316
142. Zhang M, Holman CD, Huang JP, Xie X (2007) Green tea and the prevention of breast cancer: a case–control study in Southeast China. Carcinogenesis 28:1074–1078
143. Wu AH, Butler LM (2011) Green tea and breast cancer. Mol Nutr Food Res 55:921–930
144. Iwasaki M, Inoue M, Sasazuki S, Sawada N, Yamaji T, Shimazu T et al (2010) Green tea drinking and subsequent risk of breast cancer in a population to based cohort of Japanese women. Breast Cancer Res 12(5):R88
145. Nagano J, Kono S, Preston DL, Mabuchi K (2001) A prospective study of green tea consumption and cancer incidence, Hiroshima and Nagasaki (Japan). Cancer Causes Control 12:501–508
146. Suzuki Y, Tsubono Y, Nakaya N, Koizumi Y, Tsuji I (2004) Green tea and the risk of breast cancer: pooled analysis of two prospective studies in Japan. Br J Cancer 90:1361–1363

147. Yuan JM, Koh WP, Sun CL, Lee HP, Yu MC (2005) Green tea intake, ACE gene polymorphism and breast cancer risk among Chinese women in Singapore. Carcinogenesis 26:1389–1394
148. Inoue M, Robien K, Wang R, Van Den Berg DJ, Koh WP, Yu MC (2008) Green tea intake, MTHFR/TYMS genotype and breast cancer risk: the Singapore Chinese Health Study. Carcinogenesis 29:1967–1972
149. Dai Q, Shu XO, Li H, Yang G, Shrubsole MJ, Cai H et al (2010) Is green tea drinking associated with a later onset of breast cancer? Ann Epidemiol 20:74–81
150. Sun CL, Yuan JM, Koh WP, Yu MC (2006) Green tea, black tea and breast cancer risk: a meta-analysis of epidemiological studies. Carcinogenesis 27:1310–1315
151. IARC Working Group on the Evaluation of Carcinogenic Risks to Humans (2004) Tobacco smoke and involuntary smoking. IARC Monogr Eval Carcinog Risks Hum 83:1–1438
152. Secretan B, Straif K, Baan R, Grosse Y, El Ghissassi F, Bouvard V et al (2009) A review of human carcinogens—Part E: tobacco, areca nut, alcohol, coal smoke, and salted fish. Lancet Oncol 10:1033–1034
153. Baron JA, La Vecchia C, Levi F (1990) The antiestrogenic effect of cigarette smoking in women. Am J Obstet Gynecol 162:502–514
154. Endogenous Hormones and Breast Cancer Collaborative Group (2011) Circulating sex hormones and breast cancer risk factors in postmenopausal women: reanalysis of 13 studies. Br J Cancer 105:709–722
155. Setiawan VW, Haiman CA, Stanczyk FZ, Le Marchand L, Henderson BE (2006) Racial/ethnic differences in postmenopausal endogenous hormones: the Multiethnic Cohort Study. Cancer Epidemiol Biomarkers Prev 15:1849–1855
156. General ARotS (2014) The health consequences of smoking—50 years of progress: a report of the Surgeon General. U.S. Department of Health and Human Services, Atlanta, GA
157. Catsburg C, Miller AB, Rohan TE (2015) Active cigarette smoking and risk of breast cancer. Int J Cancer 136:2204–2209
158. Dossus L, Boutron-Ruault MC, Kaaks R, Gram IT, Vilier A, Fervers B et al (2014) Active and passive cigarette smoking and breast cancer risk: results from the EPIC cohort. Int J Cancer 134:1871–1888
159. Gaudet MM, Gapstur SM, Sun J, Diver WR, Hannan LM, Thun MJ (2013) Active smoking and breast cancer risk: original cohort data and meta-analysis. J Natl Cancer Inst 105:515–525
160. Gram IT, Park SY, Kolonel LN, Maskarinec G, Wilkens LR, Henderson BE et al (2015) Smoking and risk of breast cancer in a racially/ethnically diverse population of mainly women who do not drink alcohol: the MEC Study. Am J Epidemiol 182:917–925
161. Hanaoka T, Yamamoto S, Sobue T, Sasaki S, Tsugane S, Japan Public Health Center-Based Prospective Study on Cancer and Cardiovascular Disease Study Group (2005) Active and passive smoking and breast cancer risk in middle-aged Japanese women. Int J Cancer 114:317–322
162. Nagata C, Mizoue T, Tanaka K, Tsuji I, Wakai K, Inoue M et al (2006) Tobacco smoking and breast cancer risk: an evaluation based on a systematic review of epidemiological evidence among the Japanese population. Jpn J Clin Oncol 36:387–394
163. Lin Y, Kikuchi S, Tamakoshi K, Wakai K, Kondo T, Niwa Y et al (2008) Active smoking, passive smoking, and breast cancer risk: findings from the Japan Collaborative Cohort Study for Evaluation of Cancer Risk. J Epidemiol 18:77–83
164. Chen Z, Shao J, Gao X, Li X (2015) Effect of passive smoking on female breast cancer in China: a meta-analysis. Asia Pac J Public Health 27:NP58–NP64
165. Yang Y, Zhang F, Skrip L, Wang Y, Liu S (2013) Lack of an association between passive smoking and incidence of female breast cancer in non-smokers: evidence from 10 prospective cohort studies. PLoS One 8:e77029
166. Nishino Y, Tsubono Y, Tsuji I, Komatsu S, Kanemura S, Nakatsuka H et al (2001) Passive smoking at home and cancer risk: a population-based prospective study in Japanese non-smoking women. Cancer Causes Control 12:797–802

167. Wada K, Kawachi T, Hori A, Takeyama N, Tanabashi S, Matsushita S et al (2015) Husband's smoking status and breast cancer risk in Japan: from the Takayama Study. Cancer Sci 106:455–460
168. Pharoah PD, Day NE, Duffy S, Easton DF, Ponder BA (1997) Family history and the risk of breast cancer: a systematic review and meta-analysis. Int J Cancer 71:800–809
169. Huang Z, Beeghly-Fadiel A, Gao YT, Zheng Y, Dai Q, Lu W et al (2014) Associations of reproductive time events and intervals with breast cancer risk: a report from the Shanghai Breast Cancer Study. Int J Cancer 135:186–195
170. Lee CP, Irwanto A, Salim A, Yuan JM, Liu J, Koh WP et al (2014) Breast cancer risk assessment using genetic variants and risk factors in a Singapore Chinese population. Breast Cancer Res 16:R64
171. Kurian AW (2010) BRCA1 and BRCA2 mutations across race and ethnicity: distribution and clinical implications. Curr Opin Obstet Gynecol 22:72–78
172. Kurian AW, Gong GD, Chun NM, Mills MA, Staton AD, Kingham KE et al (2008) Performance of BRCA1/2 mutation prediction models in Asian Americans. J Clin Oncol 26:4752–4758
173. Kwong A, Shin VY, Ho JC, Kang E, Nakamura S, Teo SH et al (2015) Comprehensive spectrum of BRCA1 and BRCA2 deleterious mutations in breast cancer in Asian countries. J Med Genet 53(1):15–23
174. Ghoussaini M, Pharoah PD, Easton DF (2013) Inherited genetic susceptibility to breast cancer: the beginning of the end or the end of the beginning? Am J Pathol 183:1038–1051
175. Michailidou K, Hall P, Gonzalez-Neira A, Ghoussaini M, Dennis J, Milne RL et al (2013) Large-scale genotyping identifies 41 new loci associated with breast cancer risk. Nat Genet 45:353–361, 61e1-2
176. Michailidou K, Beesley J, Lindstrom S, Canisius S, Dennis J, Lush MJ et al (2015) Genome-wide association analysis of more than 120,000 individuals identifies 15 new susceptibility loci for breast cancer. Nat Genet 47:373–380
177. Cai Q, Zhang B, Sung H, Low SK, Kweon SS, Lu W et al (2014) Genome-wide association analysis in East Asians identifies breast cancer susceptibility loci at 1q32.1, 5q14.3 and 15q26.1. Nat Genet 46:886–890
178. Zheng W, Zhang B, Cai Q, Sung H, Michailidou K, Shi J et al (2013) Common genetic determinants of breast-cancer risk in East Asian women: a collaborative study of 23 637 breast cancer cases and 25 579 controls. Hum Mol Genet 22:2539–2550
179. Kim HC, Lee JY, Sung H, Choi JY, Park SK, Lee KM et al (2012) A genome-wide association study identifies a breast cancer risk variant in ERBB4 at 2q34: results from the Seoul Breast Cancer Study. Breast Cancer Res 14:R56
180. Pike MC (1983) Hormonal risk factors, breast tissue age, and the age-incidence of breast cancer. Nature 303:767–770
181. Henderson BE, Ross RK, Pike MC, Casagrande JT (1982) Endogenous hormones as a major factor in human cancer. Cancer Res 42:3232–3239
182. Henderson BE, Feigelson HS (2000) Hormonal carcinogenesis. Carcinogenesis 21:427–433
183. Key T, Appleby P, Barnes I, Reeves G (2002) Endogenous sex hormones and breast cancer in postmenopausal women: reanalysis of nine prospective studies. J Natl Cancer Inst 94: 606–616
184. Woolcott CG, Shvetsov YB, Stanczyk FZ, Wilkens LR, White KK, Caberto C et al (2010) Plasma sex hormone concentrations and breast cancer risk in an ethnically diverse population of postmenopausal women: the Multiethnic Cohort Study. Endocr Relat Cancer 17:125–134
185. Kaaks R, Tikk K, Sookthai D, Schock H, Johnson T, Tjonneland A et al (2014) Premenopausal serum sex hormone levels in relation to breast cancer risk, overall and by hormone receptor status—results from the EPIC cohort. Int J Cancer 134:1947–1957
186. Eliassen AH, Missmer SA, Tworoger SS, Spiegelman D, Barbieri RL, Dowsett M et al (2006) Endogenous steroid hormone concentrations and risk of breast cancer among premenopausal women. J Natl Cancer Inst 98:1406–1415

187. Wu AH, Bernstein L (1998) Breast cancer among Asian Americans and Pacific Islanders. Asian Am Pac Isl J Health 6:327–343
188. Bernstein L, Ross RK (1993) Endogenous hormones and breast cancer risk. Epidemiol Rev 15:48–65
189. Randolph JF Jr, Sowers M, Gold EB, Mohr BA, Luborsky J, Santoro N et al (2003) Reproductive hormones in the early menopausal transition: relationship to ethnicity, body size, and menopausal status. J Clin Endocrinol Metab 88:1516–1522
190. Falk RT, Fears TR, Hoover RN, Pike MC, Wu AH, Nomura AM et al (2002) Does place of birth influence endogenous hormone levels in Asian-American women? Br J Cancer 87:54–60
191. Falk RT, Fears TR, Xu X, Hoover RN, Pike MC, Wu AH et al (2005) Urinary estrogen metabolites and their ratio among Asian American women. Cancer Epidemiol Biomarkers Prev 14:221–226
192. Boyd NF, Lockwood GA, Martin LJ, Knight JA, Byng JW, Yaffe MJ et al (1998) Mammographic densities and breast cancer risk. Breast Dis 10:113–126
193. Boyd NF, Rommens JM, Vogt K, Lee V, Hopper JL, Yaffe MJ et al (2005) Mammographic breast density as an intermediate phenotype for breast cancer. Lancet Oncol 6:798–808
194. Byrne C, Schairer C, Wolfe J, Parekh N, Salane M, Brinton LA et al (1995) Mammographic features and breast cancer risk: effects with time, age, and menopause status. J Natl Cancer Inst 87:1622–1629
195. Ursin G, Ma H, Wu AH, Bernstein L, Salane M, Parisky YR et al (2003) Mammographic density and breast cancer in three ethnic groups. Cancer Epidemiol Biomarkers Prev 12:332–338
196. Maskarinec G, Pagano I, Lurie G, Wilkens LR, Kolonel LN (2005) Mammographic density and breast cancer risk: the Multiethnic Cohort Study. Am J Epidemiol 162:743–752
197. Wong CS, Lim GH, Gao F, Jakes RW, Offman J, Chia KS et al (2011) Mammographic density and its interaction with other breast cancer risk factors in an Asian population. Br J Cancer 104:871–874
198. Maskarinec G, Takata Y, Kaaks R (2005) The relation between nutritional factors and insulin-like growth factor-I in premenopausal women of different ethnicity. Eur J Nutr 44:105–113
199. Chen Z, Wu AH, Gauderman WJ, Bernstein L, Ma H, Pike MC et al (2004) Does mammographic density reflect ethnic differences in breast cancer incidence rates? Am J Epidemiol 159:140–147
200. Habel LA, Capra AM, Oestreicher N, Greendale GA, Cauley JA, Bromberger J et al (2007) Mammographic density in a multiethnic cohort. Menopause 14:891–899
201. Maskarinec G, Lyu LC, Meng L, Theriault A, Ursin G (2001) Determinants of mammographic densities among women of Asian, native Hawaiian, and Caucasian ancestry. Ethn Dis 11:44–50
202. Maskarinec G, Nagata C, Shimizu H, Kashiki Y (2002) Comparison of mammographic densities and their determinants in women from Japan and Hawaii. Int J Cancer 102:29–33
203. Maskarinec G, Pagano I, Chen Z, Nagata C, Gram IT (2007) Ethnic and geographic differences in mammographic density and their association with breast cancer incidence. Breast Cancer Res Treat 104:47–56
204. Tseng M, Byrne C, Evers KA, London WT, Daly MB (2006) Acculturation and breast density in foreign-born U.S. Chinese women. Cancer Epidemiol Biomarkers Prev 15:1301–1305
205. Boyd NF, Dite GS, Stone J, Gunasekara A, English DR, McCredie MR et al (2002) Heritability of mammographic density, a risk factor for breast cancer. N Engl J Med 347:886–894
206. Pankow JS, Vachon CM, Kuni CC, King RA, Arnett DK, Grabrick DM et al (1997) Genetic analysis of mammographic breast density in adult women: evidence of a gene effect. J Natl Cancer Inst 89:549–556
207. Ursin G, Lillie EO, Lee E, Cockburn M, Schork NJ, Cozen W et al (2009) The relative importance of genetics and environment on mammographic density. Cancer Epidemiol Biomarkers Prev 18:102–112

208. Lindstrom S, Vachon CM, Li J, Varghese J, Thompson D, Warren R et al (2011) Common variants in ZNF365 are associated with both mammographic density and breast cancer risk. Nat Genet 43:185–187
209. Vachon CM, Scott CG, Fasching PA, Hall P, Tamimi RM, Li J et al (2012) Common breast cancer susceptibility variants in LSP1 and RAD51L1 are associated with mammographic density measures that predict breast cancer risk. Cancer Epidemiol Biomarkers Prev 21:1156–1166
210. Odefrey F, Stone J, Gurrin LC, Byrnes GB, Apicella C, Dite GS et al (2010) Common genetic variants associated with breast cancer and mammographic density measures that predict disease. Cancer Res 70:1449–1458
211. Lee E, Hsu C, Van den Berg D, Ursin G, Koh WP, Yuan JM et al (2012) Genetic variation in peroxisome proliferator-activated receptor gamma, soy, and mammographic density in Singapore Chinese women. Cancer Epidemiol Biomarkers Prev 21:635–644
212. Lee E, Van Den Berg D, Hsu C, Ursin G, Koh WP, Yuan JM et al (2013) Genetic variation in transforming growth factor beta 1 and mammographic density in Singapore Chinese women. Cancer Res 73:1876–1882
213. Mariapun S, Ho WK, Kang PC, Li J, Lindstrom S, Yip CH et al (2016) Variants in 6q25.1 are associated with mammographic density in Malaysian Chinese women. Cancer Epidemiol Biomarkers Prev 25:327–333
214. Research UCFHP (2014) Asians below state average for timely mammograms. www.chis.ucla.edu
215. Ryu SY, Crespi CM, Maxwell AE (2013) What factors explain disparities in mammography rates among Asian-American immigrant women? A population-based study in California. Womens Health Issues 23:e403–e410
216. Naghavi M and Global Burden of Disease Cancer Collaboration (2015) The global burden of cancer 2013. JAMA Oncol 1(4):505–527

Endometrial Cancer Among Asian Americans

Veronica Wendy Setiawan

Abstract Endometrial cancer is the most common cancer of the female reproductive organs. While the incidence rates of endometrial cancer in Asian Americans are lower relative to non-Hispanic whites, their rates are increasing steadily. Between 1990 and 2008, all Asian groups in the United States (USA) have experienced a statistically significant annual increase in endometrial cancer incidence. Migrant studies showed that US-born Asians had higher endometrial cancer incidence than among their Asian-born counterparts suggesting that environmental exposures in Asian Americans may explain these observed increases. In this chapter, we discuss the epidemiology of endometrial cancer including tumor characteristics, risk factors (lifestyle and genetics), and survivorship in Asian-American women.

Keywords Asian Americans • Endometrium • Obesity • Diabetes • Exogenous hormones

Introduction

Clinical Description of Endometrial Cancer

Endometrial cancer is a type of cancer that starts in the cells that line the uterus. The most common type of endometrial cancer is endometrioid adenocarcinomas which are cancers of the cells that form glands in the endometrium. Endometrial cancer is rare in women under 45 years of age, and approximately 75 % of cases are found in women aged 55 and older. The majority (up to 80 %) of endometrial tumors are type I which are of endometrioid histology, present at an early stage, and have good

V.W. Setiawan, Ph.D. (✉)
Department of Preventive Medicine, Keck School of Medicine, University of Southern California, 1450 Biggy Street, Room 1517G, Los Angeles, CA 90033, USA
e-mail: vsetiawa@med.usc.edu

A.H. Wu, D.O. Stram (eds.), *Cancer Epidemiology Among Asian Americans*,
DOI 10.1007/978-3-319-41118-7_9

prognosis. The much less common types (up to 20 %), type II, are of serous or clear cell histology and are associated with poor prognosis. The key symptom of endometrial cancer is abnormal vaginal bleeding which present in 90 % of endometrial cancer patients. Because the majority of endometrial cancers are found at an early stage, the overall prognosis for this cancer is generally good. The established treatments for endometrial cancer include surgery, radiation therapy, hormonal therapy, and chemotherapy which depend largely on the type of cancer and stage of the disease when it is diagnosed.

Descriptive Epidemiology

Endometrial Cancer Trends

In the USA, endometrial cancer is the most common cancer of the female reproductive organs and the fourth most common cancer in women with estimated 60,050 incident cases and 10,470 deaths in 2016 [1]. Relative to non-Hispanic whites, the incidence rates of endometrial cancer in Asian Americans are lower, but their rates are increasing [2], while the rates among non-Hispanic whites are stable [3]. Approximately 7600 cases were diagnosed per year in Asian-American women [4]. Cancer incidence data from 13 Surveillance, Epidemiology, and End Results (SEER) registries show that endometrial cancer is the fourth most frequent incident cancer in Chinese-, Filipina-, and Japanese Americans during 2004–2008. Among Asian ethnic groups, the overall incidence rates are highest in Filipina- (22.0 per 100,000) and Japanese Americans (20.0 per 100,000) which are approaching the rates in non-Hispanic whites (26.3 per 100,000) [2]. While endometrial cancer is the third most frequent cancer diagnosed in Asian Indian/Pakistani women, the rate of 16.4 (per 100,000) is lower compared to Filipina- and Japanese Americans but similar to the rates of Chinese Americans (14.3 per 100,000) [2]. Between 1990 and 2008, all Asian groups have experienced a statistically significant annual increase in endometrial cancer incidence: 1 % in Japanese, 3 % in both Asian Indians and Filipinas, and 7 % in Chinese, while the rates in non-Hispanic whites remain stable [2].

Figure 1 shows the age-adjusted incidence rates of endometrial cancer by racial/ethnic group (non-Hispanic whites and Asian-American ethnic group) from the same 13 SEER registries with additional 2 years of observation (1990–2010); patterns were similar to that described above. While the rates among Asian groups are still lower than those of non-Hispanic whites, the rates in all Asian subgroups (i.e., Japanese, Chinese, Filipinos, Koreans, Vietnamese) have continued to increase steadily. The rates in Filipino (22.9 per 100,000) and Japanese (20.3 per 100,000) women in 2008–2010 are approaching the rates of non-Hispanic white women (27.1 per 100,000). Of particular interest is the substantial increase in rate among Filipinas. Among these Asian subgroups, Korean women have the lowest rate; the incidence rate in 2008–2010 was 7.9 per 100,000. Changes in the prevalence of endometrial cancer risk factors, especially overweight and obesity, may explain these observed increases.

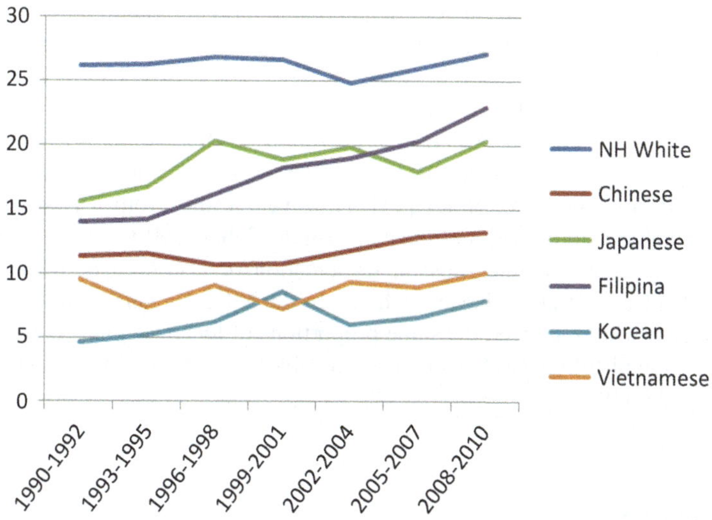

Fig. 1 Age-adjusted incidence rates of endometrial cancer per 100,000 SEER 13 1990–2010

Migrant Studies of Endometrial Cancer

Studies of women emigrating from low-risk countries to the USA and studies of descendants of these women show that the incidence of endometrial cancer is highest in whites, intermediate in Asians born in the USA, and lowest in Asian-American women born in Asia [5]. US-born Chinese and Japanese had higher endometrial cancer incidence than their Asian-born counterparts, but the rates among US-born and Asian-born Filipino women were similar [5]. While incidence rates for endometrial cancer was lower among Koreans in the USA than whites, the rates of Korean Americans were 2.9 times higher than the rates in Korea [6]. Recent data from Korea showed that between 1999 and 2012, the incidence rates of endometrial cancer have been increasing steadily, with an average annual percentage increase of 5.8 % [7].

A study covering data from 2001–2009 among Asians in the USA showed that US-born Asian women were more likely to be diagnosed with type I endometrial cancer (i.e., endometrioid histology, early stage) compared with foreign-born Asians (65 % vs. 56 %; $P<0.01$) [8]. These migrant studies suggest that possible environmental and/or cultural differences in the exposure to endometrial cancer risk factors may include differences in the prevalence of obesity, menopausal hormone use, and/or dietary patterns as discussed below.

Endometrial Cancer Characteristics in US Asians

While differences in tumor characteristics between African Americans and non-Hispanic whites are widely recognized, with African Americans more likely to be diagnosed with higher stage, grade, and more aggressive type II tumors [9–11], very little data are available in Asian-American populations [12]. Based on studies using data from the SEER program, compared to whites, Asian-American women tended to present at a younger age at diagnosis (58 years in Asians vs. 65 in whites) [12, 13]. Furthermore, recent data (1988 to 2009) showed a slightly higher prevalence of advanced stage disease (III–IV) (15.6 % vs. 13.3 %; $p=0.04$) and aggressive histology subtypes (serous/clear cell) (10.6 % vs. 9.6 %; $p=0.04$) among Asian women compared to non-Hispanic whites [13]. However, results from a Department of Defense database study [14] and the Multiethnic Cohort (MEC) [9] did not show significant difference in the stage at presentation or histology between Asians/Pacific Islanders and non-Hispanic whites. In the MEC, Japanese Americans and non-Hispanic whites showed the same proportions of localized cancers (82 %) and nonaggressive histology (91 %) and a comparable proportion of high grade tumors (20 % vs. 19 %) [9].

Risk Factors

Epidemiologic studies have identified several risk factors associated with an increased risk of endometrial cancer. Most of these factors are related to an imbalance between estrogen and progesterone exposures, including the use of unopposed estrogen therapy and obesity. The use of combined oral contraceptives (OCs), which is associated with progesterone-dominant states, reduces the risk of endometrial cancer. Other hormonal risk factors include nulliparity, early menarche, and late menopause. Smoking has been associated with reduced risk, while metabolic syndrome including type 2 diabetes has been associated with higher risk of developing endometrial cancer. The majority of these etiologic studies have been conducted in non-Hispanic white populations. There have been a few analytic epidemiologic studies of endometrial cancer in Asian Americans; these include a case–control study conducted among Japanese, Chinese, and Korean women in Hawaii [15] and the prospective Multiethnic Cohort (MEC) that included a large number of Japanese Americans [9]. There are very few large endometrial cancer studies in Asia; they include a population-based case–control study in Shanghai, China [16], and a prospective cohort study in Japan [17].

Obesity

In the USA, the majority of epidemiologic studies have been conducted in non-Hispanic whites. A few migrant studies among Asian Americans suggest potential influences of diet and lifestyle exposures on endometrial cancer etiology. Obesity is one of the strongest risk factors for endometrial cancer. The exact biological mechanism is unknown, but it is thought that the effect of excess fat on endometrial cancer is mediated through endogenous hormones. In postmenopausal women, adipose tissue is the primary source of estrogen production by aromatization of androstenedione. Obesity has been associated with increased production rates of androgens, increased peripheral conversion of androgens to estrogens, and decreased levels of progesterone and sex hormone-binding globulin. Increased exposures to estrogens unopposed by progesterone in obese women may stimulate mitotic activity of endometrial cells, leading to hyperplasia and subsequent cancer [18].

Data from the National Longitudinal Study of Adolescent Health showed that the acculturation to American diet and lifestyles, including a high-fat diet and decreases in physical activity, was associated with an increase in obesity in first-generation migrants which further increased in successive generations [19]. This is consistent with the observed increase in endometrial cancer incidence in US-born Asian women compared to immigrants. While the prevalence of overweight and obesity (BMI $\geq$ 25 kg/m^2) in US Asians remained lower than that of non-Hispanic whites, the prevalence was higher in Japanese (28.3 %) and Filipina women (33.5 %) compared to other Asian groups (Chinese 18.6 %, Vietnamese 16.9 %, Korean 17.3 %) [20].

In the MEC, the association between obesity and endometrial cancer risk was much stronger among Japanese Americans than among African Americans, non-Hispanic whites, and Latinas [21]. The relative risk for endometrial cancer comparing obese (BMI $\geq$ 30 kg/m^2) to normal weight (BMI < 25 kg/m^2) women was 4.6 (95 % CI: 2.61, 8.11) in Japanese Americans and ~3.0 in non-Hispanic whites (95 % CI: 1.71, 4.43), African Americans (95 % CI: 1.51, 6.28), and Latinos (95 % CI: 1.59, 5.94). Furthermore, Japanese Americans, who were generally leaner than women of the other MEC ethnic groups, had an increase in endometrial cancer risk with a much smaller weight gain (~5 %) than the other three ethnic groups where a greater gain (~35 %) was needed to observe similar effects. These findings suggest that a lower percentage of weight gain in Japanese women may result in sufficient hormonal changes to influence their endometrial cancer risk. It is also possible that ethnic variation in adiposity phenotype may contribute to these observations. Previous studies have shown that Asian women had a higher body fat percentage than non-Hispanic whites with a comparable BMI [22]. In the MEC, Japanese American relative to non-Hispanic whites had higher circulating levels of estrogens independent of BMI [23].

Body fat distribution might influence endometrial cancer risk. In a pilot study in the MEC that included 60 non-Hispanic white and Japanese American women who had a comprehensive body fat analysis using both DEXA and MRI, Japanese Americans had significantly greater waist to hip ratio (WHR), trunk fat mass, and visceral/abdominal fat and lower leg fat mass compared to non-Hispanic whites of similar BMI [22]. These data showed that Asian women carried greater abdominal and visceral fat when compared to non-Hispanic whites with similar overall BMI. The largest case–control study of body fat distribution and endometrial cancer in Chinese women from urban Shanghai (832 cases and 846 controls) showed that increasing WHR and waist circumference was significantly associated with endometrial cancer risk after BMI adjustment [24]. The odds ratios (OR) associated with the highest quartile versus lowest quartile of WHR and waist circumference were 2.6 and 3.9, respectively. In fact, the association of BMI with endometrial cancer was weakened substantially after waist circumference was included in the model; increasing BMI was associated with endometrial cancer risk ($P<0.01$), but after waist circumference was adjusted in the model, the trend became nonsignificant ($P=0.79$).

Estimates of population attributable risk for endometrial cancer associated with excess body weight in Asian studies ranged from 17–19 % for two studies in China [16, 25] to 33 % for a study in Korea [26]. However, the upper BMI cut point for these studies varied, ≥23 kg/m^2 in the Korean study and ≥23 or ≥25 kg/m^2 in the Chinese studies. We are not aware of published data on the population attributable risk for endometrial cancer associated with excess body weight in Asian Americans.

Hormone Use: Menstrual and Reproductive Factors

Estrogen therapy for postmenopausal women is an established risk factor associated with an increased risk for endometrial cancer [27, 28]. Women with breast cancer are at increased risk of endometrial cancer, and the risk was tripled among women who had used tamoxifen for chemoprevention for breast cancer [27], because of tamoxifen's estrogenic effect on the endometrium. Other exogenous hormones, such as combined oral contraceptive use, have been associated with reduced risk of endometrial cancer by approximately 50 % [28, 29]. In the MEC, women who used combined oral contraceptives longer than 5 years had a 40 % reduced risk of endometrial cancer (RR=0.60; 95 % CI: 0.39, 0.91) compared to women who never used oral contraceptives [9]. Early menarche and late menopause are additional known risk factors for endometrial cancer [27, 28]. In the MEC, an inverse association between increasing age at menarche and risk of endometrial cancer was observed but this was not statistically significant ($P=0.24$) after adjustment for other risk factors. Among postmenopausal women, later age at natural menopause was significantly associated with increased endometrial cancer risk (p trend=0.002). The RR comparing to age at natural menopause ≤44 years was 1.67 and 1.79 for those with age at menopause of 50–54 and ≥55 years, respectively [9].

Nulliparity is associated with a two- to threefold increased endometrial cancer risk [28], and it is believed to be related to infertility which is due to anovulation and progesterone deficiency. Risk of endometrial cancer decreases with increasing number of children. In the MEC, compared to nulliparous women, those with 3–4 children and ≥5 children had significantly lower risk of developing endometrial cancer (respective RR was 0.72 and 0.68) [9]. In a large pooled analysis of 17 epidemiologic studies, late age at last birth was associated with reduced endometrial cancer risk [30]; the risk reduction was observed among Asian women in the study (OR per 5 years increase in age at last birth=0.92, 95 % CI: 0.84, 1.02; P trend=0.09), albeit to a lesser extent compared to the risk reduction in white women (OR=0.87, 95 % CI: 0.84, 0.89; P trend <0.0001). Most studies have found that there is no significant association between age at first birth and risk of endometrial cancer. No pooled analysis data on risk of endometrial cancer and age at menarche or age at menopause in Asian women are currently available.

Diabetes

Results from recent meta-analysis of 23 studies showed a 1.6–1.9-fold higher risk of endometrial cancer in diabetic versus nondiabetic women [31]. Studies from Taiwan showed that history of diabetes was associated with 40–70 % increased risk of endometrial cancer [32–34]. Diabetes has been associated with endometrial cancer independent of BMI [35]. This is particularly important for Asians because of the high prevalence of type 2 diabetes despite their relatively low body weight. Studies have been inconclusive with respect to the role of diabetic drugs, such as metformin, in lowering risk of endometrial cancer among diabetics. Studies in the USA and UK did not support a protective effect of metformin [36, 37]. A recent study in Taiwan, however, showed that the use of metformin in Chinese women with type 2 diabetes was associated with a reduced risk of endometrial cancer with a significant dose–response relationship [38].

Physical Activity

In a recent meta-analysis of 33 studies on physical activity and endometrial cancer risk [39], high physical activity was associated with reduced risk of endometrial cancer (RR=0.80; 95 % CI: 0.75, 0.85). The inverse association was observed mainly among overweight and obese women (BMI≥25 kg/m^2) (RR=0.69; 95 % CI: 0.52, 0.91) and not among women with a BMI<25 kg/m^2 (RR=0.97; 95 % CI: 0.84, 1.13). When comparing studies that adjusted for BMI with studies that did not adjust for BMI, there was no difference in the summary risk estimates ($P=0.39$). The majority of the studies included in this meta-analysis were conducted among Caucasians in Europe and the USA. The combined analysis using data from two case–control studies from China and one from Japan yielded a RR of 0.69 (95 % CI: 0.51, 0.93) comparing high to low physical activity. Plausible mechanisms linking increased physical activity to lowered endometrial cancer risk include decreased levels of sex steroids, insulin resistance, and chronic inflammation [39]. It is possible that physical activity is indirectly associated with endometrial cancer risk by lowering body weight.

Cigarette Smoking

The inverse association between cigarette smoking and endometrial cancer is well established, with a greater reduction in risk among current smokers than former smokers compared to never smokers. Some have speculated that cigarette smoking is related to endometrial cancer risk through relationships with other known risk factors such as by lowering body weight; however, a recent study showed that the effect of smoking on endometrial cancer risk is not significantly modified by any endometrial cancer risk factor [40]. Suggested mechanism linking smoking with endometrial cancer risk is related to smoking's effect on estradiol production and metabolism [41].

Dietary Factors

The role of diet in endometrial cancer etiology is unclear. Most of the diet studies in the USA have been conducted in non-Asian populations. A few dietary factors have been associated with endometrial cancer including soy, coffee, and alcohol consumption, albeit with some inconsistencies across studies.

Soy intake is part of the traditional Asian diet. Soy foods are an almost exclusive dietary source of a class of phytoestrogens called isoflavones which are structurally similar to endogenous estrogens. It is particularly important for endometrial cancer because isoflavone possesses both estrogenic and antiestrogenic effects. A 2009 meta-analysis of 7 studies concluded that high soy intake was inversely associated with risk of endometrial cancer (RR=0.70; 95 % CI: 0.57, 0.86) [42]. However, results from two prospective cohort studies published since 2009 are not in agreement. In the MEC that included Japanese Americans, higher soy intake was associated with a reduction of risk by about 30 % [43] In contrast, in a prospective cohort study in Japan, intake of soy food and isoflavones was not associated with risk of endometrial cancer [17]. Furthermore, a study from China suggested that body mass index may be a potential modifier of the soy–endometrial cancer association [44]. Specifically, the association differed by BMI category ($OR_{\text{highest vs. lowest quartile}}=0.51$; 95 % CI: 0.31 to 0.84 for overweight and $OR_{\text{highest vs. lowest quartile}}=0.79$; 95 % CI: 0.52 to 1.20 for non-overweight women) although the test for interaction was not statistically significant [44].

Alcohol intake has been associated with increased circulating concentrations of estrogen, and it can further increase estrogen levels among postmenopausal women who are taking estrogen replacement therapy [45, 46]; therefore, it is plausible that women who consume alcoholic beverages are at increased risk of endometrial cancer. In a meta-analysis of alcohol and endometrial cancer risk [47], there was no overall association between alcohol drinking and risk in cohort studies (RR combined=1.04; 95 % CI: 0.91, 1.18) and case–control studies (OR combined=0.89; 95 % CI: 0.76, 1.05). However, in analysis by type of alcoholic beverages, an increased risk associated with hard liquor (RR combined=1.22; 95 % CI: 1.03, 1.45) was suggested.

Coffee is one of the most widely consumed beverages in the world. It contains various phytochemicals having potential antioxidant and antimutagenic properties [48]. Recent data show increasing coffee consumption is associated with reduced endometrial cancer risk [49–51]. Three Japanese studies showed a 20–30 % reduction in risk per additional cup of coffee per day [52–54]. The association of coffee with endometrial cancer risk is independent of BMI and diabetes. Tea consumption, primarily green tea, was not associated with endometrial cancer risk in studies conducted in Japan and China [49].

Family History and Genetic Susceptibility

Women with a first-degree family history of endometrial cancer had approximately a twofold increased risk of endometrial cancer compared to those without a family history [55]. Women with a first-degree relative with colorectal cancer had approximately a 17 % increased risk of endometrial cancer [55]. Twin studies have suggested that familial aggregation of endometrial cancer cases is more likely to be due to a combination of shared environmental factors than shared genetics [56]. Previous studies have also shown an increased risk of endometrial cancer associated with a family history of endometrial cancer in second (i.e., grandparents, aunts, uncles, nieces, nephews, half siblings) and third (i.e., first cousins, great grandparents) degree relatives indicating genetic causes [57–59]. None of these epidemiologic studies, however, were conducted in Asian-American women. The case–control study conducted in China found a positive association between family history of endometrial, breast, or colorectal cancer and endometrial cancer risk (OR = 2.24; 95 % CI: 1.54, 3.28) [16].

Women with hereditary non-polyposis colorectal cancer (HNPCC) or Lynch syndrome, a familial syndrome associated with germline mutation in DNA mismatch repair genes, have a higher lifetime risk of endometrial cancer (50–60 %) [60]. Other studies, however, have reported that a family history of endometrial cancer is associated with an increased risk of endometrial cancer in women from families without Lynch syndrome [59, 61, 62]. One study also has reported that a family history of early-onset colorectal cancer is associated with an increased risk of endometrial cancer [59]. These studies suggest the existence of inherited genetic defects other than mismatch repair gene mutations may predispose women to endometrial cancer. To date, genome-wide association studies (GWAS) have identified only one locus associated with endometrial cancer risk at the 17q21 (*HNF1B*) locus [63]. A follow-up fine mapping study of *HNF1B* identified additional variants associated with endometrial cancer risk which is likely to be mediated via altered gene expression [64]. A meta-analysis of existing GWAS is currently underway to identify additional loci for endometrial cancer; however, data on Asian populations are scarce.

Survivorship

The 5-year survival rates for endometrial cancer across all stages are 70 to 80 %, ranging from 90 % for patients with stage I cancer to 20 % for those with stage IV cancer. Differences in endometrial cancer survival between African-Americans and non-Hispanic whites are well documented, but there are currently limited data on survival in Asian-American populations. In a study conducted among women treated in the US Department of Defense system between 1988 and 1995, Asians/Pacific Islanders were found to have poorer survival compared to non-Hispanic whites [14]. Two SEER-based studies, however, showed that Asians diagnosed with endometrial cancer had a significantly improved overall survival compared to non-Hispanic whites [12, 13], with one study suggesting that this overall survival advantage experienced by Asians may be attributable to their younger age at the time of diagnosis [12]. The SEER study conducted using 1988–2009 data also suggested that Asian immigrants had better overall and cancer-specific survival compared to US-born Asians [13]. It was suggested that in addition to younger age at diagnosis, Asian immigrants may be more likely to retain lifestyle practices (e.g., lower body weight, diets rich in soy) from their country of origin which may have favorable impact on cancer outcome.

Concluding Remarks

Based on the 2012 Census Bureau figures, Asian women are the fastest growing immigrant populations in the USA. We observed a trend toward an increase in endometrial cancer incidence among Asian women in the USA, particularly among those born in the USA. With increasing obesity, metabolic syndrome, and physical inactivity, the incidence of endometrial cancer is expected to increase further. Studies are warranted to examine the role of diet and other environmental exposures on the risk of the development of endometrial cancer in Asian women.

Financial Disclosure None

References

1. Siegel RL, Miller KD, Jemal A (2016) Cancer Statistics, 2016. CA Cancer J Clin 66:7–30
2. Gomez SL, Noone AM, Lichtensztajn DY et al (2013) Cancer incidence trends among Asian American populations in the United States, 1990-2008. J Natl Cancer Inst 105:1096–1110
3. Duong LM, Wilson RJ, Ajani UA, Singh SD, Eheman CR (2011) Trends in endometrial cancer incidence rates in the United States, 1999-2006. J Womens Health (Larchmt) 20:1157–1163
4. Siegel R, Naishadham D, Jemal A (2012) Cancer statistics, 2012. CA Cancer J Clin 62:10–29
5. Liao CK, Rosenblatt KA, Schwartz SM, Weiss NS (2003) Endometrial cancer in Asian migrants to the United States and their descendants. Cancer Causes Control 14:357–360
6. Lee J, Demissie K, Lu SE, Rhoads GG (2007) Cancer incidence among Korean-American immigrants in the United States and native Koreans in South Korea. Cancer Control 14:78–85
7. Jung KW, Won YJ, Kong HJ et al (2015) Cancer statistics in Korea: incidence, mortality, survival, and prevalence in 2012. Cancer Res Treat 47:127–141
8. Simons E, Blansit K, Tsuei T et al (2015) Foreign- vs US-born Asians and the association of type I uterine cancer. Am J Obstet Gynecol 212(43):e41–e46
9. Setiawan VW, Pike MC, Kolonel LN, Nomura AM, Goodman MT, Henderson BE (2007) Racial/ethnic differences in endometrial cancer risk: the multiethnic cohort study. Am J Epidemiol 165:262–270
10. Allard JE, Maxwell GL (2009) Race disparities between black and white women in the incidence, treatment, and prognosis of endometrial cancer. Cancer Control 16:53–56
11. Sherman ME, Devesa SS (2003) Analysis of racial differences in incidence, survival, and mortality for malignant tumors of the uterine corpus. Cancer 98:176–186

12. Zhang MM, Cheung MK, Osann K et al (2006) Improved survival of Asians with corpus cancer compared with whites: an analysis of underlying factors. Obstet Gynecol 107:329–335
13. Mahdi H, Schlick CJ, Kowk LL, Moslemi-Kebria M, Michener C (2014) Endometrial cancer in Asian and American Indian/Alaskan native women: tumor characteristics, treatment and outcome compared to non-Hispanic white women. Gynecol Oncol 132:443–449
14. Kost ER, Hall KL, Hines JF et al (2003) Asian-Pacific Islander race independently predicts poor outcome in patients with endometrial cancer. Gynecol Oncol 89:218–226
15. Goodman MT, Hankin JH, Wilkens LR et al (1997) Diet, body size, physical activity, and the risk of endometrial cancer. Cancer Res 57:5077–5085
16. Gao J, Yang G, Wen W et al (2015) Impact of known risk factors on endometrial cancer burden in Chinese women. Eur J Cancer Prev 25(4):329–334
17. Budhathoki S, Iwasaki M, Sawada N et al (2015) Soy food and isoflavone intake and endometrial cancer risk: the Japan Public Health Center-based prospective study. BJOG 122:304–311
18. Key TJ, Pike MC (1988) The dose-effect relationship between 'unopposed' oestrogens and endometrial mitotic rate: its central role in explaining and predicting endometrial cancer risk. Br J Cancer 57:205–212
19. Popkin BM, Udry JR (1998) Adolescent obesity increases significantly in second and third generation U.S. immigrants: the National Longitudinal Study of Adolescent Health. J Nutr 128:701–706
20. McCracken M, Olsen M, Chen MS Jr et al (2007) Cancer incidence, mortality, and associated risk factors among Asian Americans of Chinese, Filipino, Vietnamese, Korean, and Japanese ethnicities. CA Cancer J Clin 57:190–205
21. Park SL, Goodman MT, Zhang ZF, Kolonel LN, Henderson BE, Setiawan VW (2010) Body size, adult BMI gain and endometrial cancer risk: the multiethnic cohort. Int J Cancer 126:490–499
22. Lim U, Ernst T, Buchthal SD et al (2011) Asian women have greater abdominal and visceral adiposity than Caucasian women with similar body mass index. Nutr Diabetes 1, e6
23. Setiawan VW, Haiman CA, Stanczyk FZ, Le Marchand L, Henderson BE (2006) Racial/ethnic differences in postmenopausal endogenous hormones: the multiethnic cohort study. Cancer Epidemiol Biomarkers Prev 15:1849–1855
24. Xu WH, Matthews CE, Xiang YB et al (2005) Effect of adiposity and fat distribution on endometrial cancer risk in Shanghai women. Am J Epidemiol 161:939–947
25. Wang D, Zheng W, Wang SM et al (2012) Estimation of cancer incidence and mortality attributable to overweight, obesity, and physical inactivity in China. Nutr Cancer 64:48–56
26. Park S, Kim Y, Shin HR et al (2014) Population-attributable causes of cancer in Korea: obesity and physical inactivity. PLoS One 9, e90871
27. Amant F, Moerman P, Neven P, Timmerman D, Van Limbergen E, Vergote I (2005) Endometrial cancer. Lancet 366:491–505
28. Sorosky JI (2012) Endometrial cancer. Obstet Gynecol 120:383–397
29. Collaborative Group on Epidemiological Studies on Endometrial Cancer (2015) Endometrial cancer and oral contraceptives: an individual participant meta-analysis of 27 276 women with endometrial cancer from 36 epidemiological studies. Lancet Oncol 16(9):1061–1070
30. Setiawan VW, Pike MC, Karageorgi S et al (2012) Age at last birth in relation to risk of endometrial cancer: pooled analysis in the epidemiology of endometrial cancer consortium. Am J Epidemiol 176:269–278
31. Liao C, Zhang D, Mungo C, Tompkins DA, Zeidan AM (2014) Is diabetes mellitus associated with increased incidence and disease-specific mortality in endometrial cancer? A systematic review and meta-analysis of cohort studies. Gynecol Oncol 135:163–171
32. Chiou WK, Huang BY, Chou WY, Weng HF, Lin JD (2011) Incidences of cancers in diabetic and non-diabetic hospitalized adult patients in Taiwan. Asian Pac J Cancer Prev 12:1577–1581
33. Lo SF, Chang SN, Muo CH et al (2013) Modest increase in risk of specific types of cancer types in type 2 diabetes mellitus patients. Int J Cancer 132:182–188
34. Chen HF, Liu MD, Chen P et al (2013) Risks of breast and endometrial cancer in women with diabetes: a population-based cohort study. PLoS One 8, e67420

35. Setiawan VW, Yang HP, Pike MC et al (2013) Type I and II endometrial cancers: have they different risk factors? J Clin Oncol 31:2607–2618
36. Becker C, Jick SS, Meier CR, Bodmer M (2013) Metformin and the risk of endometrial cancer: a case-control analysis. Gynecol Oncol 129:565–569
37. Ko EM, Sturmer T, Hong JL, Castillo WC, Bae-Jump V, Funk MJ (2015) Metformin and the risk of endometrial cancer: a population-based cohort study. Gynecol Oncol 136:341–347
38. Tseng CH (2015) Metformin and endometrial cancer risk in Chinese women with type 2 diabetes mellitus in Taiwan. Gynecol Oncol 138:147–153
39. Schmid D, Behrens G, Keimling M, Jochem C, Ricci C, Leitzmann M (2015) A systematic review and meta-analysis of physical activity and endometrial cancer risk. Eur J Epidemiol 30:397–412
40. Felix AS, Yang HP, Gierach GL, Park Y, Brinton LA (2014) Cigarette smoking and endometrial carcinoma risk: the role of effect modification and tumor heterogeneity. Cancer Causes Control 25:479–489
41. Viswanathan AN, Feskanich D, De Vivo I et al (2005) Smoking and the risk of endometrial cancer: results from the Nurses' Health Study. Int J Cancer 114:996–1001
42. Myung SK, Ju W, Choi HJ, Kim SC (2009) Soy intake and risk of endocrine-related gynaecological cancer: a meta-analysis. BJOG 116:1697–1705
43. Ollberding NJ, Lim U, Wilkens LR et al (2012) Legume, soy, tofu, and isoflavone intake and endometrial cancer risk in postmenopausal women in the multiethnic cohort study. J Natl Cancer Inst 104:67–76
44. Xu WH, Zheng W, Xiang YB et al (2004) Soya food intake and risk of endometrial cancer among Chinese women in Shanghai: population based case-control study. BMJ 328:1285
45. Purohit V, Brenner DA (2006) Mechanisms of alcohol-induced hepatic fibrosis: a summary of the Ron Thurman Symposium. Hepatology 43:872–878
46. Ginsburg ES (1999) Estrogen, alcohol and breast cancer risk. J Steroid Biochem Mol Biol 69:299–306
47. Sun Q, Xu L, Zhou B, Wang Y, Jing Y, Wang B (2011) Alcohol consumption and the risk of endometrial cancer: a meta-analysis. Asia Pac J Clin Nutr 20:125–133
48. Bohn SK, Blomhoff R, Paur I (2014) Coffee and cancer risk, epidemiological evidence, and molecular mechanisms. Mol Nutr Food Res 58:915–930
49. Yang TO, Crowe F, Cairns BJ, Reeves GK, Beral V (2015) Tea and coffee and risk of endometrial cancer: cohort study and meta-analysis. Am J Clin Nutr 101:570–578
50. Merritt MA, Tzoulaki I, Tworoger SS et al (2015) Investigation of dietary factors and endometrial cancer risk using a nutrient-wide association study approach in the EPIC and Nurses' Health Study (NHS) and NHSII. Cancer Epidemiol Biomarkers Prev 24:466–471
51. Hashibe M, Galeone C, Buys SS et al (2015) Coffee, tea, caffeine intake, and the risk of cancer in the PLCO cohort. Br J Cancer 113:809–816
52. Shimazu T, Inoue M, Sasazuki S et al (2008) Coffee consumption and risk of endometrial cancer: a prospective study in Japan. Int J Cancer 123:2406–2410
53. Hirose K, Niwa Y, Wakai K, Matsuo K, Nakanishi T, Tajima K (2007) Coffee consumption and the risk of endometrial cancer: evidence from a case-control study of female hormone-related cancers in Japan. Cancer Sci 98:411–415
54. Koizumi T, Nakaya N, Okamura C et al (2008) Case-control study of coffee consumption and the risk of endometrial endometrioid adenocarcinoma. Eur J Cancer Prev 17:358–363
55. Win AK, Reece JC, Ryan S (2015) Family history and risk of endometrial cancer: a systematic review and meta-analysis. Obstet Gynecol 125:89–98
56. Lichtenstein P, Holm NV, Verkasalo PK et al (2000) Environmental and heritable factors in the causation of cancer—analyses of cohorts of twins from Sweden, Denmark, and Finland. N Engl J Med 343:78–85
57. Seger HM, Soisson AP, Dodson MK, Rowe KG, Cannon-Albright LA (2011) Familial clustering of endometrial cancer in a well-defined population. Gynecol Oncol 122:75–78

58. Gruber SB, Thompson WD (1996) A population-based study of endometrial cancer and familial risk in younger women. Cancer and Steroid Hormone Study Group. Cancer Epidemiol Biomarkers Prev 5:411–417
59. Bharati R, Jenkins MA, Lindor NM et al (2014) Does risk of endometrial cancer for women without a germline mutation in a DNA mismatch repair gene depend on family history of endometrial cancer or colorectal cancer? Gynecol Oncol 133:287–292
60. Vasen HF, Watson P, Mecklin JP et al (1994) The epidemiology of endometrial cancer in hereditary nonpolyposis colorectal cancer. Anticancer Res 14:1675–1678
61. Lorenzo Bermejo J, Buchner FL, Hemminki K (2004) Familial risk of endometrial cancer after exclusion of families that fulfilled Amsterdam, Japanese or Bethesda criteria for HNPCC. Ann Oncol 15:598–604
62. Cook LS, Nelson HE, Stidley CA et al (2013) Endometrial cancer and a family history of cancer. Gynecol Oncol 130:334–339
63. Spurdle AB, Thompson DJ, Ahmed S et al (2011) Genome-wide association study identifies a common variant associated with risk of endometrial cancer. Nat Genet 43:451–454
64. Painter JN, O'Mara TA, Batra J et al (2015) Fine-mapping of the HNF1B multicancer locus identifies candidate variants that mediate endometrial cancer risk. Hum Mol Genet 24: 1478–1492

58. Gruber SB, Thompson WD (1996) A population-based study of endometrial cancer and familial risk in younger women. Cancer and Steroid Hormone Study Group. Cancer Epidemiol Biomarkers Prev 5:411–417
59. Bharati R, Jenkins MA, Lindor NM et al (2014) Does risk of endometrial cancer for women without a germline mutation in a DNA mismatch repair gene depend on family history of endometrial cancer or colorectal cancer? Gynecol Oncol 133:287–292
60. Vasen HF, Watson P, Mecklin JP et al (1994) The epidemiology of endometrial cancer in hereditary nonpolyposis colorectal cancer. Anticancer Res 14:1675–1678
61. Lorenzo Bermejo J, Büchner FL, Hemminki K (2004) Familial risk of endometrial cancer after exclusion of families that fulfilled Amsterdam, Japanese or Bethesda criteria for HNPCC. Ann Oncol 15:598–604
62. Cook LS, Nelson HE, Stidley CA et al (2013) Endometrial cancer and a family history of cancer. Gynecol Oncol 130:334–339
63. Spurdle AB, Thompson DJ, Ahmed S et al (2011) Genome-wide association study identifies a common variant associated with risk of endometrial cancer. Nat Genet 43:451–454
64. Painter JN, O'Mara TA, Batra J et al (2015) Fine-mapping of the HNF1B multicancer locus identifies candidate variants that mediate endometrial cancer risk. Hum Mol Genet 24:1478–1492

Liver Cancer Among Asian Americans

Channa R. Jayasekera and Mindie H. Nguyen

Abstract Asian Americans represent a highly heterogeneous racial group in the USA, defined by the US Census as persons having origins in any of the original peoples of the Far East, Southeast Asia, or the Indian subcontinent. Currently accounting for 5.6 % of the US population, over two-thirds of the Asian American population is foreign born, and it has been the fastest-growing racial group with an average growth rate of 45.6 % between 2000 and 2010. The five largest Asian American subpopulations are those of Chinese (28 %), Filipino (19.7 %), Indian (18.3 %), Vietnamese (10 %), and Korean (9.8 %) origin. Just under half of the Asian American population resides in the Western USA, followed by 21 % in the South, 20 % in the Northeast, and 11 % in the Midwest.

Primary liver cancer, which includes hepatocellular carcinoma and cholangiocarcinoma, is among the three cancers with rising incidence and is the fastest-growing cause of cancer-related death in the USA. Asian Americans represent one of the highest-risk groups for both incidence and mortality due to primary liver cancer in the USA. This chapter provides an overview of the epidemiology, clinical outcomes, and avenues for further research on primary liver cancer among Asian Americans.

Keywords Ethnicity • HCC • HBV • HCV • Epidemiology • Treatment

AASLD	American Association for the Study of Liver Diseases
AFP	Alpha-fetoprotein
BCLC	Barcelona Clinic Liver Cancer
CDC	Centers for Disease Control and Prevention
HBIG	Hepatitis B immune globulin
HBV	Hepatitis B virus

C.R. Jayasekera, M.D., M.Sc.
The Barry S Levin Department of Transplantation, California Pacific Medical Center, San Francisco, CA 94115, USA

M.H. Nguyen, M.D., M.A.S. (✉)
Division of Gastroenterology and Hepatology, Stanford University Medical Center, 750 Welch Road, Suite 210, Stanford, CA 94305, USA
e-mail: mindiehn@stanford.edu

A.H. Wu, D.O. Stram (eds.), *Cancer Epidemiology Among Asian Americans*,
DOI 10.1007/978-3-319-41118-7_10

HCC	Hepatocellular carcinoma
HCV	Hepatitis C virus
MELD	Model for end-stage liver disease
SEER	Surveillance, Epidemiology, and End Results
TACE	Trans-arterial chemoembolization
TARE	Trans-arterial radioembolization
UCSF	University of California, San Francisco
USPSTF	United States Preventive Services Task Force

Epidemiology

Primary liver cancer, over 85 % of which is hepatocellular carcinoma (HCC) with the remainder due to cholangiocarcinoma and rarer cancers such as hepatoblastoma, is the seventh leading contributor to cancer burden in the USA [1]. This chapter will focus primarily on HCC among Asian Americans.

Hepatocellular Carcinoma Incidence

HCC is one of the three cancers with rising incidence in the USA, where it is also the fastest-growing cause of cancer-related death over the past two decades [2, 3]. Data collected by the Surveillance, Epidemiology, and End Results Program (SEER) and other national registries show that Asian Americans have the highest age-adjusted incidence of HCC compared to other groups in the USA [2, 4]. The age-adjusted incidence of HCC (per 100,000 persons) during 2006–2010 for Asian American men and women combined stands at 11.7 compared to 9.5 in Hispanics, 7.5 in African Americans, and 4.2 in non-Hispanic whites [2] (Fig. 1). In analyses stratified

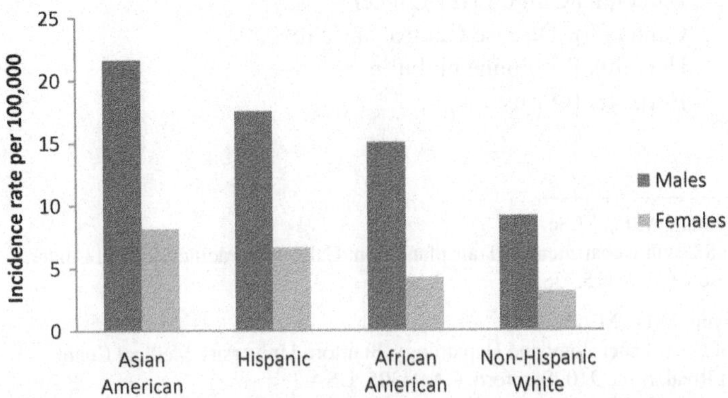

Fig. 1 Age-adjusted incidence of hepatocellular carcinoma (per 100,000) by race and gender [1]

by age groups, Asian Americans have the highest HCC incidence in the 35–49 age group and over 65 age group (4.7 and 54.7 per 100,000 persons, respectively). The incidence of HCC in the 50–64 age group (23.5 per 100,000 people) is slightly lower than that of Hispanics (24.3) and African Americans (26.9) [2]. While HCC incidence rates in the general US population increased during the 2000–2010 period, the rate of rise is decreasing (5.4 % per year during 2000–2007 and 2.3 % per year during 2007–2010). Among Asian American men and women, the annual incidence of HCC appears to have plateaued during the 2000–2010 period [2].

The incidence of liver cancer in Asian Americans is notable for significant within-group disparities. Data (2004–2008) from SEER registries showed that age-adjusted incidence of liver cancer was the leading cancer in Kampuchean (Cambodian) men (52.7 per 100,000) and second leading cancer among Laotian (64.5 per 100,000) and Vietnamese men (58.5 per 100,000), while it is not among the top five leading cancer sites in Asian Indian/Pakistani or Japanese men [5]. This large range in liver cancer incidence among Asian American ethnic groups is corroborated by data from the statewide California Cancer Registry (Table 1). This registry notes a nearly sevenfold difference in liver cancer incidence among the different Asian ethnic subgroups, highest in Vietnamese men (57.0) and lowest among Asian Indian/Pakistani men (7.9). Patterns are also comparable between Asian-American men and women (Table 1). While there is an apparent plateauing in HCC incidence in the general Asian American population in the 2000s, the trends of Asian American subpopulations over the 1990–2008 period demonstrate a mixed picture with declines in some populations and increases in others (Fig. 2) [2, 5].

Figure 1 also demonstrates the markedly higher incidence of liver cancer in men than in women; Asian American men have an age-adjusted incidence of 21.2 per 100,000, compared to 8.0 per 100,000 in Asian American women. This male to female ratio of approximately 2.7:1 in Asian Americans is comparable to that observed in non-Hispanic whites (3.0:1), African Americans (3.6:1), American Indian/Alaska Natives (2.2:1), and Hispanic/Latinos (2.8:1) [1]. Stage at diagnosis, an important predictor of outcome, appears to be comparable between racial groups in the USA [4]. In a study based on the large National Cancer Database, the distribution by pathologic stage among Asian American HCC patients (37.9 % stage I, 29.8 % stage II, 24.9 % stage III, and 7.4 % stage IV) did not differ from that of African American and White patients with HCC [6].

Table 1 Age-adjusted incidence of hepatocellular carcinoma (per 100,000) in California, 2004–2008 (Personal communication, Gomez)

	Males	Females
White non-Hispanic	8.2	7.0
Asian Indian/Pakistani	7.9	4.3
Chinese	23.8	7.9
Filipino	16.5	5.2
Japanese	11.0	9.0
Korean	29.1	10.8
Laotian	41.1	–
Vietnamese	57.0	19.5

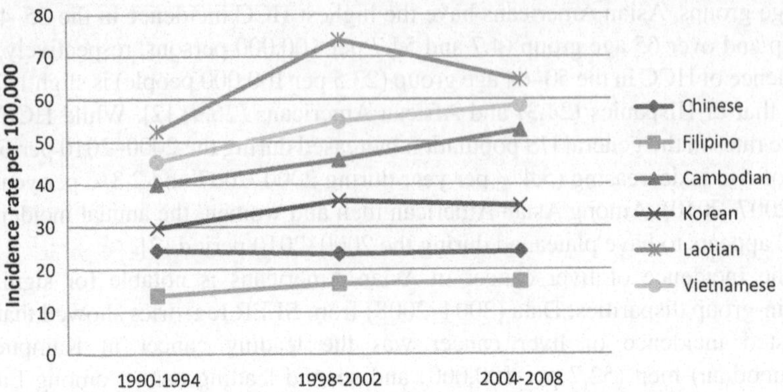

Fig. 2 Trends in age-adjusted incidence (per 100,000) of hepatocellular carcinoma by Asian American subpopulation men [5]

Hepatocellular Carcinoma-Related Mortality

Trends in liver cancer mortality follow those in incidence, attesting to the dismal outcomes seen with this malignancy. Five-year survival among patients with liver cancer remains relatively unchanged over the past decade, at approximately 17 % [7, 8]. Outcomes of HCC are highly dependent on stage of disease at diagnosis. Five-year survival rates are 30 % for patients with localized disease, 11 % for those with regionally advanced disease, and 3 % for those with distant metastatic disease [8]. The cumulative survival can be much higher for patients who receive optimal treatment. For example, based on SEER registry data, patients who met criteria for and underwent partial hepatectomy or liver transplantation had 5-year survival rates of 65 % and 77 %, respectively [9]. Other potentially curative, local tissue destruction therapies such as radiofrequency ablation have demonstrated 5-year survival rates over 50 % [10]. These comparatively high survival rates demonstrate that earlier detection and better access to appropriate care may dramatically improve liver cancer survival.

Asian Americans, owing to their higher incidence of disease, have the highest liver cancer mortality rates compared to other race/ethnic groups in the USA. Mortality rates in men (14.5 per 100,000) and women (6.1 per 100,000) are more than double the mortality rates in non-Hispanic white men (7.3 per 100,000) and women (3.0 per 100,000) (Fig. 3) [8].

Between 2000 and 2010, overall liver cancer mortality increased by 2.1 % per year in the USA; the steepest rise was observed in the 50–64 age group (5.6 % per year). Asian Americans showed an overall decline in liver cancer mortality during this time period (−1.6 % per year). The declining trend in liver cancer mortality in Asian Americans was seen in all age groups, but the magnitude of decline differed

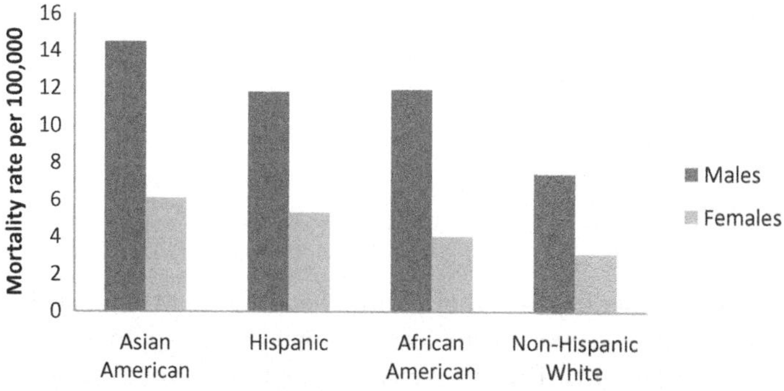

Fig. 3 Hepatocellular carcinoma-related mortality rate (per 100,000) by race and gender [1]

by age; it was steepest in the 35–49 age group (−4.3 % per year), intermediate in the 50–64 age group (−2.4 % per year), and weakest in the 65+ age group (−0.8 % per year) [2]. The increase in HCC mortality for the overall US population may be a reflection of the aging hepatitis C virus birth cohort which is not a major component of the Asian-American population at risk for HCC. Multivariate survival analysis of HCC patients with localized stage cancer, in fact, shows that Asian Americans have higher 5-year survival rates (hazard ratio 0.66) compared to non-Hispanic whites and African Americans [9].

Significant within-group mortality disparities also exist among the specific Asian American subgroups. Results from SEER between 1998 and 2002 showed that liver cancer mortality rates (per 100,000) in men were highest among Vietnamese (33.8), intermediate in Korean (26.3) and Chinese (20.3), and substantially lower in Asian Indian (5.3) and Japanese men [11]. In an analysis of 6028 Californians of Asian ancestry with HCC diagnosed in 1988 to 2007, survival outcome was found to differ among the nine Asian American ethnic groups. The cause-specific mortality risks were higher among Laotian/Hmong (adjusted HR = 1.51, 95 % CI 1.28–1.79) and Kampuchean (Cambodians) (HR = 1.24, 95 CI 1.02–1.48) than the other Asian American ethnic groups (adjusted HRs were less than 1.0) [12]. These disparities are likely reflections of poorer access to care, and thereby higher rates of delayed diagnosis and ineligibility for potentially curative therapies, among Laotian and Kampuchean (Cambodian) patients compared to other Asian American subpopulations.

Risk Factors for Hepatocellular Carcinoma

The risk factors for HCC include cirrhosis of any etiology—including alcoholic cirrhosis, chronic hepatitis B and C, nonalcoholic steatohepatitis, autoimmune liver diseases, and metabolic liver diseases such as alpha-1 antitrypsin deficiency, hereditary hemochromatosis, and Wilson's disease—as well as chronic hepatitis B without cirrhosis. Cirrhosis is believed to underlie approximately 80 % of cases of HCC in the general population [7, 13].

Hepatitis B and C

A viral etiology—either hepatitis B or C virus—is believed to underlie the approximately 90 % of HCC in Asian Americans, as opposed to approximately 65 % of non-Asian Americans [14]. The relative contributions of chronic hepatitis B and C differ considerably by racial groups with chronic hepatitis B accounting for approximately 50 % of cases in Asian Americans, 16 % in African Americans, and 6 % in non-Hispanic whites and chronic hepatitis C accounting for approximately 50 % in non-Hispanic whites and African Americans and 30 % in Asian Americans [15]. Similarly, data from the United Network for Organ Sharing (UNOS) indicate that among Asian Americans who underwent liver transplantation for HCC, 50 % had underlying chronic hepatitis B, compared with 14 % of African Americans, 7 % of non-Hispanic whites, and 4 % of Hispanic/Latinos [16].

In addition to hepatitis B virus, the importance of hepatitis C virus in the development of HCC in Asian Americans has also been well borne out. In a retrospective analysis of over 500 Asian Americans with HCC in California, Lin et al. demonstrated that chronic hepatitis B was the underlying etiology of 78 % of HCC among Chinese patients, 61 % of Korean patients, and 47 % of Southeast Asian-origin patients (Vietnamese, Filipino, Indonesian, Kampuchean (Cambodians), Malaysian, Burmese, Laotian, Singaporean), but hepatitis C virus was also found to be a significant cause of HCC accounting for 38 % of HCC in Southeast Asians, 28 % in Koreans, and 14 % in HCC among Chinese [17]. In addition, in the aforementioned UNOS analysis, 39 % of Asian Americans undergoing liver transplantation for HCC in the USA also had underlying hepatitis C virus infection [16]. Thus, both hepatitis B and hepatitis C virus are important etiologic entities in certain Asian-American subpopulations.

In individuals with chronic hepatitis C, HCC almost always occurs in the presence of advanced fibrosis or cirrhosis. While hepatitis B virus is an independent risk factor for HCC irrespective of the presence of cirrhosis, the majority of cases of HCC in hepatitis B virus-infected persons also tend to occur in the presence of cirrhosis [18]. For instance, among Asian Americans where the dominant risk factor for HCC is chronic hepatitis B, the prevalence of underlying cirrhosis appears to be in the 50–80 % range, suggesting that cirrhosis and hepatitis B virus have a synergistic influence in the development of HCC [17, 19, 20]. Other risk factors that independently accelerate the development of HCC in hepatitis B-infected patients include elevated serum alanine aminotransferases, advanced age, male gender, concurrent alcohol intake, family history, and, importantly, hepatitis B viral DNA levels. For example, individuals with hepatitis B DNA levels greater than 10^6 copies/mL have a sixfold risk of developing HCC compared with those who have undetectable, medically suppressed hepatitis B DNA levels [21]. Additional consideration with regard to both hepatitis B and C virus in Asian Americans is the chronicity of infection—wherein Asian Americans are more likely to have acquired these infections early on in life, and the longer duration of infection is believed to elevate the risk of HCC [3, 22]. In addition to HCC, recent evidence suggests that hepatitis B and C virus are also risk factors for intrahepatic cholangiocarcinoma and mixed hepatocellular carcinoma [23].

The high prevalence of these chronic viral hepatitides as the dominant drivers of HCC in Asian Americans highlights the importance of vaccination against hepatitis B, screening for chronic hepatitis B and C, appropriate treatment of chronic hepatitis B and C, and appropriate surveillance for liver cancer in patients with cirrhosis or chronic hepatitis B in this population [24]. These aspects will be discussed further in the prevention subsection of this chapter.

Non-viral Etiologies

While non-viral etiologies account for a smaller share of liver cancer among Asian Americans, several lines of evidence suggest that nonalcoholic fatty liver disease—a condition strongly associated with metabolic syndrome (coexistence of at least three of the following: central obesity, hypertension, impaired fasting glucose or diabetes, hypertriglyceridemia, or low levels of high-density lipoprotein)—may play an increasingly important role in this population. For instance, while Asian Americans have a lower average body mass index compared to other racial groups in the USA, the prevalence of metabolic syndrome has been recently found to be unexpectedly higher than their non-Hispanic white counterparts in a large cohort of over 40,000 patients in California [25, 26]. Nonalcoholic fatty liver disease also has been found to account for a considerable proportion of chronic liver disease in several Asian countries, although robust data regarding the prevalence of nonalcoholic fatty liver disease among Asian populations in the USA are lacking [27, 28]. Finally, whether nonalcoholic fatty liver disease progresses to liver cancer at the same rate in Asian Americans as in other racial groups is also uncertain at this time.

Treatment

Treatment Modalities and Outcomes

Treatment of HCC is broadly categorized in modalities that aim to cure and those that aim to palliate. The most robust criteria, and that which is recommended by the American Association for the Study of Liver Disease for treatment decision-making in HCC, is the Barcelona Clinic Liver Cancer (BCLC) classification (Fig. 4) [29–31]. The BCLC classification considers the extent of disease on computed tomography or magnetic resonance imaging (number of tumors present within and outside

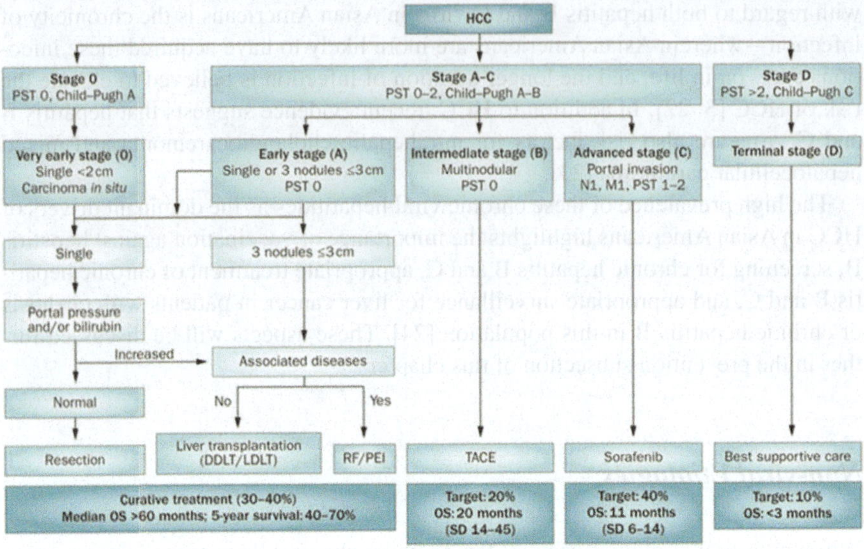

Fig. 4 The Barcelona Clinic Liver Cancer (BCLC) classification (Image copyright of: [29])

the liver, the size of the intrahepatic tumors), the severity of underlying liver disease, and the patient performance status as guides to therapy. Stages 0 (very early) and A (early) portend a relatively good prognosis where therapies with curative intent—liver transplantation, partial hepatectomy, radiofrequency ablation, or percutaneous ethanol injection—have been shown to provide clinical benefit. Liver transplantation, when performed within criteria defined by Mazzaferro et al. (the Milan Criteria) or by Yao et al. (the UCSF Criteria), has demonstrated the best 5-year survival rates, ranging between 70 and 80 % [32, 33]. Partial hepatectomy for resection of solitary lesions less than 2 cm in diameter provides approximately a 60 % 5-year survival although with a substantially higher rate of HCC recurrence [34]. Local tumor destructive therapies such as radiofrequency ablation—also considered potentially curative—have achieved 5-year survival rates over 50 % [11]. However, less than 25 % of patients in the USA are diagnosed at stages 0 and A, and the overall 5-year survival of patients in the USA is consequently close to 17 % [2, 7, 8, 33]. With adjunctive treatment modalities such as trans-arterial chemoembolization (TACE) and trans-arterial radioembolization (TARE), some patients who present beyond stage A may be "down-staged" in order to be within eligibility criteria for curative-intent therapies, and this strategy is successful in approximately 40–50 % of patients [36–38].

Disparities exist in the age at diagnosis, treatment modalities employed, and clinical outcomes between Asian Americans and other major ethnic groups and between the different Asian-American subpopulations. In large retrospective cohorts, Asian Americans excluding Pacific Islanders were shown to present at later age, but with lower rates of liver decompensation, comparable BCLC stages, and equal likelihood of meeting Milan or UCSF criteria, compared to non-Asian Americans [14, 39]. Despite these apparently favorable presenting characteristics and despite lower rates of tobacco and alcohol use and lower body mass index—factors that may influence better treatment outcomes—Asian Americans meeting Milan or UCSF criteria for liver transplantation were more likely to not receive liver transplantation or to be declined for transplant listing due to comorbidities, nonadherence, and psychosocial issues [39–41]. Based on the large National Cancer Database of the American College of Surgeons and other smaller cohorts, Asian Americans, however, appear to have an equal or higher likelihood of receiving partial hepatectomy or local tumor destructive therapies [6, 10, 39]. Data on within-group treatment disparities in the Asian-American community are limited, but preliminary analyses from California appear to show lower rates of receiving any therapy with curative intent in Vietnamese and Filipino patients who met Milan criteria, compared to patients of Chinese origin [42].

Despite the lower likelihood of receiving curative-intent therapy, 5-year survival rates among Asian Americans with HCC, on the whole, appear to exceed those of their white and African American counterparts. Devaki et al., using SEER registry data, demonstrated that among patients with localized HCC who received any therapy or no therapy, Asian Americans had a cumulative 5-year survival rate of 53 %, compared with 42 % in whites and 29 % in African Americans. Moreover, 5-year survival rates after receipt of these curative therapies did not differ between Chinese, Korean, Vietnamese, and Japanese patients included in this analysis [43].

Public Health Challenges and Prevention

Asian Americans with HCC, as a group, are unique in that approximately 90 % of the burden of disease stems from chronic hepatitis B and C—infections that can be readily screened and treated. Furthermore, at-risk individuals can be readily vaccinated against in the case of hepatitis B as means of preventing the development of HCC. Moreover, in patients with chronic hepatitis B or C and/or cirrhosis, the justification of routine screening for HCC meets the tenets set by the World Health Organization (Wilson and Jungner Criteria) that the burden of disease is significant, early disease is insidious and thereby requires formal testing, the natural history of disease is well understood such that patients can be risk-stratified and treated systematically, there are effective treatments available, and screening is likely cost-effective [44, 45]. In this context, while screening guidelines for both viral hepatitis and HCC have been developed, a key factor in the rates of delayed diagnosis of viral infection and poor adherence to HCC surveillance as well as nonreceipt of timely or appropriate therapy for viral hepatitis and HCC among Asian Americans may be inherently poorer healthcare access and cultural differences in health beliefs. These will be discussed further in this section.

Vaccination Against Infection with Hepatitis B Virus

The hepatitis B virus vaccination series has been available since 1982 and is included in the Centers for Disease Control and Prevention's (CDC) standard vaccination guidelines in the USA. It is also increasingly being implemented as mandatory by vaccination programs globally. The vaccination schedule includes three doses of the monovalent hepatitis B virus vaccine given at birth, at 1–2 months of age, and at 6–18 months of age. In addition, children of mothers with chronic hepatitis B should be administered the hepatitis B immune globulin (HBIG) within 12 h of birth. The combination of the vaccination series and birth dose of HBIG prevents approximately 95 % of hepatitis B virus transmission from infected mothers to their newborns [46]. While it is believed that concerted, community-based, multilingual efforts to engage higher-risk groups such as recent Asian immigrants have contributed substantially to expanding hepatitis B virus vaccination over the past 20 years, millions of at-risk individuals in the USA remain unvaccinated [47, 48].

Screening for Hepatitis B Virus

Chronic hepatitis B portends an annual cumulative risk of approximately 0.5 % of developing HCC in the absence of cirrhosis and between 3 and 10 % in the setting of cirrhosis [15]. Given that most cases of chronic hepatitis B in Asian Americans are contracted at birth or in early childhood, the American Association for the Study of Liver Diseases (AASLD) currently recommends a one-time hepatitis B virus serologic screen in Asian-American males over 40 years and Asian-American females over 50 years [49]. The CDC has adopted a broader definition of those at risk, recommending testing all persons born in regions of high and intermediate hepatitis B endemicity and those who were born in the USA to parents born in those regions [50]. Most recently, in early 2014, the US Preventive Services Task Force (USPSTF) also initiated recommendation for hepatitis B virus screening in foreign-born individuals from regions with hepatitis B virus prevalence of 2 % or higher [51]. While there has been considerable focus on this issue with nationwide efforts such as the Department of Health and Human Services' National Viral Hepatitis Action Plan, it is believed that the majority of hepatitis B-infected Asian Americans remain undiagnosed [47]. For instance, in a study of over 3100 Asian Americans screened for hepatitis B in California, 65 % of those found to have chronic infection were unaware of their status [52].

Screening for Hepatitis C Virus

The annual cumulative risk of HCC in patients with chronic hepatitis C without cirrhosis or advanced fibrosis is considered to be very low but is 3–5 % per year in the setting of cirrhosis [53, 54]. Despite the considerable hepatitis C burden in some subgroups of Asian Americans, much of which is likely contracted in early childhood via iatrogenic exposure, there are no specific, dedicated screening guidelines for the Asian American population. Instead, the AASLD, CDC, and USPSTF recommend a one-time hepatitis C screen in individuals born between 1945 and 1965 (the "baby boomer" birth cohort) and in patients with specific risk factors such as drug abuse, hemodialysis, etc. [55–57]. The specific risk factors for hepatitis C virus infection in Asian Americans are poorly understood, but it is well documented that immigrants from countries with high or intermediate endemicity—which includes much of Asia—have high rates of chronic hepatitis C and that iatrogenic exposure during routine dental and medical practices is the most likely transmission route. Given that infection with hepatitis C virus is likely underdiagnosed among first-generation Asian immigrants, screening for hepatitis C virus in these individuals—particularly those originating in countries with hepatitis C virus endemicity—may be one strategy to improve case detection in this higher-risk group [58, 59].

Antiviral Therapy for Chronic Hepatitis B and C

A proportion of individuals with chronic hepatitis B would require initiation of long-term (likely lifelong) antiviral therapy depending on serum alanine aminotransferase levels, serum hepatitis B HBV DNA levels, the degree of liver inflammation and fibrosis, and the presence of cirrhosis or HCC. The strongest evidentiary support for hepatitis B viral suppression as a means of preventing HCC comes from a randomized trial of lamivudine versus placebo in patients ($N=651$) with high hepatitis B virus DNA levels and advanced fibrosis or cirrhosis (stage 3–4). This trial was terminated early at 32 months of median follow-up due to the rate of HCC among treated patients being 3.9 % versus 7.4 % in the placebo arm [60]. Entecavir and tenofovir as long-term oral therapies have demonstrated superior efficacy, resistance, safety, and tolerability profiles compared with lamivudine, adefovir, telbivudine, and injectable interferon, and there have been cohort studies suggesting benefits with reduced HCC incidence in treated patients, especially those with cirrhosis [61–64]. However, studies in the USA comprising mostly of Asian Americans have suggested that there is significant under-evaluation and undertreatment of patients who have been diagnosed with infection with hepatitis B virus [65–69].

Hepatitis C treatment has seen dramatic changes in recent years. In comparison to onerous regimens of injectable interferon with oral ribavirin for 6–12 months, chronic hepatitis C can now be treated with remarkably high efficacy (virologic cure often exceeding 90 %), safety, and tolerability with 3–6-month courses of all oral regimens with direct-acting antivirals in most patients [70]. Although pan-genotypic regimens are likely to be approved before 2017, hepatitis C treatment currently remains tailored by genotype—a factor that must be considered in Asian American patients who predominantly carry genotypes 1, 3, and 6, which are endemic in their countries of origin [71].

HCC Surveillance

Among patients with risk factors for HCC, the benefit of HCC surveillance has been demonstrated mostly by observational studies and one randomized trial in Chinese patients with chronic hepatitis B. This randomized trial utilized biannual liver ultrasonography and alpha-fetoprotein (AFP) versus no screening in 18,816 patients aged 35–59 in Shanghai, China, where biannual screening was found to detect far more subclinical HCC (52 vs. 0) and reduce HCC mortality by 37 % [69]. Subsequent analyses have demonstrated insufficient sensitivity and specificity of AFP for diagnosis of HCC, and therefore, the AASLD currently recommends biannual imaging with liver ultrasonography as the sole surveillance modality [72]. However, the sensitivity of liver ultrasonography alone is poor, and most other practice guidelines recommend the combination of both liver ultrasonography and serum AFP biannually for HCC surveillance. This combination approach appears to be more widely preferred in the USA [45, 73]. Rates of surveillance with ultrasonography by community medical practitioners however have been exceptionally low, with a meta-analysis by Singal et al. revealing that only 18.4 % of patients with clear HCC risk factors underwent appropriate screening.

Based on SEER registry data, Asian Americans appear to have the highest—albeit still grossly below target—rate of HCC diagnosed via screening (28.1 %) compared with Hispanic (16.8 %), white (14.9 %), and African American (12.2 %) patients [74]. Adherence to HCC screening in a cohort of 1333 patients with chronic hepatitis B was found to be even poorer in patients without cirrhosis compared to those with cirrhosis, and consequently, in a cohort of approximately 500 hepatitis B virus-related HCC patients, most of whom were Asian Americans, patients without cirrhosis were more likely to present with symptoms and had poorer survival compared to those with cirrhosis [75, 76].

Conclusions

Individuals of Asian origin are the highest-risk ethnic group for HCC in the USA. Chronic hepatitis B and C remain the leading risk factors for HCC in this group, accounting for approximately 90 % of cases. Despite available screening and treatment guidelines, a large proportion of individuals with chronic hepatitis B and C remain undiagnosed and/or untreated. Screening for HCC in Asian Americans with risk factors (e.g., cirrhosis, chronic hepatitis B), while better than other groups, remains poor. Asian Americans appear to present at comparable HCC stages to other population groups but the least likely to receive liver transplantation, the treatment modality with the highest rates of recurrence-free survival. Nevertheless, possibly owing to higher rates of other curative-intent therapies such as partial hepatectomy and radiofrequency ablation and better performance status at presentation, Asian Americans demonstrate a higher than average 5-year overall survival rate.

Financial Disclosure 1. **Authors' Declaration of Personal Interests**:
(i) Channa Jayasekera has no declarations to disclose.
(ii) Mindie H. Nguyen has served as a consultant for Bristol-Myers Squibb and Gilead Sciences Inc. and has received funding from Bristol-Myers Squibb, Novartis Pharmaceuticals, and Roche.
2. **Declaration of Funding Interests**:
None to disclose.

References

1. Siegel R, Naishadham D, Jemal A (2013) Cancer statistics, 2013. CA Cancer J Clin 63:11–30. doi:10.3322/caac.21166
2. Altekruse SF, Henley SJ, Cucinelli JE, McGlynn KA (2014) Changing hepatocellular carcinoma incidence and liver cancer mortality rates in the united states. Am J Gastroenterol 109:542–553. doi:10.1038/ajg.2014.11
3. El-Serag HB, Kanwal F (2014) Epidemiology of hepatocellular carcinoma in the United States: Where are we? Where do we go? Hepatology 60:1767–1775. doi:10.1002/hep.27222
4. Wong R, Corley DA (2008) Racial and ethnic variations in hepatocellular carcinoma incidence within the United States. Am J Med 121:525–531. doi:10.1016/j.amjmed.2008.03.005
5. Gomez SL, Noone A-M, Lichtensztajn DY et al (2013) Cancer incidence trends among Asian American populations in the united states, 1990–2008. J Natl Cancer Inst 105:1096–1110. doi:10.1093/jnci/djt157
6. Hoehn RS, Hanseman DJ, Wima K et al (2015) Does race affect management and survival in hepatocellular carcinoma in the United States? Surgery 158(5):1244–1251. doi:10.1016/j.surg.2015.03.026
7. El-Serag HB (2011) Hepatocellular carcinoma. N Engl J Med 365:1118–1127. doi:10.1056/NEJMra1001683
8. Siegel RL, Miller KD, Jemal A (2015) Cancer statistics, 2015. CA Cancer J Clin 65(1):5–29. doi:10.3322/caac.21254, Epub 2015 Jan 5
9. Devaki P, Wong RJ, Marupakula V et al (2014) Approximately one-half of patients with early-stage hepatocellular carcinoma meeting Milan criteria did not receive local tumor destructive or curative surgery in the post-MELD exception era. Cancer 120:1725–1732. doi:10.1002/cncr.28639
10. Huang J, Yan L, Cheng Z et al (2010) A randomized trial comparing radiofrequency ablation and surgical resection for HCC conforming to the Milan criteria. Ann Surg 252:903–912. doi:10.1097/SLA.0b013e3181efc656
11. Miller BA, Chu KC, Hankey BF, Ries LAG (2008) Cancer incidence and mortality patterns among specific Asian and Pacific Islander populations in the U.S. Cancer Causes Control 19(3):227–256
12. Kwong SL, Stewart SL, Aoki CA, Chen MS (2010) Disparities in hepatocellular carcinoma survival among Californians of Asian ancestry, 1988 to 2007. Cancer Epidemiol Biomarkers Prev 19:2747–2757. doi:10.1158/1055-9965.EPI-10-0477
13. Fattovich G, Stroffolini T, Zagni I, Donato F (2004) Hepatocellular carcinoma in cirrhosis: incidence and risk factors. Gastroenterology 127:S35–S50
14. Wong PY, Xia V, Imagawa DK et al (2011) Clinical presentation of hepatocellular carcinoma (HCC) in Asian-Americans versus Non-Asian-Americans. J Immigr Minor Health 13:842–848. doi:10.1007/s10903-010-9395-8
15. Di Bisceglie AM (2009) Hepatitis B and hepatocellular carcinoma. Hepatology 49:S56–S60. doi:10.1002/hep.22962

16. Artinyan A, Mailey B, Sanchez-Luege N et al (2010) Race, ethnicity, and socioeconomic status influence the survival of patients with hepatocellular carcinoma in the United States. Cancer 116:1367–1377. doi:10.1002/cncr.24817
17. Lin H, Ha NB, Ahmed A et al (2013) Both HCV and HBV are major causes of liver cancer in southeast Asians. J Immigr Minor Health 15:1023–1029. doi:10.1007/s10903-013-9871-z
18. Yang JD, Kim WR, Coelho R et al (2011) Cirrhosis is present in most patients with hepatitis B and hepatocellular carcinoma. Clin Gastroenterol Hepatol 9:64–70. doi:10.1016/j.cgh.2010.08.019
19. Chang ET, Keegan THM, Gomez SL et al (2007) The burden of liver cancer in Asians and Pacific islanders in the greater San Francisco Bay area, 1990 through 2004. Cancer 109:2100–2108. doi:10.1002/cncr.22642
20. Pollack HJ, Kwon SC, Wang SH et al (2014) Chronic hepatitis B and liver cancer risks among Asian immigrants in New York city: results from a large, community-based screening, evaluation, and treatment program. Cancer Epidemiol Biomarks Prev 23:2229–2239. doi:10.1158/1055-9965.EPI-14-0491
21. Chen C-J, Iloeje UH, Yang H-I (2007) Long-term outcomes in hepatitis B: the REVEAL-HBV study. Clin Liver Dis 11:797–816. doi:10.1016/j.cld.2007.08.005, viii
22. Nguyen MH, Whittemore AS, Garcia RT et al (2004) Role of ethnicity in risk for hepatocellular carcinoma in patients with chronic hepatitis C and cirrhosis. Clin Gastroenterol Hepatol 2:820–824
23. Razumilava N, Gores GJ (2014) Cholangiocarcinoma. Lancet 383:2168–2179. doi:10.1016/S0140-6736(13)61903-0
24. Tong MJ, Pan CQ, Hann H-W et al (2011) The management of chronic hepatitis B in Asian Americans. Dig Dis Sci 56:3143–3162. doi:10.1007/s10620-011-1841-5
25. Palaniappan LP, Wong EC, Shin JJ et al (2011) Asian Americans have greater prevalence of metabolic syndrome despite lower body mass index. Int J Obes 35:393–400. doi:10.1038/ijo.2010.152
26. Wong RJ (2014) Obesity and non-alcoholic fatty liver disease: disparate associations among Asian populations. World J Hepatol 6:263. doi:10.4254/wjh.v6.i5.263
27. Farrell GC, Wong VW-S, Chitturi S (2013) NAFLD in Asia—as common and important as in the West. Nat Rev Gastroenterol Hepatol 10:307–318. doi:10.1038/nrgastro.2013.34
28. Wong VW (2013) Nonalcoholic fatty liver disease in Asia: a story of growth: nonalcoholic fatty liver disease in Asia. J Gastroenterol Hepatol 28:18–23. doi:10.1111/jgh.12011
29. Villanueva A, Hernandez-Gea V, Llovet JM (2012) Medical therapies for hepatocellular carcinoma: a critical view of the evidence. Nat Rev Gastroenterol Hepatol 10:34–42. doi:10.1038/nrgastro.2012.199
30. Llovet JM, Brú C, Bruix J (1999) Prognosis of hepatocellular carcinoma: the BCLC staging classification. Semin Liver Dis 19:329–338. doi:10.1055/s-2007-1007122
31. Marrero JA, Fontana RJ, Barrat A et al (2005) Prognosis of hepatocellular carcinoma: comparison of 7 staging systems in an American cohort. Hepatology (Baltimore, Md) 41:707–716. doi:10.1002/hep.20636
32. Mazzaferro V, Regalia E, Doci R et al (1996) Liver transplantation for the treatment of small hepatocellular carcinomas in patients with cirrhosis. N Engl J Med 334:693–700. doi:10.1056/NEJM199603143341104
33. Yao FY, Ferrell L, Bass NM et al (2001) Liver transplantation for hepatocellular carcinoma: expansion of the tumor size limits does not adversely impact survival. Hepatology (Baltimore, Md) 33:1394–1403. doi:10.1053/jhep.2001.24563
34. Akoad ME, Pomfret EA (2015) Surgical resection and liver transplantation for hepatocellular carcinoma. Clin Liver Dis 19:381–399. doi:10.1016/j.cld.2015.01.007
35. Altekruse SF, McGlynn KA, Reichman ME (2009) Hepatocellular carcinoma incidence, mortality, and survival trends in the united states from 1975 to 2005. J Clin Oncol 27:1485–1491. doi:10.1200/JCO.2008.20.7753
36. De Luna W, Sze DY, Ahmed A et al (2009) Transarterial chemoinfusion for hepatocellular carcinoma as downstaging therapy and a bridge toward liver transplantation. Am J Transplant 9:1158–1168. doi:10.1111/j.1600-6143.2009.02576.x

37. Parikh ND, Waljee AK, Singal AG (2015) Downstaging hepatocellular carcinoma: a systematic review and pooled analysis. Liver Transpl 21(9):1142–1152. doi:10.1002/lt.24169
38. Yao FY, Kinkhabwala M, LaBerge JM et al (2005) The impact of pre-operative loco-regional therapy on outcome after liver transplantation for hepatocellular carcinoma. Am J Transpl 5:795–804. doi:10.1111/j.1600-6143.2005.00750.x
39. Yip B, Wantuck JM, Kim LH et al (2014) Clinical presentation and survival of Asian and non-Asian patients with HCV-related hepatocellular carcinoma. Dig Dis Sci 59:192–200. doi:10.1007/s10620-013-2948-7
40. Wong RJ, Devaki P, Nguyen L et al (2014) Ethnic disparities and liver transplantation rates in hepatocellular carcinoma patients in the recent era: results from the surveillance, epidemiology, and end results registry: liver transplantation trends in HCC patients. Liver Transpl 20:528–535. doi:10.1002/lt.23820
41. Yu JC, Neugut AI, Wang S et al (2010) Racial and insurance disparities in the receipt of transplant among patients with hepatocellular carcinoma. Cancer 116:1801–1809. doi:10.1002/cncr.24936
42. Jayasekera CR, Kim LH, Wantuck JM, et al (2014) Heterogeneity in risk factors and treatment allocation, but comparable clinical presentation and survival with hepatocellular carcinoma (HCC) among the three largest Asian sub-populations in California. The Liver Meeting: American Association for the Study of Liver Diseases, Boston, MA. Abstract 1419.
43. Tong MJ, Chavalitdhamrong D, Lu DSK et al (2010) Survival in Asian Americans after treatments for hepatocellular carcinoma: a seven-year experience at UCLA. J Clin Gastroenterol 44:e63–e70. doi:10.1097/MCG.0b013e3181b4b68b
44. Wilson JMG, Jungner G (1968) Principles and practice of screening for disease. World Health Organization, Geneva, Switzerland
45. Zhao C, Nguyen MH (2016) Hepatocellular Carcinoma Screening and Surveillance: Practice Guidelines and Real-Life Practice. J Clin Gastroenterol 50(2):120–33
46. Pan CQ, Duan Z-P, Bhamidimarri KR et al (2012) An algorithm for risk assessment and intervention of mother to child transmission of hepatitis B virus. Clin Gastroenterol Hepatol 10:452–459. doi:10.1016/j.cgh.2011.10.041
47. Cohen C, Caballero J, Martin M et al (2013) Eradication of hepatitis B: a nationwide community coalition approach to improving vaccination, screening, and linkage to care. J Community Health 38:799–804. doi:10.1007/s10900-013-9699-4
48. Wong WF, LaVeist TA, Sharfstein JM (2015) Achieving health equity by design. JAMA 313:1417. doi:10.1001/jama.2015.2434
49. Lok ASF, McMahon BJ (2009) Chronic hepatitis B: update 2009. Hepatology (Baltimore, Md) 50:661–662. doi:10.1002/hep.23190
50. Weinbaum CM, Williams I, Mast EE et al (2008) Recommendations for identification and public health management of persons with chronic hepatitis B virus infection. MMWR Recomm Rep 57:1–20
51. USPSTF (2014) Final recommendation statement: hepatitis B virus infection: screening, 2014. United States Preventative Services Task Force, Rockville
52. Lin SY, Chang ET, So SK (2007) Why we should routinely screen Asian American adults for hepatitis B: a cross-sectional study of Asians in California. Hepatology (Baltimore, Md) 46:1034–1040. doi:10.1002/hep.21784
53. Bruix J, Sherman M (2011) Management of hepatocellular carcinoma: an update. Hepatology 53:1020–1022. doi:10.1002/hep.24199
54. Lok AS, Seeff LB, Morgan TR et al (2009) Incidence of hepatocellular carcinoma and associated risk factors in hepatitis C-related advanced liver disease. Gastroenterology 136:138–148. doi:10.1053/j.gastro.2008.09.014
55. American Association for the Study of Liver Diseases, Infectious Diseases Society of America. Recommendations for Testing, Managing, and Treating Hepatitis C [Internet]. 2016 [cited 2016 May 7]. Available from: http://www.hcvguidelines.org/full-report-view.
56. Moyer VA, U.S. Preventive Services Task Force (2013) Screening for hepatitis C virus infection in adults: U.S. Preventive services task force recommendation statement. Ann Intern Med 159:349–357. doi:10.7326/0003-4819-159-5-201309030-00672

57. Smith BD, Morgan RL, Beckett GA et al (2012) Recommendations for the identification of chronic hepatitis C virus infection among persons born during 1945–1965. MMWR Recomm Rep 61:1–32
58. Kin KC, Lin B, Chaung KT et al (2013) Less-established risk factors are common in Asian Americans with hepatitis C virus: a case-controlled study. Dig Dis Sci 58:3342–3347. doi:10.1007/s10620-013-2884-6
59. Nguyen LH, Nguyen MH (2013) Systematic review: Asian patients with chronic hepatitis C infection. Aliment Pharmacol Ther 37:921–936. doi:10.1111/apt.12300
60. Liaw Y-F, Sung JJY, Chow WC et al (2004) Lamivudine for patients with chronic hepatitis B and advanced liver disease. N Engl J Med 351:1521–1531. doi:10.1056/NEJMoa033364
61. Ayoub WS, Keeffe EB (2011) Review article: current antiviral therapy of chronic hepatitis B. Aliment Pharmacol Ther 34:1145–1158. doi:10.1111/j.1365-2036.2011.04869.x
62. Gordon SC, Lamerato LE, Rupp LB et al (2014) Antiviral therapy for chronic hepatitis B virus infection and development of hepatocellular carcinoma in a US population. Clin Gastroenterol Hepatol 12:885–893. doi:10.1016/j.cgh.2013.09.062
63. Hosaka T, Suzuki F, Kobayashi M et al (2013) Long-term entecavir treatment reduces hepatocellular carcinoma incidence in patients with hepatitis B virus infection. Hepatology 58:98–107. doi:10.1002/hep.26180
64. Lin D, Yang HI, Nguyen NH, Hoang JK, Kim Y, Vu VD, Le AK, Chaung KT, Nguyen VG, Trinh HN, Li J, Zhang JQ, Hsing AW, Chen CJ, Nguyen MH (2015) Antiviral Therapy for Chronic Hepatitis B (CHB) Reduces the Incidence of Hepatocellular Carcinoma (HCC) Regardless of Cirrhosis Status: Analysis with Adjustment for REACH-B Risk Score. Hepatology 62(Suppl):S315
65. Kim LH, Nguyen VG, Trinh HN et al (2014) Low treatment rates in patients meeting guideline criteria in diverse practice settings. Dig Dis Sci 59:2091–2099. doi:10.1007/s10620-014-3283-3
66. Ku KC, Li J, Ha NB et al (2013) Chronic hepatitis B management based on standard guidelines in community primary care and specialty clinics. Dig Dis Sci 58:3626–3633. doi:10.1007/s10620-013-2889-1
67. Sarkar M, Shvachko VA, Ready JB et al (2014) Characteristics and management of patients with chronic hepatitis B in an integrated care setting. Dig Dis Sci 59:2100–2108. doi:10.1007/s10620-014-3142-2
68. Wu Y, Johnson KB, Roccaro G et al (2014) Poor adherence to AASLD guidelines for chronic hepatitis B management and treatment in a large academic medical center. Am J Gastroenterol 109:867–875. doi:10.1038/ajg.2014.72
69. Zhang B-H, Yang B-H, Tang Z-Y (2004) Randomized controlled trial of screening for hepatocellular carcinoma. J Cancer Res Clin Oncol 130:417–422. doi:10.1007/s00432-004-0552-0
70. Dore GJ, Feld JJ (2015) Hepatitis C virus therapeutic development: in pursuit of "perfectovir". Clin Infect Dis 60:1829–1836. doi:10.1093/cid/civ197
71. Messina JP, Humphreys I, Flaxman A et al (2014) Global distribution and prevalence of hepatitis C virus genotypes. Hepatology 61(1):77–87. doi:10.1002/hep.27259
72. Bruix J, Sherman M (2005) Management of hepatocellular carcinoma. Hepatology 42:1208–1236. doi:10.1002/hep.20933
73. Yapali S, Talaat N, Lok AS (2014) Management of hepatitis B: our practice and how it relates to the guidelines. Clin Gastroenterol Hepatol 12:16–26. doi:10.1016/j.cgh.2013.04.036
74. Singal AG, Yopp A, S Skinner C et al (2012) Utilization of hepatocellular carcinoma surveillance among American patients: a systematic review. J Gen Intern Med 27:861–867. doi:10.1007/s11606-011-1952-x
75. Chen VL, Kim LH, Nguyen P, Zhao C, Nguyen MH (2016) Diagnosis by Screening Rather Than Symptoms in Hepatitis B Virus (HBV)-Associated Hepatocellular Carcinoma (HCC) is Associated with Earlier Stage, More Curative Treatment Options, and Improved Survival, Regardless of Cirrhosis Status. Clin Gastroenterol Hepatol 14(6):887–895.e1
76. Wang C, Zhao C, Le AK, Nguyen L, Trinh HN, Li J, Hoang J, Nguyen N, Nguyen MH. Poor adherence and poor persistency of consistent adherence to AASLD guidelines for hepatocellular carcinoma (HCC) screening and surveillance in chronic hepatitis B (CHB) patients at both university and community clinics: A multicenter U.S. cohort study. Medicine 2016. In press

Gastric Cancer Among Asian Americans

Afsaneh Barzi, Dongyun Yang, and Anna H. Wu

Abstract Gastric cancer is the third leading cause of cancer mortality worldwide. It remains the eighth most commonly diagnosed cancer among Asian American men and women in the United States (USA) with considerable heterogeneity in incidence rates across Asian American subgroups, highest in Korean American men. Because of the lack of routine screening for gastric cancer in the USA, patients are usually diagnosed at a late stage because of symptoms. While infection with *Helicobacter pylori* is the primary risk factor for gastric cancer, only a small proportion of those infected go on to develop gastric cancer, which means that better understanding of the interactions between *H. pylori* infection and other lifestyle factors (e.g., cigarette smoking, dietary factors) are needed to better characterize persons who eventually develop gastric cancer. Treatment benefits can vary by ethnicity and region of the world, possibly due to host-related factors. Continued efforts to improve treatment outcome by considering race/ethnicity, country of birth, and other parameters should be a priority.

Keywords Gastric cancer • Asian Americans • *Helicobacter pylori* • Smoking • Diet • Screening • Treatment

Introduction

Gastric cancer is generally categorized by anatomic subsite as either in the cardia of the stomach, including the gastroesophageal junction, or more distally (non-cardia), including the fundus, corpus, and antrum. Although cardia and non-cardia gastric cancers appear to have different etiologies, and the incidence of cardia cancers may

---

A. Barzi, M.D., Ph.D. (✉) • D. Yang, Ph.D.
University of Southern California, Norris Comprehensive Cancer Center,
1441 Eastlake Avenue, Suite 3440, Los Angeles, CA 90089, USA
e-mail: barzi@usc.edu

A.H. Wu, Ph.D.
Department of Preventive Medicine, Keck School of Medicine of USC,
University of Southern California, Los Angeles, CA, USA

A.H. Wu, D.O. Stram (eds.), *Cancer Epidemiology Among Asian Americans*,
DOI 10.1007/978-3-319-41118-7_11

have increased (or did not decline) in recent years, non-cardia cancers still constitute the majority (estimated at 80–90 %) of gastric cancers worldwide [1]. Gastric cancers include a collection of histologies including adenocarcinoma, lymphoma, and gastrointestinal stromal tumors. Adenocarcinomas, cancers arising from the epithelium of the stomach, comprise about 90–95 % of the cases [2, 3]. This chapter is focused on gastric adenocarcinoma, herein called gastric cancer, and includes both cardia and non-cardia gastric cancers. Although many studies did not distinguish between gastric cardia vs. non-cardia gastric cancers, the differences between gastric cardia versus non-cardia will be mentioned if the data are available.

Incidence and Mortality Trends

Incidence Patterns

The incidence of gastric cancer has declined dramatically over the last half of the twentieth century. However, it remains the fifth most commonly diagnosed cancer worldwide with over 951,000 new cases (6.8 % of the total incidence) and the third most common cause of cancer death with over 723,000 deaths (8.8 % of the total deaths) [4]. The incidence rate of gastric cancer has declined steadily since the 1950s in North America and Europe and more recently in East Asia and Latin America [4]. Gastric cancer rates vary worldwide, highest in East Asia including Korea, Japan, and China (age-adjusted incidence rates are 35.4 per 100,000 men, 13.8 per 100,000 women) and lowest in Western Africa (3.3 per 100,000 men and 2.6 per 100,000 women) and North America (5.5 per 100,000 men and 2.7 per 100,000 women) [4]. Migration studies show a consistent decline in gastric cancer incidence within two generations when individuals migrate from a high-risk country to a low-risk country, particularly among Asian migrants to the USA [5]. Gastric cancer incidence is about two times higher in men than in women across both high-risk and low-risk regions in the world [4].

An estimated 24,590 new gastric cancer cases and 10,720 gastric cancer deaths are expected in the USA in 2015 [6]. Rates of gastric cancer also vary by race/ethnicity and sex in the USA [6]. In 2008–2012, the age-adjusted incidence rates (per 100,000) were lowest for non-Hispanic white men (8.3) and women (3.7). Rates among Asian/Pacific Islander (API) men (14.5) and API women (8.8) are comparable to those in non-Hispanic black men (14.6) and women (8.4) as well as those in Hispanic men (14.2) and women (8.4) [7].

Gastric cancer incidence rates vary considerably among Asian ethnic groups living in the USA [8, 9]. Gastric cancer remains one of the five most commonly occurring malignancies among Chinese, Japanese, Korean, and Vietnamese men and among Japanese and Korean women in the USA [8]. SEER-based registry studies show that in the most recent study period (2004–2008), incidence (per 100,000) was highest among Korean American men (52.5); intermediate among Japanese (24.2), Vietnamese (21.2), and Chinese (16.3) men; and considerably lower in Laotian, Filipino, Kampuchean (Cambodian), and Asian Indian/Pakistani men (<10) [8].

A similar pattern was observed among Asian-American women; rates were highest in Korean-American women (27.4) which were 50–60 % higher than the rates in Japanese, Vietnamese, and Chinese American women [8]. During the past two decades (1990–2008), significant annual percent declines in gastric cancer incidence were observed among Chinese, Vietnamese, and Japanese men, ranging from −1.3 % per year to −3.2 % per year, and comparable declines were found among their female counterparts in the USA [8]. However, the decline in gastric cancer incidence is much less among Korean American men (−0.6 %) and women (0.3 %) during this same time period [8].

Mortality Patterns

Gastric cancer mortality follows a pattern similar to incidence rates. In the USA, mortality rates (per 100,000) are highest in non-Hispanic blacks (9.2 in men and 4.4 in women), followed by API (7.9 in men and 4.7 in women) and Hispanics (7.2 in men and 4.2 in women), and lowest in whites (3.6 in men and 1.8 in women) [7]. Data from the Los Angeles County Cancer Surveillance Program (CSP) for 1988 to 2006 ($n=13{,}084$) showed that median survival was better in Asian (16.3 months) than whites (8.4 months) with gastric cancer ($P<0.001$); the hazard ratio (HR) in Asians compared to whites was 0.76 (95 % CI 0.72–0.82) after adjusting for age, gender, tumor location, histology, grade, stage, and treatment [10]. The more favorable survival in Asian Americans was also found in a California Cancer Registry (CCR)-based study that included 47,647 patients diagnosed between 1988 and 2005. Compared to non-Hispanic whites, Asian Americans had lower adjusted HRs for localized (HR=0.63, 95 % CI 0.55–0.71), regional (HR=0.81, 95 % CI=0.76–0.85), and distant/remote (HR=0.92, 95 % CI 0.87–0.97) stage at diagnosis as well as for all stages combined (HR=0.81, 95 % CI 0.78–0.83) [11]. A SEER-17 registry-based study of 49,058 gastric cancer patients diagnosed between 1998 and 2008 found that Asian Americans had significantly better overall survival for all stages and better disease-specific survival in stage I and II, but not stage III or IV when compared to whites [12]. Survival may also differ between different Asian American ethnicities. For example, in the Los Angeles County-CSP study of 1817 Asian Americans treated for gastric cancer between 1988–2006, median survival was longest among Koreans (22.4 months) but shortest among Filipinos (10.3 months) [13].

Pathology

Lauren classified gastric adenocarcinomas into intestinal and diffuse type. Intestinal-type tumors composed of moderately to well-differentiated gland-like structures, and diffuse-type tumors composed of solitary cells or small groups of cells infiltrating normal gastric tissues, without formation of glands [14]. These two types have different morphological features, risk factors, clinical presentations, and outcomes. The differences stem from intrinsic biological differences between these two histologies [15]. The intestinal type resembles the adenocarcinomas arising in the intestinal tracts and is more frequently associated with *Helicobacter pylori* (*H. pylori*) infection, whereas diffuse-type cancers arise when there is a germ line or somatic mutations resulting in loss of expression of E-cadherin, an adhesion molecule that maintains the organization of the epithelial cells [16].

Lauren classification is not routinely used and reported in Western countries; therefore, it is difficult to ascertain differences in the incidence of these two types between Asian Americans and non-Hispanic whites. For example, in the CCR-SEER-based study mentioned above, 21.1 % of gastric cancers were classified as diffuse, 4.6 % as intestinal, but information was missing on 74.1 % [11]. In another SEER-based study that specifically recoded the histologic classification of gastric cancer into the intestinal and diffuse, the comparison was between whites, blacks, and other race groups combined, which included Asian Americans [17].

Risk Factors

There is a wealth of literature on gastric cancer risk factors but only a few of these studies were conducted among Asian Americans, and most of the work was led by Nomura and colleagues at the University of Hawaii. They conducted three cohort studies in Hawaii. The first was a cohort of 7990 Japanese men from the Hawaiian island of Oahu who were enrolled from 1965 to 1968, provided detailed information on diet and other lifestyle factors, and donated blood specimens, and some also participated in a physical examination [18]. The second cohort study enrolled 11,907 randomly selected Japanese residents of Hawaii (6297 women and 5610 men) who completed a short dietary questionnaire at enrollment between 1975–1980 [19]. The third cohort is the large Multiethnic Cohort (MEC), an ongoing population-based prospective study with >215,000 men and women; over 50,000 are Japanese men and women from Hawaii and California (mainly Los Angeles County) and were enrolled between 1993 and 1996 [20]. Several case–control studies that included Asians in the USA have also been conducted [21, 22]. In particular, a population-based case–control study was conducted among 300 gastric cancer cases and 446 control subjects in Hawaii in the 1990s; most of the participants (233 cases and 330 controls) were Japanese, Filipino, Korean, and Chinese Americans [21]. A subset of these participants (212 cases and 336 controls) provided blood specimens, representing one of the few studies in Asian Americans to investigate risk factors separately for those who were positive for *H. pylori*/CagA infection (160 cases, 164 controls) and negative for *H. pylori*/CagA (52 cases, 172 controls) infection [23].

Helicobacter pylori (H. pylori)

Since the discovery of *Helicobacter pylori* (*H. pylori*), a gram-negative microaerophilic spiral bacteria in 1979–1982 by Marshall and Warren [24, 25], the epidemiology of *H. pylori* has been extensively studied [26–30] culminating in its classification by the International Agency on Research in Cancer (IARC) in 1994 as a class I human carcinogen and a major cause of gastric cancer [31]. The evidence on *H. pylori* and gastric was confirmed in 2009 by a second IARC working group which more precisely quantified the association between *H. pylori* and non-cardia gastric cancer [32]. It is now known that *H. pylori* can colonize the gastric mucosa for years, and their presence is strongly associated with chronic, diffuse, and superficial gastritis of the fundus and antrum. *H. pylori* has an etiologic role in gastritis and may progress over several decades to chronic atrophic gastritis, an established precursor of gastric carcinoma [33].

One of the first prospective studies on *H. pylori* infection and risk of gastric cancer was conducted among 5908 Japanese-American men in Hawaii [34]. In this nested case–control study, 94 % of the 109 men with gastric cancer and 76 % of the 109 matched control men tested positive for *H. pylori* antibodies in pre-diagnostic blood samples that had been stored for more than 20 years (adjusted odds ratio (OR) 6.0, 95 % CI 2.1–17.3) [34]. This significant risk association was observed for non-cardia gastric cancer which represented 95 % of gastric cancers in this cohort of men [34]. A subsequent analysis investigated the association of distal gastric cancer with *H. pylori* and particularly the cytotoxin-associated gene A (CagA) type of *H. pylori* infection, which is present in 60 to 70 % of *H. pylori* strains and has been found to elicit a more marked inflammatory response [35]. This analysis of 261 Japanese American men with gastric cancer and an equal number of control men found an adjusted OR of 3.0 (95 % CI 1.8–5.0) for *H. pylori* and 1.9 (95 % CI 1.3–2.8) for colonization by a cagA+ *H. pylori* strain. Persons who were *H. pylori* and CagA positive had an OR of 4.1 (95 % CI 2.2–7.7) for intestinal gastric cancer compared with those who were seronegative for both *H. pylori* and CagA antibodies [36]. This study in Japanese-American men was included in an international pooled analysis of 12 studies which found an overall OR of 3.0 (95 % CI 2.3–3.8) for non-cardia gastric cancers and no association with gastric cardia cancers (OR = 1.0, 95 % CI 0.7–1.4). When the analysis was restricted to cases occurring at least 10 years after diagnosis of *H. pylori*, the OR for non-cardia gastric cancer increased to 5.93 (95 % CI 3.41–10.37) [37]. The attributable fraction for *H. pylori* infection in non-cardia gastric cancers is between 74.7 to 89.0 % [1, 38]. The declining incidence of gastric cancer has been attributed to the reduction of *H. pylori* infection in successive birth cohorts in Asian countries, which is presumably related to changing childhood environment, improved food preservation practices, and other factors [39, 40].

Although infection with *H. pylori* is an established risk factor for non-cardia gastric cancers, only a small proportion of those infected go on to develop gastric cancer, which means that better understanding of the interactions between host factors, environmental factors, and *H. pylori* infection is needed to better characterize persons who eventually develop this cancer.

Tobacco Smoking

There is convincing evidence that tobacco smoking moderately increases the risk of both cardia and non-cardia gastric cancers. Japanese-American men who were current smokers had a significant 2.7 (95 % CI 1.8–4.1) risk of gastric cancer compared with never smokers [18]. In the MEC, Japanese Americans who were current smokers had a higher risk of gastric cancer (RR = 1.75, 95 % CI 1.2–2.5); this magnitude of smoking effect was comparable across different racial/ethnic groups [41]. In the MEC as in other studies, the effect of smoking tended to be stronger in men than in the women. In a pooled analysis of 42 case–control and cohort studies [42], the risk of gastric cancer was 1.62 (95 % CI 1.50–1.75) among male current smokers and 1.20 (95 % CI 1.01–1.43) among female current smokers compared to never smokers. Smoking is associated with increased risk of both cardia (RR = 1.87, 95 % CI 1.31–2.67) and non-cardia (RR = 1.60, 95 % CI 1.41–1.80) gastric cancer [42]. The smoking-gastric cancer association was similar in studies conducted in Asia (RR = 1.57, 95 % CI 1.47–1.68), Europe (RR = 1.72, 95 % CI 1.13–2.61), and the USA (RR = 1.84, 95 % CI 1.25–2.70) [42].

The extent to which infection with *H. pylori* modifies the smoking-gastric cancer association has been studied in only a few studies. In a cross-sectional study of whites and nonwhites using NHANES data, the prevalence of H. *pylori* infection was higher in current smokers (prevalence OR = 1.9 (95 % CI 1.4–2.5) and former smokers (prevalence OR = 1.3 (95 % CI 1.0–1.7) compared with never smokers [43]. In a case–control study conducted in Hawaii which included mostly Asian Americans, the increased risk of gastric cancer among smokers was statistically significant among those who were *H. pylori* and/or CagA+ positive ($p = 0.0004$) but not among those who were *H. pylori* and/or CagA+ negative ($p = 0.21$) [23]. These observations are supportive of the suggestion of increased inflammatory reaction to *H. pylori* infection among smokers [44] and that smokers are more likely to have persistent *H. pylori* infection due to adverse effects of smoking on the immune system [45]. The combined deleterious effects of tobacco smoking and *H. pylori* infection may be particularly important for some Asian-American subgroups such as Korean Americans who are at high risk for both risk factors. In combination with a high *H. pylori* infection rate, the current smoking prevalence among Korean-American men and women is about two to three times higher than other Asian Americans [46], which may explain, in part, the slower decline and persistently higher rates of gastric cancer among Korean men and women in the USA [8].

Alcohol

Alcohol intake appears to be unrelated to risk of cardia gastric cancer but may be positively associated with risk of non-cardia gastric cancer, particularly among heavy alcohol consumers. In the cohort study of Japanese-American men in Hawaii, risk of gastric cancer was not significantly increased among alcohol drinkers

(RR = 1.1) after adjusting for age and smoking history [18]. Risk was unrelated to increasing amount of alcohol intake from all sources or specifically from beer, wine, or hard liquor [18]. In a case–control study of mostly Asians in Hawaii, alcohol use was also not associated with gastric cancer risk [21], irrespective of *H. pylori*/CagA+ status [23].

The null findings in Asian Americans are compatible with the overall evidence from meta-analyses of case–control and cohort studies [47–49]. However, a weak positive association cannot be ruled out for non-cardia gastric cancer and for heavy alcohol drinking. For example, in the meta-analysis conducted by Tramacere et al. [48], the overall RR based on 44 case–control and 15 cohort studies was 1.07 (95 % CI = 1.01–1.13); a positive association was found for non-cardia (RR = 1.07, 95 % CI = 0.91–1.26) but not for cardia (RR = 0.94, 95 % CI = 0.78–1.13) gastric cancers. In the subset of 13 studies on heavy alcohol drinking (four or more drinks per day), the overall RR was 1.20 (95 % CI 1.01–1.44) which was stronger for non-cardia (RR = 1.17, 95 % CI 0.78–1.75) than for cardia (RR = 0.99, 95 % CI 0.67–1.47) gastric cancers. A possible effect of heavy alcohol intake among never smokers was evident in a population-based cohort of older men in Shanghai, China [50]. It will be informative in future meta-analysis to pool the results of studies that allow investigation of the effect of alcohol in the presence and absence of smoking. Nitrosamines present in alcoholic beverages [51], acetaldehyde, a metabolic intermediate of ethanol and an animal carcinogen [52], and alcohol intake may enhance the deleterious effects of tobacco carcinogens. Alcohol may also influence the pathogenesis of gastric cancer development by enhancing the penetration of tobacco carcinogens [51].

Dietary Factors

Many studies have investigated the role of diet and risk of gastric cancer. In general, the associations with specific dietary factors were stronger in case–control studies than in cohort studies. Depending on the specific dietary factor of interest, the associations were generally more evident for non-cardia gastric cancer.

Total Meat and Processed Meat

The intake of red meat is a potential risk factor for gastric cancer, for both cardia and non-cardia gastric cancer, but the positive findings were based primarily on case–control studies. In a meta-analysis conducted by Zhu et al. [53], the risk of gastric cancer was increased in association with high intake of red meat (RR = 1.45, 95 % CI 1.22–1.73), for both cardia (RR = 1.26, 95 % CI 1.05–1.52) and non-cardia (RR = 1.26, 95 % CI 0.92–1.71) gastric cancer. The RR was 1.56 (95 % CI 0.93–2.63) for studies conducted in Asia and 1.52 (95 % CI 1.16–2.00) in European populations. However, there was no significant association with red meat intake in the four cohort studies (RR = 1.02, 95 % CI 0.90–1.17). In contrast, in the same meta-analysis, the risk of gastric cancer was increased in association with intake of processed meat (RR = 1.45, 95 % CI 1.26–1.65); this was also observed in the cohort studies (RR = 1.18, 95 % CI 1.00–1.38). The processed meat association appeared to be observed for non-cardia gastric cancer (RR = 1.27, 95 % CI 1.07–1.52) but not for cardia cancer (RR = 0.95, 0.76–1.19). The risk association appeared to be similar for studies conducted in Asian and Western populations; the respective RRs were 1.58 (95 % CI 1.06–2.37) and 1.50 (95 % CI 1.18–1.91) [53].

In the case–control study of gastric cancer among Asian and non-Asian residents in Hawaii, gastric cancer in men was increased significantly by twofold among those with high intake of processed meat and bacon, but this was not observed in women [21]. In a subset of participants with information on *H. pylori*/CagA status [23], high intake of processed meat and bacon was associated with significant increase risks among those who were *H. pylori* CagA positive (ORs for low, medium, and high intake of bacon were 1.0, 0.8, 1.7, *P* trend = 0.02). Although results were similar among those who were *H. pylori*/CagA negative, the finding was weaker (respective ORs were 1.0, 0.9, and 1.4, *P* trend = 0.26), which may be related to the modest sample size. The increased risk associated with red and processed meat intake and gastric cancer may involve heme iron, more abundant in red meat than white meat [54], and may contribute to endogenous formation of carcinogenic N-nitroso compounds which have been linked to gastric cancer [55]. N-nitroso compounds are also formed in processed meat containing high amount of salt, nitrate, and nitrite compounds [56].

Fruits and Vegetables

In a meta-analysis of cohort studies of intake of fruit and vegetables and risk of gastric cancer, high intake of fruit was inversely associated with risk of gastric cancer (RR = 0.90, 95 % CI 0.83–0.98), but a weaker association was observed with intake of vegetables (RR = 0.96, 95 % CI 0.88–1.06) [57]. The inverse association with intake of fruit was observed for both cardia (RR = 0.88, 95 % CI 0.76–1.02) and non-cardia gastric cancer (RR = 0.89, 95 % CI 0.77–1.02), whereas the inverse association with intake of vegetables was only observed for non-cardia (RR = 0.94, 95% CI 0.81–1.09) but not for cardia gastric cancer (RR = 1.06, 95 % CI 0.90–1.25).

In cohort studies conducted of Japanese men in Hawaii [5, 18, 58] and of Japanese men and women in Hawaii [19], high assumption of fruits and/or vegetables (≥80 g/day or ≥7 times per week) was associated with 40 % lower risk of gastric cancer compared to the lowest level of intakes. In the case–control study conducted among mostly Asians in Hawaii, high intake of total vegetables, dark-green vegetables, and yellow vegetables was significantly inversely associated with risk in both men and women [21]. However, in analysis by *H. pylori*/Cag status [23], significant inverse trends in association with intake of total and green vegetables and cruciferous vegetables were found only among *H. pylori*/CagA positive individuals but not among *H. pylori*/CagA negative persons. Further investigation of the role of cruciferous vegetables may be warranted since it was suggested to be inversely associated with gastric cancer risk in a meta-analysis [59].

Salt

High intake of salt in cooking, processing, and preserving meat has been implicated as a gastric cancer risk factor. Experimental data suggest that high salt intake can cause mucosal damage and inflammation [60, 61]. In a meta-analysis of prospective studies, compared to low salt intake, gastric cancer risk was increased with moderately high (OR = 1.41, 95 % CI 1.03–1.93) and very high salt intake (OR = 1.68, 95 % CI 1.17–1.41) [62]. Although the evidence on high salt intake and risk was strong in studies conducted in Japan, the association was less consistent in an investigation among Japanese in Hawaii which may be related, in part, to the relatively modest number of gastric cancer cases ($n = 108$) [19]. Further investigation of the role of salt intake among more than 50,000 Japanese Americans in the ongoing MEC will be informative [41].

Clinical Features

In countries such as Japan and Korea where routine screening is offered, many patients are diagnosed with cancer before development of symptoms. In contrast, in the USA, the majority of gastric cancer patients present with symptoms and have advanced disease at the time of presentation. Symptoms at presentation are typically nonspecific and include weight loss, abdominal pain, nausea, vomiting, and difficulty swallowing [63]. With disease progression, many patients develop gastric outlet obstruction, ascites, and other presentation of metastatic disease such as jaundice. Knowledge of the higher incidence of gastric cancer among Asian Americans forces clinicians to be more attentive to the early signs in patients of Asian descent and therefore allows earlier diagnosis and possibly better outcome.

Diagnosis

In the unscreened population, patients are diagnosed based on their symptoms, which prompt providers to use diagnostic tools such as endoscopy or CT scan. Diagnosis is usually made using endoscopy to visualize the tumor and take a tissue sample for histological confirmation. Alternatively patients with metastatic disease may have a CT scan with findings of liver metastases or peritoneal involvement. To confirm the diagnosis and to start treatment, it is required to have histologic confirmation of gastric cancer. In contrast, the screened patients are asymptomatic at diagnosis and endoscopic examination combined with biopsy results will identify gastric cancer.

With histological diagnosis, patients undergo staging workup which includes imaging techniques such as CT and/or PET scans. The goal of staging workup is to identify subjects who are possible candidates for surgery or in the case of metastatic disease to initiate palliative chemotherapy. Although there is no uniform way to stage gastric cancer, a rational approach is to obtain a CT scan of the abdomen and chest to assess the extent of the disease and whether metastatic disease to liver or peritoneum is present. In the absence of metastatic disease by a CT scan, many providers will require a combined PET/CT scan to confirm the lack of occult evidence for metastatic disease before determining treatment [64]. In patients who are candidates for perioperative chemotherapy, an endoscopic ultrasound will assess the depth of the tumor and establish the clinical stage [65]. Given that CT and even PET/CT have limited capability to identify peritoneal disease, recent data support the use of diagnostic laparoscopy for direct visualization as well as peritoneal washing for assessment of peritoneum prior to the planned laparotomy [66].

East–West Differences

As noted above, Asian Americans with gastric cancer appear to have more favorable outcome than non-Hispanic whites. Overall survival of patients with gastric cancer in Japan and Korea is better than that in Western countries [67, 68]. The reasons for this observed difference are not completely clear. Although better surgery in eastern countries with removal of the tumor and a higher number of lymph nodes has been suggested as a possible explanation for better outcomes, a large randomized Dutch trial failed to show improvement in survival with extended lymph node removal in Western populations [69, 70]. The possibility exists that the biology of gastric cancer in eastern and Western populations may differ, contributing to differences in outcome.

Prognosis of gastric cancer depends on the stage at the time of diagnosis. There are, in fact, differences in the staging classification between Western countries and Japan [71, 72]. Staging in Western countries is outcome driven, while the Japanese staging system provides guidance for treatment. These differences in staging may result in some of the reported outcome differences between Western countries and Japan [73].

In Western countries, the conventional staging system is TNM (tumor, node, metastasis). Using TNM criteria tumors are staged broadly from stage I–IV. Japanese staging classification has three locations for cancer: upper, middle, and lower. Additionally, visual appearance of cancers (superficial, mass, ulcerative, infiltrative ulcerative, diffuse infiltrative, and unclassifiable) is recorded on the pathology report. Lymph nodes are reported by their station (location of the lymph nodes and their proximity to major organs surrounding stomach) and provide a guide to the required degree of surgical resection based on the location of the tumor. However, we are not aware of any studies that used both TNM and the Japanese stage classification in the same study to directly compare the two methods.

Treatment

Patients with gastric cancer require multidisciplinary care by a group of specialists including gastroenterologist, surgeon, medical oncologist, and radiation oncologist. Extent of the disease dictates the type and number of specialists involved in patient care. For example, for patients with early-stage disease (i.e., no distant metastasis and no involvement of structures surrounding stomach) who are candidates for surgical resection, the team will include a surgeon, medical oncologist, and radiation oncologist while for those with late-stage diagnosis who are candidates for palliative treatment, the team may include a medical oncologist, gastroenterologist, and palliative care specialist. In the following section, the modalities of treatment as well as the role of each of the specialist are discussed. It is important to point out that models of care in the USA differ from the practice in Asian countries including Japan, Korea, and China. In the USA, only medical oncologists administer chemotherapy, while in Asian countries, surgeons frequently administer chemotherapy, making the coordination of care less cumbersome.

Surgical Interventions

For patients with early-stage disease, surgery is the treatment of choice. Currently the only way to achieve cure is to have surgical removal of the tumor and regional lymph nodes. Endoscopic removal of the tumor (endoscopic mucosal resection (EMR) or endoscopic submucosal dissection (ESD)) is an acceptable approach in selected patients with low likelihood of nodal involvement [74, 75]. Although endoscopic removal of the tumor is minimally invasive, the follow-up is extensive and requires regular endoscopy. The data for endoscopic removal of gastric cancer is from Asian countries as this procedure is not commonly performed in the USA and Europe [76]. In the USA, the frequency of this procedure is unknown and patients are not candidates due to a higher stage at diagnosis. For patients with higher-stage gastric cancer, surgery may involve total or partial gastrectomy. Partial gastrectomy is an option for patients with cancers in the distal part of the stomach. Recent data show that laparoscopic surgeries are generally safe, require shorter duration of hospital stay, and provide equivalent outcomes [77, 78].

There are also differences in the timing and extent of surgical approach between Western countries compared to practices in Korea and Japan [79]. In Western countries many patients undergo perioperative chemotherapy (neo-adjuvant chemotherapy followed by surgery and then adjuvant chemotherapy) on the basis of favorable results from several randomized trials showing the effectiveness of this approach compared to surgery alone. However, the approach in Korea and Japan is primarily up-front surgery.

Adjuvant and Neo-adjuvant Therapies

Results of multiple clinical trials have established that in patients who undergo surgery for gastric cancer, surgery alone is no longer an accepted standard of care. However, there is no consensus on the best approach to manage these patients. Two large trials conducted in Asia have established that adjuvant chemotherapy with fluoropyrimidine alone or in combination with platinum significantly improved overall survival. The Japanese trial established that 1-year treatment with S1 (an oral fluoropyrimidine) improved the 3-year survival rate from 70 % in the surgery alone arm to 80 % in the surgery + S1 arm [80]. The second trial from Korea and China showed that 6 months of treatment with capecitabine + oxaliplatin (fluoropyrimidine + platinum) improved the 3-year survival rate from 59 % in the surgery arm to 74 % in the surgery and chemotherapy arm [81]. Despite these findings, adjuvant chemotherapy alone is not an accepted modality in Western countries because of differences in patient identification and surgical techniques and that S1 is not available in the USA and has limited availability in Europe [82]. In the following section, we describe the landscape of adopted modalities of adjuvant and neo-adjuvant therapies in the Western world.

Chemotherapy alone around the time of surgery and chemotherapy combined with radiation (chemoradiation) after surgery are both efficacious strategies established in different randomized clinical trials, but there is no head-to-head comparison between these two strategies.

As for chemotherapy, it is administered in the perioperative setting with surgical intervention sandwiched between chemotherapies [83, 84]. Results from the MAGIC trial, one of the largest chemotherapy trials, showed that chemotherapy improved the likelihood of survival. In this trial, the probability of 5-year survival was 36 % in recipients of perioperative chemotherapy compared to 23 % in those who received surgery alone (HR for death, 0.75; 95 % CI: 0.60 to 0.93) [83]. In the French trial, another large chemotherapy trial in Western countries, the 5-year survival rate was 38 % in recipients of perioperative chemotherapy compared to 24 % for surgery alone (HR for death: 0.69; 95 % CI 0.50 to 0.9) [84]. The most active agents used in these trials are believed to be 5-FU and cisplatin [84]. However, at best only 50 % of the patients are able to complete the treatment due to toxicities [83, 84]. Interestingly, a small study did not confirm these findings in Korean population; the findings were presented in abstract in the ASCO annual meeting in 1996 and never published in manuscript [85].

Chemotherapy combined with radiation or chemoradiation is a treatment modality initially studied in USA [86]. Although the initial study revealed a 35 %

reduction in the rate of death from gastric cancer in recipients of chemoradiation, the study was criticized for suboptimal surgery and the fact that radiation compensated for inadequate lymph node dissection. Furthermore, a retrospective study using Oregon Cancer registry suggests a lower rate of survival benefit for chemoradiation in gastric cancer patients [87]. Thus the overall benefit of chemoradiation may be less than the reported rates in randomized trials. Regarding the chemotherapy agent that is used with radiation, standard chemotherapy is a 5-FU-based treatment in the adjuvant setting followed by concurrent 5-FU with radiation. The addition of platinum agent to 5-FU may be beneficial in a subset of patients with node-positive disease based on a recent analysis for a study that was conducted in Asia [88].

It is evident that the interaction between race/ethnicity and treatment selection and efficacy in the literature is not well defined. This is because the randomized trials for assessment of efficacy are conducted in different areas of the world with different population characteristics. In international trials analysis of subgroups is not always possible due to limited numbers and therefore inadequate prediction power. We hope that with improvement in the understanding of the racial/ethnic differences in risk factors, predisposition, and outcomes, future efforts for conduct of the international trials would take the racial/ethnic factors into account at the time of trial design and provide the information that can improve our understanding of the treatment-specific differences among different racial/ethnic populations.

Palliative Treatments

For patients who are not candidates for curative therapies, palliative treatments, including chemotherapy, radiation, palliative surgeries, and hospice and end-of-life care are other options. Chemotherapy plays a significant role in prolongation of survival and palliation of symptoms. In a recent meta-analysis, combination chemotherapy is associated with 63% improvement in survival from a median of 4.3 months to 11 months [89]. Although there is no consensus on the best regimen in the first-line setting, platinum-containing regimens are considered standard of care, and oxaliplatin-containing regimens are widely used in the USA [90, 91].

Radiation plays a role in alleviating symptoms of obstruction for gastroesophageal junctional cancers, cessation of bleeding, or alleviating symptoms at metastatic sites such as bone lesions.

Palliative surgeries such as gastrojejunal bypass or placement of tubes for relief of intractable vomiting and feeding are available to selected patients with incurable disease. Finally, all patients should receive supportive care for their symptoms of pain, depression, nausea, and vomiting. Hospice is an appropriate disposition for patients who have poor performance status and are not candidates for aggressive interventions.

Two targeted agents have established role in gastric cancers. Trastuzumab confers a survival benefit in patients with HER2 positive cancers [92]. Additionally, ramucirumab is shown to have survival benefit in the second-line setting as a single agent or in combination with chemotherapy [93, 94]. The data for ramucirumab suggests that there is a preferential benefit for Caucasian patients, while Asian patients achieve a lower degree of benefit from these interventions [95].

Screening and Prevention

Although there is a debate in whether screening reduces mortality from gastric cancer, Korea, Japan, and Venezuela have screening programs for gastric cancer at a population level [96–99]. The modality of screening varies between different countries. In Korea upper endoscopy every 2 years starting at age 40 is the standard of care, and it has proven to be cost-effective from a societal perspective [100].

Many professional societies recommend treatment for incidental finding of *H. pylori*; however, a randomized trial to assess the role of treatment in prevention of gastric cancer found no statistically significant reduction in the risk of gastric cancer in the treated population [101].

Conclusion

Despite decline in the incidence of gastric cancer, it remains one of the major causes of cancer mortality worldwide with significant variation in the geographic, racial, and socioeconomic distribution. Gastric cancer is heterogeneous with multiple genetic and environmental risk factors, variable disease presentation, and outcome; furthermore, practices for diagnosis and management of the disease are diverse across the world. In recent years, we have learned that treatment benefits can vary by race/ethnicity and region of the world, possibly due to host-related factors and differences in disease etiology. The consistent difference in outcome in Asian patients compared to non-Asian patients after controlling for stage at diagnosis emphasizes the importance of considering race/ethnicity and specifically Asian ethnicity in international trials.

Efforts to better understand the disease course and risk factors will provide a framework to better classification of this cancer into homogenous categories and lead the way for uniform approach to the diagnosis and management of the disease with significant impact on outcome. Continued efforts to improve outcomes through consideration of race, ethnicity, and country of birth in their diagnostic algorithm are needed.

Financial Disclosure Authors' declaration of personal interests:

None

Declaration of funding interests:

None

References

1. de Martel C, Ferlay J, Franceschi S, Vignat J, Bray F, Forman D, Plummer M (2012) Global burden of cancers attributable to infections in 2008: a review and synthetic analysis. Lancet Oncol 13(6):607–615
2. Edge SB, Byrd DR, Compton CC, Fritz AG, Greene FL, Trotti A (2010) AJCC cancer staging handbook, 7th edn. Springer, New York
3. Karpeh MS, Kelsen DP, Tepper JE (2001) Section 3 cancer of the stomach. In: DeVita VT, Hellman S, Rosenberg SA (eds) Cancer principles & practice of oncology, 6th edn. Lippincott Williams & Wilkins, Philadelphia, PA, pp 1092–1126, Chapter 33.3
4. Torre LA, Bray F, Siegel RL, Ferlay J, Lortet-Tieulent J, Jemal A (2015) Global cancer statistics, 2012. CA Cancer J Clin 65(2):87–108
5. Nomura AMY, Stemmermann GN, Chyou PH (1995) Gastric-cancer among the Japanese in Hawaii. Jpn J Cancer Res 86(10):916–923
6. Siegel RL, Miller KD, Jemal A (2015) Cancer statistics, 2015. CA Cancer J Clin 65(1):5–29
7. NIH National Cancer Institute Surveillance E, and End Results Program (2015) Table 24.15 Cancer of the Stomach (Invasive) SEER Incidence and U.S. Mortality Age-Adjusted Rates and Trends By Race/Ethnicity and Sex. Bethesda, MD 20892–9760. http://seer.cancer.gov/csr/1975_2012/browse_csr.php?sectionSEL=24&pageSEL=sect_24_table.15.html
8. Gomez SL, Noone A-M, Lichtensztajn DY, Scoppa S, Gibson JT, Liu L, Morris C, Kwong S, Fish K, Wilkens LR, Goodman MT, Deapen D, Miller BA (2013) Cancer incidence trends among Asian American populations in the United States, 1990–2008. J Natl Cancer Ins 105(15):1096–1110
9. Miller BA, Chu KC, Hankey BF, Ries LAG (2008) Cancer incidence and mortality patterns among specific Asian and Pacific Islander populations in the US. Cancer Causes Control 19(3):227–256
10. Kim J, Sun CL, Mailey B, Prendergast C, Artinyan A, Bhatia S, Pigazzi A, Ellenhorn JD (2010) Race and ethnicity correlate with survival in patients with gastric adenocarcinoma. Ann Oncol 21(1):152–160
11. Kunz PL, Gubens M, Fisher GA, Ford JM, Lichtensztajn DY, Clarke CA (2012) Long-term survivors of gastric cancer: a California population-based study. J Clin Oncol 30(28): 3507–3515
12. Howard JH, Hiles JM, Leung AM, Stern SL, Bilchik AJ (2015) Race influences stage-specific survival in gastric cancer. Am Surg 81(3):259–267
13. Kim J, Mailey B, Senthil M, Artinyan A, Sun C-L, Bhatia S (2009) Disparities in gastric cancer outcomes among Asian Ethnicities in the USA. Ann Surg Oncol 16(9):2433–2441
14. Lauren P (1965) The two histological main types of gastric carcinoma: diffuse and so-called intestinal-type carcinoma. An attempt at a histo-clinical classification. Acta Pathol Microbiol Scand 64:31–49
15. Tan IB, Ivanova T, Lim KH, Ong CW, Deng N, Lee J, Tan SH, Wu J, Lee MH, Ooi CH, Rha SY, Wong WK, Boussioutas A, Yeoh KG, So J, Yong WP, Tsuburaya A, Grabsch H, Toh HC, Rozen S, Cheong JH, Noh SH, Wan WK, Ajani JA, Lee JS, Tellez MS, Tan P (2011) Intrinsic

subtypes of gastric cancer, based on gene expression pattern, predict survival and respond differently to chemotherapy. Gastroenterology 141(2):476–485, 485.e1–11

16. Graziano F, Humar B, Guilford P (2003) The role of the E-cadherin gene (CDH1) in diffuse gastric cancer susceptibility: from the laboratory to clinical practice. Ann Oncol 14(12):1705–1713
17. Wu H, Rusiecki JA, Zhu K, Potter J, Devesa SS (2009) Stomach carcinoma incidence patterns in the United States by histologic type and anatomic site. Cancer Epidemiol Biomark Prev 18(7):1945–1952
18. Nomura A, Grove JS, Stemmermann GN, Severson RK (1990) A prospective-study of stomach-cancer and its relation to diet, cigarettes, and alcohol-consumption. Cancer Res 50(3):627–631
19. Galanis DJ, Kolonel LN, Lee J, Nomura A (1998) Intakes of selected foods and beverages and the incidence of gastric cancer among the Japanese residents of Hawaii: a prospective study. Int J Epidemiol 27(2):173–180
20. Kolonel LN, Henderson BE, Hankin JH, Nomura AMY, Wilkens LR, Pike MC, Stram DO, Monroe KR, Earle ME, Nagamine FS (2000) A multiethnic cohort in Hawaii and Los Angeles: Baseline characteristics. Am J Epidemiol 151(4):346–357
21. Nomura AMY, Hankin JH, Kolonel LN, Wilkens LR, Goodman MT, Stemmermann GN (2003) Case–control study of diet and other risk factors for gastric cancer in Hawaii (United States). Cancer Causes Control 14(6):547–558
22. Wu AH, Wan P, Bernstein L (2001) A multiethnic population-based study of smoking, alcohol and body size and risk of adenocarcinomas of the stomach and esophagus (United States). Cancer Causes Control 12(8):721–732
23. Epplein M, Nomura AMY, Hankin JH, Blaser MJ, Perez-Perez G, Stemmermann GN, Wilkens LR, Kolonel LN (2008) Association of Helicobacter pylori infection and diet on the risk of gastric cancer: a case–control study in Hawaii. Cancer Causes Control 19(8): 869–877
24. Marshall B (1983) Unidentified curved bacilli on gastric epithelium in active chronic gastritis. Lancet 1(8336):1273–1275
25. Marshall BJ, Warren JR (1984) Unidentified curved bacilli in the stomach of patients with gastritis and peptic-ulceration. Lancet 1(8390):1311–1315
26. Correa P, Fox J, Fontham E, Ruiz B, Lin YP, Zavala D, Taylor N, Mackinley D, Delima E, Portilla H, Zarama G (1990) Helicobacter-pylori and gastric-carcinoma—serum antibody prevalence in populations with contrasting cancer risks. Cancer 66(12):2569–2574
27. Munoz N (1994) Is Helicobacter-pylori a cause of gastric-cancer—an appraisal of the seroepidemiological evidence. Cancer Epidemiol Biomark Prev 3(5):445–451
28. Munoz N, Pisani P (1994) Helicobacter-pylori and gastric-cancer. Eur J Gastroenterol Hepatol 6(12):1097–1103
29. Parsonnet J, Friedman GD, Vandersteen DP, Chang Y, Vogelman JH, Orentreich N, Sibley RK (1991) Helicobacter-pylori infection and the risk of gastric-carcinoma. N Engl J Med 325(16):1127–1131
30. Talley NJ, Zinsmeister AR, Weaver A, Dimagno EP, Carpenter HA, Perezperez GI, Blaser MJ (1991) Gastric adenocarcinoma and Helicobacter-pylori infection. J Natl Cancer Inst 83(23):1734–1739
31. IARC Working Group (1994) Schistosomes, liver flukes and *Helicobacter pylori*. Lyon, France: IARC Monographs on the Evaluation of Carcinogenic Risks to Humans 61:1–241. Lyon, 7–14 June 1994
32. IARC Working Group monographs (2012) *Helicobacter pylori*. Lyon, France: International Agency for Research on Cancer (Volume 100B:385–435). http://monographs.iarc.fr/ENG/Monographs/vol100B/mono100B-15.pdf
33. IARC *Helicobacter pylori* Working Group (2014) *Helicobacter pylori* Eradication as a Strategy for Preventing Gastric Cancer. Lyon, France: International Agency for Research on Cancer (IARC Working Group Reports, No. 8). http://www.iarc.fr/en/publications/pdfsonline/wrk/wrk8/index.php

34. Nomura A, Stemmermann GN, Chyou PH, Kato I, Perezperez GI, Blaser MJ (1991) Helicobacter-Pylori infection and gastric-carcinoma among Japanese-Americans in Hawaii. N Engl J Med 325(16):1132–1136
35. Crabtree JE, Taylor JD, Wyatt JI, Heatley RV, Shallcross TM, Tompkins DS, Rathbone BJ (1991) Mucosal IGA recognition of Helicobacter-pylori 120-KDA protein, peptic-ulceration, and gastric pathology. Lancet 338(8763):332–335
36. Nomura AMY, Lee J, Stemmermann GN, Nomura RY, Perez-Perez GI, Blaser MJ (2002) Helicobacter pylori CagA seropositivity and gastric carcinoma risk in a Japanese American population. J Infect Dis 186(8):1138–1144
37. Webb PM, Law M, Varghese C, Forman D, Yuan JM, Yu M, Ross R, Limberg PJ, Mark SD, Taylor PR, Dawsey SM, Qiao YL, Aromaa A, Knekt P, Kosunen TU, Heinonen OP, Virtamo J, Tulinius H, Watanabe Y, Ozasa K, Kurata JH, Hansen S, Melby KK, Aase S, Jellum E, Vollset SE, Siman JH, Forsgren A, Berglund G, Floren CH, Lin JT, Chen CJ, Wald NJ, Parsonnet J, Friedman GD, Blaser MJ, Nomura A, Stemmermann GN, Helicobacter Canc Collaborative G (2001) Gastric cancer and Helicobacter pylori: a combined analysis of 12 case control studies nested within prospective cohorts. Gut 49(3):347–353
38. Plummer M, Franceschi S, Vignat J, Forman D, de Martel C (2015) Global burden of gastric cancer attributable to Helicobacter pylori. Int J Cancer 136(2):487–490
39. Hirayama Y, Kawai T, Otaki J, Kawakami K, Harada Y (2014) Prevalence of Helicobacter pylori infection with healthy subjects in Japan. J Gastroenterol Hepatol 29:16–19
40. Yim JY, Kim N, Choi SH, Kim YS, Cho KR, Kim SS, Seo GS, Kim HU, Baik GH, Sin CS, Cho SH, Oh BH (2007) Seroprevalence of Helicobacter pylori in South Korea. Helicobacter 12(4):333–340
41. Nomura AMY, Wilkens LR, Henderson BE, Epplein M, Kolonel LN (2012) The association of cigarette smoking with gastric cancer: the multiethnic cohort study. Cancer Causes Control 23(1):51–58
42. Ladeiras-Lopes R, Pereira AK, Nogueira A, Pinheiro-Torres T, Pinto I, Santos-Pereira R, Lunet N (2008) Smoking and gastric cancer: systematic review and meta-analysis of cohort studies. Cancer Causes Control 19(7):689–701
43. Cardenas VM, Graham DY (2005) Smoking and Helicobacter pylori infection in a sample of US adults. Epidemiology 16(4):586–590
44. Shimoyama T, Everett SM, Fukuda S, Axon ATR, Dixon MF, Crabtree JE (2001) Influence of smoking and alcohol on gastric chemokine mRNA expression in patients with Helicobacter pylori infection. J Clin Pathol 54(4):332–334
45. Johnson JD, Houchens DP, Kluwe WM, Craig DK, Fisher GL (1990) Effects of mainstream and environmental tobacco-smoke on the immune-system in animals and humans—a review. Crit Rev Toxicol 20(5):369–395
46. Li S, Kwon SC, Weerasinghe I, Rey MJ, Trinh-Shevrin C (2013) Smoking among Asian Americans: acculturation and gender in the context of tobacco control policies in New York City. Health Promot Pract 14(5 Suppl):18S–28S
47. Shimazu T, Tsuji I, Inoue M, Wakai K, Nagata C, Mizoue T, Tanaka K, Tsugane S, Research Group for the Development and Evaluation of Cancer Prevention Strategies in Japan (2008) Alcohol drinking and gastric cancer risk: An evaluation based on a systematic review of epidemiologic evidence among the Japanese population. Jpn J Clin Oncol 38(1):8–25
48. Tramacere I, Negri E, Pelucchi C, Bagnardi V, Rota M, Scotti L, Islami F, Corrao G, La Vecchia C, Boffetta P (2012) A meta-analysis on alcohol drinking and gastric cancer risk. Ann Oncol 23(1):28–36
49. Tramacere I, Pelucchi C, Bagnardi V, Rota M, Scotti L, Islami F, Corrao G, Boffetta P, La Vecchia C, Negri E (2012) A meta-analysis on alcohol drinking and esophageal and gastric cardia adenocarcinoma risk. Ann Oncol 23(2):287–297
50. Moy KA, Fan YH, Wang RW, Gao YT, Yu MC, Yuan JM (2010) Alcohol and tobacco use in relation to gastric cancer: a prospective study of men in Shanghai, China. Cancer Epidemiol Biomark Prev 19(9):2287–2297

51. IARC Working Group (2010) IARC Monographs on the Evaluation of Carcinogenic Risks to Humans VOLUME 96 Alcohol Consumption and Ethyl Carbamate. Lyon, France: International Agency for Research on Cancer. http://monographs.iarc.fr/ENG/Monographs/vol96/mono96.pdf.
52. Seitz HK, Meier P (2007) The role of acetaldehyde in upper digestive tract cancer in alcoholics. Transl Res 149(6):293–297
53. Zhu H, Yang X, Zhang C, Zhu C, Tao G, Zhao L, Tang S, Shu Z, Cai J, Dai S, Qin Q, Xu L, Cheng H, Sun X (2013) Red and processed meat intake is associated with higher gastric cancer risk: a meta-analysis of epidemiological observational studies. PLoS One 8(8), e70955
54. Cross AJ, Pollock JRA, Bingham SA (2003) Haem, not protein or inorganic iron, is responsible for endogenous intestinal N-nitrosation arising from red meat. Cancer Res 63(10):2358–2360
55. Ward MH, Cross AJ, Abnet CC, Sinha R, Markin RS, Weisenburger DD (2012) Heme iron from meat and risk of adenocarcinoma of the esophagus and stomach. Eur J Cancer Prev 21(2):134–138
56. Tricker AR (1997) N-nitroso compounds and man: sources of exposure, endogenous formation and occurrence in body fluids. Eur J Cancer Prev 6(3):226–268
57. Wang QB, Chen Y, Wang XL, Gong GQ, Li GP, Li CY (2014) Consumption of fruit, but not vegetables, may reduce risk of gastric cancer: results from a meta-analysis of cohort studies. Eur J Cancer 50(8):1498–1509
58. Chyou PH, Nomura AMY, Hankin JH, Stemmermann GN (1990) A case-cohort study of diet and stomach-cancer. Cancer Res 50(23):7501–7504
59. Wu Q-J, Yang Y, Wang J, Han L-H, Xiang Y-B (2013) Cruciferous vegetable consumption and gastric cancer risk: a meta-analysis of epidemiological studies. Cancer Sci 104(8): 1067–1073
60. Bergin IL, Sheppard BJ, Fox JG (2003) Helicobacter pylori infection and high dietary salt independently induce atrophic gastritis and intestinal metaplasia in commercially available outbred Mongolian gerbils. Dig Dis Sci 48(3):475–485
61. Furihata C, Ishida S, Ohta H, Tokuyama T, Katsuyama T, Ogita Z (1996) Cytotoxicity of NaCl, a stomach tumor promoter, and prevention by rice extract in stomach mucose of F344 rats. Cancer Detect Prev 20(3):193–198
62. D'Elia L, Rossi G, Ippolito R, Cappuccio FP, Strazzullo P (2012) Habitual salt intake and risk of gastric cancer: A meta-analysis of prospective studies. Clin Nutr 31(4):489–498
63. Wanebo HJ, Kennedy BJ, Chmiel J, Steele G Jr, Winchester D, Osteen R (1993) Cancer of the stomach. A patient care study by the American College of Surgeons. Ann Surg 218(5): 583–592
64. Lim JS, Yun MJ, Kim MJ, Hyung WJ, Park MS, Choi JY, Kim TS, Lee JD, Noh SH, Kim KW (2006) CT and PET in stomach cancer: preoperative staging and monitoring of response to therapy. Radiographics 26(1):143–156
65. Choi J, Kim SG, Im JP, Kim JS, Jung HC, Song IS (2010) Comparison of endoscopic ultrasonography and conventional endoscopy for prediction of depth of tumor invasion in early gastric cancer. Endoscopy 42(9):705–713
66. Leake PA, Cardoso R, Seevaratnam R, Lourenco L, Helyer L, Mahar A, Law C, Coburn NG (2012) A systematic review of the accuracy and indications for diagnostic laparoscopy prior to curative-intent resection of gastric cancer. Gastric Cancer 15(Suppl 1):S38–S47
67. Matsuda T, Saika K (2013) The 5-year relative survival rate of stomach cancer in the USA, Europe and Japan. Jpn J Clin Oncol 43(11):1157–1158
68. Park J-M, Kim YH (2008) Current approaches to gastric cancer in Korea. Gastrointest Cancer Res 2(3):137–144
69. Bonenkamp JJ, Hermans J, Sasako M, van de Velde CJ, Welvaart K, Songun I, Meyer S, Plukker JT, Van Elk P, Obertop H, Gouma DJ, van Lanschot JJ, Taat CW, de Graaf PW, von Meyenfeldt MF, Tilanus H, Dutch Gastric Cancer Group (1999) Extended lymph-node dissection for gastric cancer. N Engl J Med 340(12):908–914

70. Hartgrink HH, van de Velde CJ, Putter H, Bonenkamp JJ, Klein Kranenbarg E, Songun I, Welvaart K, van Krieken JH, Meijer S, Plukker JT, van Elk PJ, Obertop H, Gouma DJ, van Lanschot JJ, Taat CW, de Graaf PW, von Meyenfeldt MF, Tilanus H, Sasako M (2004) Extended lymph node dissection for gastric cancer: who may benefit? Final results of the randomized Dutch gastric cancer group trial. J Clin Oncol 22(11):2069–2077
71. Japanese Gastric Cancer A (2011) Japanese classification of gastric carcinoma: 3rd English edition. Gastric Cancer 14(2):101–112
72. Verdecchia A, Mariotto A, Gatta G, Bustamante-Teixeira MT, Ajiki W (2003) Comparison of stomach cancer incidence and survival in four continents. Eur J Cancer 39(11): 1603–1609
73. Sayegh ME, Sano T, Dexter S, Katai H, Fukagawa T, Sasako M (2004) TNM and Japanese staging systems for gastric cancer: how do they coexist? Gastric Cancer 7(3):140–148
74. Choi IJ, Lee JH, Kim YI, Kim CG, Cho SJ, Lee JY, Ryu KW, Nam BH, Kook MC, Kim YW (2015) Long-term outcome comparison of endoscopic resection and surgery in early gastric cancer meeting the absolute indication for endoscopic resection. Gastrointest Endosc 81(2):333–341.e1
75. Gotoda T (2006) Endoscopic resection of early gastric cancer: the Japanese perspective. Curr Opin Gastroenterol 22(5):561–569
76. Ribeiro-Mourao F, Pimentel-Nunes P, Dinis-Ribeiro M (2010) Endoscopic submucosal dissection for gastric lesions: results of an European inquiry. Endoscopy 42(10):814–819
77. Ding J, Liao GQ, Liu HL, Liu S, Tang J (2012) Meta-analysis of laparoscopy-assisted distal gastrectomy with D2 lymph node dissection for gastric cancer. J Surg Oncol 105(3): 297–303
78. Vinuela EF, Gonen M, Brennan MF, Coit DG, Strong VE (2012) Laparoscopic versus open distal gastrectomy for gastric cancer: a meta-analysis of randomized controlled trials and high-quality nonrandomized studies. Ann Surg 255(3):446–456
79. Yamamoto M, Rashid OM, Wong J (2015) Surgical management of gastric cancer: the East vs. West perspective. J Gastrointest Oncol 6(1):79–88
80. Sakuramoto S, Sasako M, Yamaguchi T, Kinoshita T, Fujii M, Nashimoto A, Furukawa H, Nakajima T, Ohashi Y, Imamura H, Higashino M, Yamamura Y, Kurita A, Arai K, Grp AG (2007) Adjuvant chemotherapy for gastric cancer with S-1, an oral fluoropyrimidine. N Engl J Med 357(18):1810–1820
81. Bang YJ, Kim YW, Yang HK, Chung HC, Park YK, Lee KH, Lee KW, Kim YH, Noh SI, Cho JY, Mok YJ, Kim YH, Ji J, Yeh TS, Button P, Sirzén F, Noh SH, CLASSIC trial investigators (2012) Adjuvant capecitabine and oxaliplatin for gastric cancer after D2 gastrectomy (CLASSIC): a phase 3 open-label, randomised controlled trial. Lancet 379(9813):315–21. doi:10.1016/S0140-6736(11)61873-4
82. Lawler M, Johnston PG (2011) The approval of Teysuno (TM)/S-1 by the European Medicines Agency: a potentially important advance for gastric cancer patients. Oncologist 16(10): E1–E4
83. Cunningham D, Allum WH, Stenning SP, Thompson JN, Van de Velde CJ, Nicolson M, Scarffe JH, Lofts FJ, Falk SJ, Iveson TJ, Smith DB, Langley RE, Verma M, Weeden S, Chua YJ, Participants MT (2006) Perioperative chemotherapy versus surgery alone for resectable gastroesophageal cancer. N Engl J Med 355(1):11–20
84. Ychou M, Boige V, Pignon JP, Conroy T, Bouche O, Lebreton G, Ducourtieux M, Bedenne L, Fabre JM, Saint-Aubert B, Geneve J, Lasser P, Rougier P (2011) Perioperative chemotherapy compared with surgery alone for resectable gastroesophageal adenocarcinoma: an FNCLCC and FFCD multicenter phase III trial. J Clin Oncol 29(13):1715–1721
85. Kang Y, Choi D, Im Y et al (1996) A phase III randomized comparison of neoadjuvant chemotherapy followed by surgery versus surgery for locally advanced stomach cancer. Proc Am Soc Clin Oncol 15:215, Abstract 503
86. Macdonald JS, Smalley SR, Benedetti J, Hundahl SA, Estes NC, Stemmermann GN, Haller DG, Ajani JA, Gunderson LL, Jessup JM, Martenson JA (2001) Chemoradiotherapy after

surgery compared with surgery alone for adenocarcinoma of the stomach or gastroesophageal junction. N Engl J Med 345(10):725–730
87. Enestvedt CK, Diggs BS, Shipley DK, Thomas CR, Billingsley KG (2009) A population-based analysis of surgical and adjuvant therapy for resected gastric cancer: are patients receiving appropriate treatment following publication of the intergroup 0116 results? Gastrointest Cancer Res 3(6):233–238
88. Lee J, do Lim H, Kim S, Park SH, Park JO, Park YS, Lim HY, Choi MG, Sohn TS, Noh JH, Bae JM, Ahn YC, Sohn I, Jung SH, Park CK, Kim KM, Kang WK (2012) Phase III trial comparing capecitabine plus cisplatin versus capecitabine plus cisplatin with concurrent capecitabine radiotherapy in completely resected gastric cancer with D2 lymph node dissection: the ARTIST trial. J Clin Oncol Off J Am Soc Clin Oncol 30(3):268–273
89. Wagner AD, Unverzagt S, Grothe W, Kleber G, Grothey A, Haerting J, Fleig WE (2010) Chemotherapy for advanced gastric cancer. Cochrane Database Syst Rev 3, CD004064
90. Cunningham D, Starling N, Rao S, Iveson T, Nicolson M, Coxon F, Middleton G, Daniel F, Oates J, Norman AR, Upper Gastrointestinal Clinical Studies Group of the National Cancer Research Institute of the United Kingdom (2008) Capecitabine and oxaliplatin for advanced esophagogastric cancer. N Engl J Med 358(1):36–46
91. Van Cutsem E, Moiseyenko VM, Tjulandin S, Majlis A, Constenla M, Boni C, Rodrigues A, Fodor M, Chao Y, Voznyi E, Risse ML, Ajani JA, V325 Study Group (2006) Phase III study of docetaxel and cisplatin plus fluorouracil compared with cisplatin and fluorouracil as first-line therapy for advanced gastric cancer: a report of the V325 Study Group. J Clin Oncol 24(31):4991–4997
92. Bang YJ, Van Cutsem E, Feyereislova A, Chung HC, Shen L, Sawaki A, Lordick F, Ohtsu A, Omuro Y, Satoh T, Aprile G, Kulikov E, Hill J, Lehle M, Ruschoff J, Kang YK, ToGA Trial Investigators (2010) Trastuzumab in combination with chemotherapy versus chemotherapy alone for treatment of HER2-positive advanced gastric or gastro-oesophageal junction cancer (ToGA): a phase 3, open-label, randomised controlled trial. Lancet 376(9742): 687–697
93. Fuchs CS, Tomasek J, Yong CJ, Dumitru F, Passalacqua R, Goswami C, Safran H, dos Santos LV, Aprile G, Ferry DR, Melichar B, Tehfe M, Topuzov E, Zalcberg JR, Chau I, Campbell W, Sivanandan C, Pikiel J, Koshiji M, Hsu Y, Liepa AM, Gao L, Schwartz JD, Tabernero J, Investigators RT (2014) Ramucirumab monotherapy for previously treated advanced gastric or gastro-oesophageal junction adenocarcinoma (REGARD): an international, randomised, multicentre, placebo-controlled, phase 3 trial. Lancet 383(9911):31–39
94. Wilke H, Muro K, Van Cutsem E, Oh SC, Bodoky G, Shimada Y, Hironaka S, Sugimoto N, Lipatov O, Kim TY, Cunningham D, Rougier P, Komatsu Y, Ajani J, Emig M, Carlesi R, Ferry D, Chandrawansa K, Schwartz JD, Ohtsu A, RAINBOW Study Group (2014) Ramucirumab plus paclitaxel versus placebo plus paclitaxel in patients with previously treated advanced gastric or gastro-oesophageal junction adenocarcinoma (RAINBOW): a double-blind, randomised phase 3 trial. Lancet Oncol 15(11):1224–1235
95. Barzi A, Thara E (2014) Angiogenesis in esophageal and gastric cancer: a paradigm shift in treatment. Expert Opin Biol Ther 14(9):1319–1332
96. Leung WK, Wu MS, Kakugawa Y, Kim JJ, Yeoh KG, Goh KL, Wu KC, Wu DC, Sollano J, Kachintorn U, Gotoda T, Lin JT, You WC, Ng EK, Sung JJ, Asia Pacific Working Group on Gastric Cancer (2008) Screening for gastric cancer in Asia: current evidence and practice. Lancet Oncol 9(3):279–287
97. Miyamoto A, Kuriyama S, Nishino Y, Tsubono Y, Nakaya N, Ohmori K, Kurashima K, Shibuya D, Tsuji I (2007) Lower risk of death from gastric cancer among participants of gastric cancer screening in Japan: a population-based cohort study. Prev Med 44(1):12–19
98. Pisani P, Oliver WE, Parkin DM, Alvarez N, Vivas J (1994) Case–control study of gastric cancer screening in Venezuela. Br J Cancer 69(6):1102–1105
99. Yoo KY (2008) Cancer control activities in the Republic of Korea. Jpn J Clin Oncol 38(5):327–333

100. Cho E, Kang MH, Choi KS, Suh M, Jun JK, Park EC (2013) Cost-effectiveness outcomes of the national gastric cancer screening program in South Korea. Asian Pac J Cancer Prev 14(4):2533–2540
101. Wong BC, Lam SK, Wong WM, Chen JS, Zheng TT, Feng RE, Lai KC, Hu WH, Yuen ST, Leung SY, Fong DY, Ho J, Ching CK, Chen JS, China Gastric Cancer Study Group (2004) Helicobacter pylori eradication to prevent gastric cancer in a high-risk region of China: a randomized controlled trial. JAMA 291(2):187–194

Cervical Cancer Among Asian Americans

Patti E. Gravitt, Ruby H.N. Nguyen, and Grace X. Ma

Abstract Cervical cancer is a leading cause of female cancers worldwide. Infection with one or more of the carcinogenic types of human papillomavirus (HPV) is considered to be a necessary, but insufficient cause of cervical cancer. Other coinfections, cigarette smoking, and hormonal influences of pregnancy and oral contraceptive use appear to synergistically increase the risk of HPV-associated cervical cancer progression. Geographical and ethnic variation in cervical cancer incidence may thus reflect differences in exposure to HPV due to different sexual mores or susceptibility to infection, differences in prevalence of cofactors, or differences in the availability or effectiveness of cervical cancer prevention programs such as Pap smear and HPV screening. Although the incidence of cervical cancer in Asian Americans is lower than the other racial/ethnic groups in the USA, incidence rates are heterogeneous among different Asian ethnic groups, which may be related to the level of endemicity of high-risk HPV types in the Asian countries of origin, with some variation in findings potentially related to selective socioeconomic migration of immigrants. It is unclear how screening influences cervical cancer survival because Asian Americans lag systematically behind the general US population in screening uptake. The lack of knowledge of the benefits of early detection and screening guidelines, cultural factors, and access barriers is associated with the low screening rates. Similar disparities, and their driving forces, result in insufficient HPV immunization,

P.E. Gravitt, Ph.D., M.S. (✉)
Department of Pathology, University of New Mexico Health Sciences Center,
Albuquerque, NM 87131, USA

Department of Global Health, George Washington University, Milken Institute School of Public Health, 950 New Hampshire Ave, NW, Washington, DC 20052, USA
e-mail: pgravitt@gwu.edu

R.H.N. Nguyen, Ph.D.
Division of Epidemiology and Community Health, School of Public Health, University of Minnesota, Minneapolis, MN 55454, USA
e-mail: nguyen@umn.edu

G.X. Ma, Ph.D.
Lewis Katz School of Medicine, Temple University,
1415 N Broad St, Suite 116, Philadelphia, PA 19122, USA
e-mail: grace.ma@temple.edu

A.H. Wu, D.O. Stram (eds.), *Cancer Epidemiology Among Asian Americans*,
DOI 10.1007/978-3-319-41118-7_12

similar to the low screening coverage reported in Asian-American communities. Future dissemination of effective culturally appropriate educational intervention programs for the reduction of access barriers shows great promise in reducing previous cervical cancer disparities in Asian-American women.

Keywords Asian American • Cervical cancer • Gynecologic cancer • Human papillomavirus • Disparities

Cervical Cancer Incidence and Mortality

Cervical cancer is the fourth leading cause of cancer incidence and mortality worldwide [1]; the age-adjusted incidence (world standard) is 14.0 per 100,000 with an estimated 528,000 new cases diagnosed in 2012. Incidence rates averaged 12.7 per 100,000 in Asia, which is intermediate of the high rates in Africa (27.6) and the low rates in North America (6.6). Cervical cancer incidence varied substantially within Asia, higher in South-Central (19.3) and Southeast (16.3) Asia and lower in Eastern (7.9) and Western (4.4) Asia. Cervical cancer ranks fourth as a cause of cancer death in women worldwide. The age-adjusted mortality rate is 6.5 per 100,000 in Asia, also intermediate of the high death rates in Africa (17.5) and the low rates in North America (2.6) [1].

In the USA, cervical cancer incidence rates (per 100,000) are considerably lower in Asian American (6.4) and non-Hispanic white women (7.1) than in African American (10.2) and Hispanic (10.5) women [2]. Squamous cell and adenocarcinoma are the two main histologic types of cervical cancer; the former accounts for approximately 70 % of the cervical cancers in Asian Americans compared to 64 % in non-Hispanic whites and 75 % in Hispanic and African American women [3].

As cervical cancer incidence varies in Asia, there are distinct differences in cervical cancer incidence across Asian ethnic subgroups in the USA. Wang and colleagues [3] conducted one of the first comprehensive analysis of cervical cancer incidence by specific Asian groups using 1996–2004 data from the five SEER registries (Hawaii, Los Angeles, Seattle-Puget Sound, San Francisco-Oakland, and San Jose-Monterey) with the highest proportion of Asian Americans or Pacific Islanders. This analysis showed that cervical cancer incidence was highest among Vietnamese (18.9), intermediate in Koreans (11.9) and Filipinos (10.0), and lower in Japanese (6.7), Chinese (5.8), and Asian India/Pakistan (4.5). This heterogeneity in cervical cancer incidence among Asian ethnic groups is also evident in two other updates that used additional SEER registry data [4, 5] and extended the analyses to include smaller Asian ethnic groups, such as Kampuchean (Cambodians) and Laotians. A 2013 study included cancers diagnosed in ten SEER registries during 1990 to 2008 and identified the top five cancer sites during each of three study periods (1990–1994, 1998–2002, and 2004–2008) by specific Asian ethnic groups. Cervical cancer was one of the top five cancer sites for Kampuchean and Laotian women in the USA during each of the three study periods; the respective rates were 16.7 and 17.1 per 100,000 during the most recent study period (2004–2008) [5]. Although cervical cancer incidence was also high for Koreans during 1990–1994 (18.6 per 100,000), rates for this group had declined in excess of 50 % by 2004–2008 (8.1 per 100,000). Similarly, cervical cancer rates for Vietnamese women were reduced from 38.6 to 13.1 per 100,000 between the study periods 1990–1994 to 2004–2008 (Gomez, personal communication).

Thus, cervical cancer rates have been declining steadily in Asian Americans as in other race/ethnic groups in the USA. From 2000–2009, there was a significant −3.0 % average annual decline in cervical cancer rates among Asian/Pacific Islanders, which was comparable to the changes observed in African American (−3.0 % per year) and Hispanic (−3.9 % per year) women [6]. However, the rates of decline are not uniform across the different Asian ethnic groups. In an analysis that estimated the average annual percent change in cervical cancer incidence between 1990–2004 in six Asian ethnic groups residing in California (Chinese, Filipino, Japanese, Korean, South Asian, Vietnamese), the decline was highest in Vietnamese (−8.7 % per year) and lowest in South Asian women (−1.0 % per year) [7]. In the nationwide SEER study mentioned above, the annual decline was −8.5 % per year in Vietnamese, −7.3 % per year in Laotian, but only −2.3 % per year in Kampuchean women [5].

In Japanese and non-Hispanic white women, cervical cancer incidence peaked at ages 45–64 years, but in the other Asian ethnic groups, the incidence continued to increase with increasing age [3]. A recent study showed that differences in invasive cervical cancer incidence in African Americans versus non-Hispanic whites were likely underestimated because SEER rates do not adjust for hysterectomy status [8]. Thus, more complete data regarding age-specific hysterectomy prevalence among the Asian ethnic subgroups are needed to calculate a hysterectomy-corrected estimate of the cervical cancer rates to allow for more accurate comparison.

Racial/ethnic differences in cervical cancer mortality largely mirrored these differences in incidence patterns. In the study conducted by Jemal and colleagues [6], cervical cancer mortality (per 100,000) was lowest in Asian Pacific Islanders (2.0) and non-Hispanic whites (2.2), intermediate in Hispanics (3.0), and highest in African Americans (4.3). The average annual percent decline in mortality rates was highest in Asian Pacific Islanders (−4.0 %) and lowest in non-Hispanic whites (−1.9 %).

Risk Factors

Natural History of Cervical Cancer: Overview

Substantial progress has been made in our understanding of the etiology of cervical cancer. Nearly 100 % of invasive cervical cancer is caused by infection with one of approximately 14 high-risk or oncogenic types of human papillomavirus, two of which—HPV16 and HPV18—account for well over half of all invasive cervical cancer worldwide (Fig. 1).

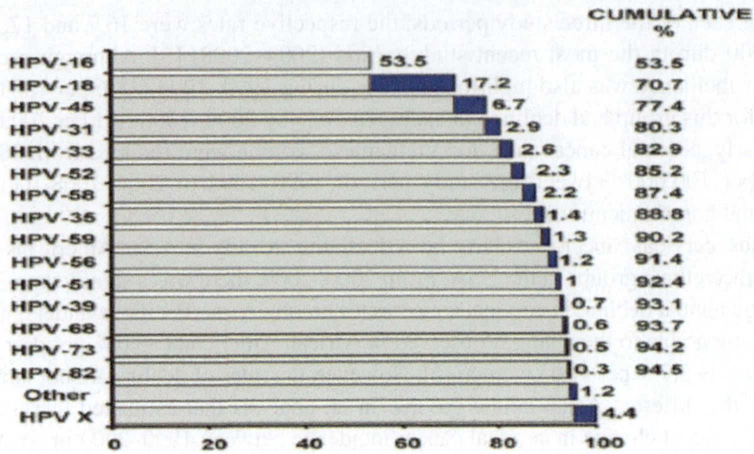

Fig. 1 Oncogenic types of human papillomavirus genotypes and worldwide attributable fraction of CxCa; Clifford et al. Vaccine 24S3 (2006) S3/26-S3/34

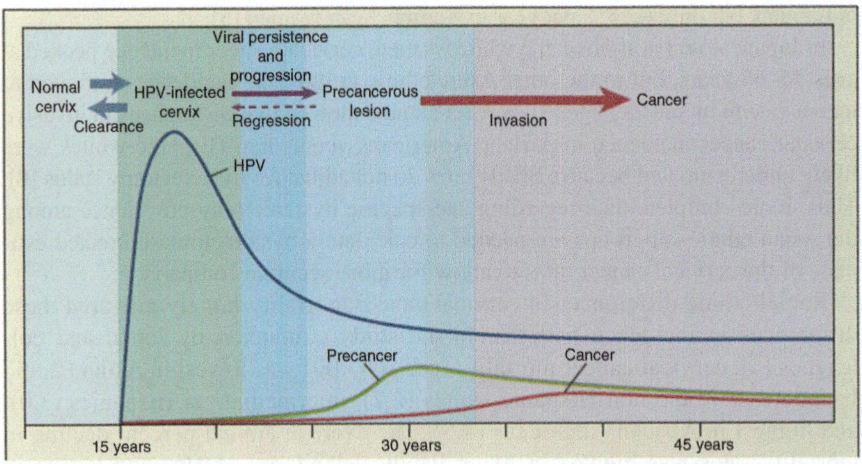

Fig. 2 The natural history of HPV and cervical cancer. Schiffman M, Castle P (2005) N Engl J Med 353(20):2101–2104

Over the past 20 years, several large epidemiologic studies have been conducted in many global regions to define the natural history of HPV infection leading to cervical cancer (Fig. 2). HPV is transmitted predominately through sexual contact, with peak prevalence observed among young women around the age of sexual debut. Natural history studies have observed that most (~90 %) of HPV infections detected at the cervix will become undetectable within 2 years of first detection (reviewed in [9]). Uncertainty remains as to whether the loss of HPV detection within 1–2 years of acquisition reflects viral eradication or clearance or control of virus below limits of detection (i.e., HPV latency) [10]). However, it is clear that

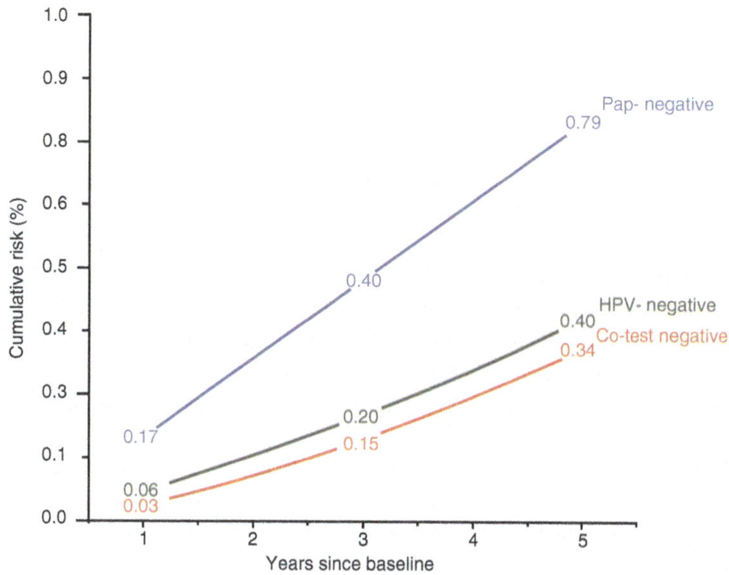

Fig. 3 Cumulative risks of cervical intraepithelial neoplasia grade 2 or more severe among women aged 30–64 years. Blue line indicates cumulative risk of CIN2+ among women with negative Pap cytology (regardless of HPV result), black-line women with a negative HPV test (regardless of Pap result) and red-line women with both HPV and Pap negative test results. Reprinted with permission from Gage JC, Schiffman M, Katki HA, Castle PE, Fetterman B, Wentzensen N, Poitras NE, Lorey T, Cheung LC, Kinney WK (2014) Reassurance against future risk of precancer and cancer conferred by a negative human papillomavirus test. JNCI 106(8):pii:jhu153. doi: 10.1093/jnci/dju153

persistent detection of oncogenic types of HPV is the strongest predictor for progression to high-grade squamous intraepithelial lesions and cancer [9]. Figure 3 represents the 5-year cumulative risk of high-grade squamous intraepithelial lesions and cancer progression following negative Pap cytology, HPV testing, or Pap+HPV co-testing screening results, demonstrating the high negative predictive value over the short term following an HPV negative test result [11]. These observations form the basis for the utility of HPV testing in cervical cancer screening programs [12]. As expected from this natural history model, the burden of HPV correlates significantly with the cervical cancer burden in populations [13].

Cervical Cancer and Human Papillomavirus (HPV) Genotype Distribution in Asia

Infection with HPV is established as a necessary cause of invasive and preinvasive cervical cancer. The generally lower rates of cervical cancer incidence in Asian Americans compared to Hispanic and African American women likely reflect differences in the prevalence of HPV infection in Asia compared to Africa, the Caribbean, Central America, and South America [1], since the relative risk of cervical cancer associated with HPV infection is similar across world regions [14]. Similarly, the heterogeneity in cervical cancer incidence among specific Asian ethnic groups in the USA may reflect rates of HPV infection and cervical cancer in the countries of origin in Asia. A recent meta-analysis estimated the prevalence and genotype distribution of HPV in women with normal cytology and across a range of cervical disease lesions and invasive cervical cancer by world geographic region [7]. Table 1 summarizes the overall prevalence of HPV in women with normal cytology (reflects the general population prevalence of detectable HPV) and women with invasive cervical cancer. Among women with normal cytology, overall HPV prevalence was lowest in Western/Central Asia (8 %), intermediate in Eastern Asia (12 %) and Europe (9 %), and considerably higher in Africa (22 %) and South/Central America (24 %) [7].

HPV16 accounts for the majority of cervical cancers in all world regions (53–73 %), with a minor exception of Asia where a lower HPV16 prevalence in Eastern Asia (68 %) compared to Western/Central Asia (82 %) has been reported. Some variation in genotype-specific prevalence of non-HPV16 cancers can be observed. Specifically, HPV52 and HPV58 are overrepresented in cervical cancers in Eastern Asia compared to other world regions (Fig. 4). The higher relative contribution of HPV58 in cervical cancers in Eastern Asia is supported by the similar 16-year cumulative risk of cervical cancer among HPV58/non-HPV16 positive women (10.3 %) and HPV16 positive women (13.5 %) in a large cohort study conducted in Taiwan [15]. It is not clear whether prevalence of HPV52 and HPV58 is also observed in higher frequency among Asian Americans.

In addition to these macro-level genotype-specific differences observed in invasive cervical cancer across geographical region, efforts have been directed to study intratypic HPV variants as these genetic variants may affect the clinical outcome of HPV infection. In fact, significant intratypic variation in HPV16 has been well described [16, 17]. The Asian variants of HPV16 have been consistently found to confer a higher relative risk of progression to high-grade squamous intraepithelial lesions and cancer compared with the more commonly detected European variant [18–20]. The higher carcinogenicity of the Asian HPV16 variant is supported by several in vitro studies demonstrating enhanced ability compared with E variant to

Table 1 Human papillomavirus prevalence in women with normal cervical cytology and invasive cervical cancer by geographic region [7]

Region	Normal cytology (%)	Invasive cervical cancer (%)
Eastern Asia	12	91
Western/Central Asia	8	90
Europe	9	90
North America	21	90
Africa	22	90
South/Central America	24	86

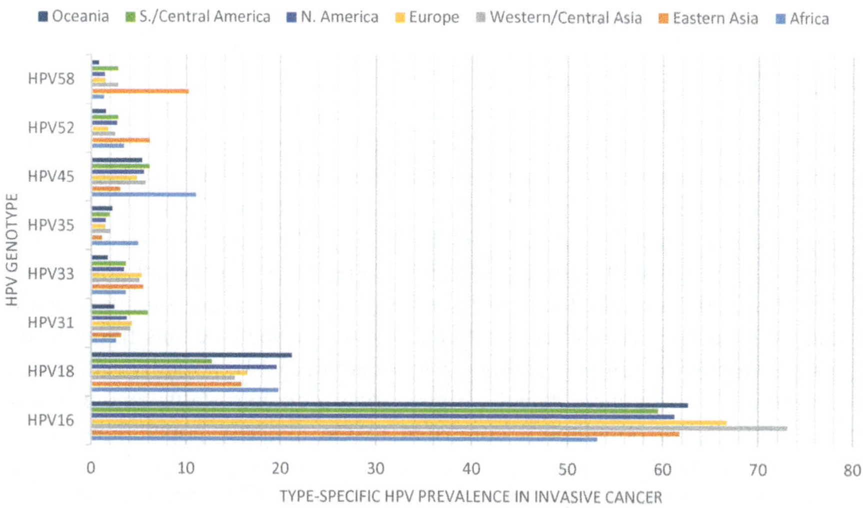

Fig. 4 Type-specific prevalence of HPV16, 18, 31, 33, 35, 45, 52, and 58 in invasive cervical cancer by geographic region. Adapted from [7]

Table 2 Cervical cancer rates and HPV16/18 prevalence among women with normal cytology (representative of population prevalence of HPV 16/18) in Asian ethnic subgroup countries of origin [25]

Country	Country-specific invasive cervical cancer rates (per 100,000)	HPV 16/18 prevalence in women with normal cytology (%)
China	9.4	3.8
India	20.2	5.0
Japan	14.5	1.9
Korea	13.5	6.3
Laos	9.8	3.0
Philippines	13.9	2.9
Vietnam	11.3	2.1

drive life cycle in raft cultures to cancer: more severe dysplasia and higher E6/E7 expression [21–23]. In addition, the Asian HPV16 variant is found at higher frequency in adenocarcinoma compared to squamous cell carcinomas of the cervix, consistent with the higher proportion of adenocarcinomas in cervical cancers diagnosed in Asian American women compared with African American and Hispanic women [24].

Similar to the heterogeneity of cervical cancer incidence among Asian ethnic subgroups in the USA, there is also significant heterogeneity across the Asian countries of origin. Table 2 reports the data in the summary reports for China, India, Japan, Korea, Laos, the Philippines, and Vietnam compiled by the Institut Catala d'Oncologia (ICO) Information Centre on HPV and Cancer [25]. In general, cervical cancer rates are positively correlated with the population prevalence of HPV16/18, a phenomenon that has been better demonstrated globally using HPV seroprevalence data [26]. In this respect, differences in cervical cancer rates among the Asian immigrants in the USA may reflect the overall HPV endemicity in the country of origin. The patterns observed in Vietnamese and Chinese-American women may reflect this phenomenon, where the higher rates of invasive cervical cancer in Vietnam and lower rates in China parallel their respective rates in the USA [27–29]. However, other countries show distinct differences in rates in the country of origin compared to immigrant populations in the USA. For example, the reported rates of cervical cancer are quite high in India [25], yet the invasive cervical cancer rates in South Asians living in the USA are among the lowest by Asian specific ethnicity [3], possibly reflecting a socioeconomic difference, namely, higher socioeconomic status among immigrant South Asian populations compared to the majority populations in the country of origin.

The most consistent predictors or HPV infection relate to measures of sexual activity [29]. Little is known about sexual practices related to HPV acquisition and transmission among Asian Americans and in Asians living in the country of origin. This is likely due to cultural taboos that restrict the assessment of sexual activity in many studies and the reluctance of participants to discuss sexual behaviors even when these questions are asked. In addition, other factors including cultural isolation and practices of male partners may contribute significantly to the HPV burden in many regions. For example, an earlier study among cytologically normal women in Hanoi and Ho Chi Minh City in Vietnam observed a nearly fivefold difference in HPV prevalence (10.6 % in Ho Chi Minh versus 2.0 % in Hanoi), despite common sampling and HPV testing protocols [30]. It is speculated that the relative isolation of North Vietnam during its war with America and the resultant socialist isolation may contribute to the lower HPV prevalence in this population at the turn of the twenty-first century. It is likely, however, that regional and cultural differences in the norms of sexual behavior influence the overall HPV prevalence in Asian populations, a phenomenon that may persist for generations even after immigration.

Other Risk Factors

While HPV is the central cause of cervical cancer, only a small proportion of women infected with HPV develop invasive cervical cancer. Cofactors including other sexually transmitted infections, smoking, reproductive factors, and the use of oral contraceptives (OCs) are likely to act in conjunction with HPV infection in the pathogenesis of cervical cancer [31–38]. Although information on cofactors and risk of cervical cancer in Asian-American women is largely absent, studies from Thailand, the Philippines, India, Japan, Taiwan, and elsewhere in Asia have found that the influence of these cofactors on risk of cervical cancer is generally consistent with the results obtained in studies conducted in western populations. Even if risk associations with these cofactors are similar by geographic or ethnic subgroups, differences in the prevalence of these cofactors may contribute to differences in cervical cancer rates.

Cervical Cancer Prevention Through Screening and HPV Immunization in Asian Americans

There are two types of tests for cervical cancer screening: the Pap test and the HPV test.

The Pap test can find early cell changes that are not yet cancer. Cell changes can be treated and prevented from becoming cervical cancer. The Pap test also can find cervical cancer at a stage that is easy to treat. The HPV test finds certain HPV infections that can lead to cell changes. These cell changes can progress to cervical cancer if not treated. Cell changes can be surgically removed from the cervix and prevented from becoming cervical cancer [12]. Over the past 30 years, there has been a steady decrease in cervical cancer incidence and mortality in the USA [39] due to the development of the Pap test. The US Preventive Service Task Force [40] currently recommends screening women ages 21–65 years with cytology or the Pap test every 3 years or, for women ages 30–65 years who want to lengthen the screening interval, screening with a combination of the Pap test and HPV test every 5 years.

Despite the proven survival benefits associated with screening and early detection of cervical cancer, the screening rate among Asian-American women lags far behind that of the general US population [41–49]. Specifically, Asian-American women have the lowest rates of screening (66 %) compared with Hispanic (74 %), Native Americans (82 %), African American (78 %), and non-Hispanic white women (78 %) [50]. Furthermore, cervical cancer screening rates among Asian-American women fall well below the Healthy People 2020 national objectives, which calls for 93 % of women aged 21–65 to be screened for the Pap test every 3 years [51].

Studies suggest that various factors, including lack of knowledge, psychosocial and cultural beliefs, and access barriers, are associated with nonadherence to cervical cancer screening among Asian-American women [41, 47–49, 52, 53]. Many Asian-American women do not know the recommended guidelines for cervical cancer screening and lack of knowledge about HPV infections [49, 54]. For example, Korean-American women with limited knowledge of cervical cancer had lower rates of screening, whereas women who were familiar with screening guidelines were three times more likely to have had a Pap test [52, 55]. Vietnamese women who believed that a Pap test can detect cervical cancer early were twice as likely to have had a Pap test compared to women who did not hold this belief [49]. Many Asian-American women have reported that they avoided the Pap test due to embarrassment. Indeed, shyness and cultural beliefs about modesty are often negatively associated with cervical cancer screening [54]. Ma and colleagues [49] reported that physician recommendation for screening and having health insurance was positively associated with cervical cancer screening. Furthermore, noncompliance with guidelines tended to be high even among Asian Americans who were ever screened [48] and that the reasons associated with noncompliance with screening guidelines may differ from those associated with never having been screened.

The few interventions that have been developed for Asian-American women demonstrate that targeting factors including transportation, language barrier, insurance, knowledge, and others can yield significant increases in screening rates. However, it is important to note that the effectiveness of educational interventions is often attenuated if access barriers are not adequately addressed. For example, to reach a larger number of individuals in the community, several programs have utilized media-based approaches. Results suggested that the media campaign had significantly increased intention to undergo cervical cancer screening, but it did not result in meaningful differences in actual screening rates [56]. Interventions employing a combined approach have been found to yield greater impact on cervical cancer screening rates [46, 57–62]. Access barriers, including the cost of screening, lack of insurance, and language difficulties, pose formidable challenges and are the most often cited factors influencing screening behavior [41, 48, 63].

Therefore, interventions that include essential components, such as the use of community-based approaches, culturally and linguistically appropriate educational tools and resources, as well as navigation assistance, are more likely to be successful in increasing cervical cancer screening rates.

The development of HPV vaccines increases the potential of prevention of cervical cancer and mitigates the long-standing disparities in cervical cancer [64]. As described above, some Asian-American subgroups (e.g., Vietnamese and Korean) have persistently higher incidence rates of cervical cancer. The two highly efficacious vaccines (Gardasil® and Cervarix®) against HPV genotypes 16 and 18, which cause 70 % of the HPV infections that cause cancer, afford an important opportunity to reduce cervical cancer disparities. These vaccines are currently recommended for adolescents ages 11–12 years, with catch-up vaccination to age 26 years for females and 21 years for males, in a three-dose regimen over a 6-month period [65–67]. Reducing disparities in cervical cancer depends on adequate vaccine uptake by those at greatest risk.

The National Immunization Survey conducted using telephone interviews in six languages shows that 44 % of US girls 13–17 years old had at least one dose, 29 % had one, and only 11 % completed the entire three-dose course [68]. The CDC estimates that 32 % of girls aged 13–17 had received all three HPV vaccine doses and that dose completion was significantly lower among the uninsured (14 %) [6]. In a community sample of 113 Vietnamese women who had at least one HPV vaccine dose, only 11 (10 %) had all three doses [68]. In a separate study of Chinese-American women, only 19 % had heard of HPV [69]. Further, Chinese-American girls and women with limited English language proficiency had low HPV awareness and HPV vaccine acceptance rates. Due to various cultural factors, language barriers, and healthcare access barriers, it would be more difficult for Chinese Americans to understand the importance of the HPV vaccination.

Preliminary results from Ma and colleagues showed that knowledge, attitudinal, cultural, and access barriers specific to Asian populations prevent the uptake of HPV vaccination. Asian Americans, especially the low income and underserved, have generally lower levels of knowledge about HPV infection and vaccination, increased parental reluctance to vaccinate children due to the association with sexually transmitted diseases, a lower perception of benefits, and increased barrier to access to preventive services. Therefore, evidence-based and culturally relevant interventions are needed to increase adherence to the recommended regimen for the diverse Asian-American populations. The availability of the new technology for cervical cancer prevention and control provides a unique opportunity to address cervical cancer disparities in Asian Americans.

Overall, community-based cervical cancer screening programs have demonstrated promise in addressing existing cervical cancer disparities by increasing awareness and knowledge and promoting recommended screening behaviors. The lessons learned from this body of research will be instrumental in guiding future community-based programs to reduce cancer health disparities among Asian American women.

Conclusion

Historical differences in cervical cancer prevalence among Asian-American women may be associated with high-risk HPV-type endemicity in the country of origin or disparities in knowledge or access barriers in the USA. Little is known about the natural history of HPV infection and cervical cancer in these understudied women. However, there is strong evidence that culturally appropriate primary prevention with educational interventions, in the presence of reduction in access barriers, can increase both screening for cervical testing and HPV vaccination rates in multiple Asian-American subgroups.

Financial Disclosures

Authors' declaration of personal interests: PEG, RHNN, and GXM have no personal interest in preparing this chapter.

Declaration of funding interests: PEG, RHNN, and GXM had no specific funding support related to the preparation of this manuscript.

References

1. Ferlay J, Soerjomataram I, Dikshit R, Eser S, Mathers C, Rebelo M et al (2015) Cancer incidence and mortality worldwide: sources, methods and major patterns in GLOBOCAN 2012. Int J Cancer 136:E359–E386
2. Siegel RL, Miller KD, Jemal A (2015) Cancer statistics, 2015. CA Cancer J Clin 65:5–29
3. Wang SS, Carreon JD, Gomez SL, Devesa SS (2010) Cervical cancer incidence among 6 Asian ethnic groups in the United States, 1996 through 2004. Cancer 116:949–956
4. Miller BA, Chu KC, Hankey BF, Ries LA (2008) Cancer incidence and mortality patterns among specific Asian and Pacific islander populations in the U.S. Cancer Causes Control 19:227–256

5. Gomez SL, Noone AM, Lichtensztajn DY, Scoppa S, Gibson JT, Liu L et al (2013) Cancer incidence trends among Asian American populations in the United States, 1990–2008. J Natl Cancer Inst 105:1096–1110
6. Jemal A, Simard EP, Dorell C, Noone AM, Markowitz LE, Kohler B et al (2013) Annual Report to the Nation on the Status of Cancer, 1975–2009, featuring the burden and trends in human papillomavirus (HPV)-associated cancers and HPV vaccination coverage levels. J Natl Cancer Inst 105:175–201
7. Guan P, Howell-Jones R, Li N, Bruni L, de Sanjose S, Franceschi S et al (2012) Human papillomavirus types in 115,789 HPV-positive women: a meta-analysis from cervical infection to cancer. Int J Cancer 131:2349–2359
8. Rositch AF, Nowak RG, Gravitt PE (2014) Increased age and race-specific incidence of cervical cancer after correction for hysterectomy prevalence in the United States from 2000 to 2009. Cancer 120:2032–2038
9. Moscicki AB, Schiffman M, Burchell A, Albero G, Giuliano AR, Goodman MT et al (2012) Updating the natural history of human papillomavirus and anogenital cancers. Vaccine 30(Suppl 5):F24–F33
10. Gravitt PE (2011) The known unknowns of HPV natural history. J Clin Invest 121:4593–4599
11. Gage JC, Schiffman M, Katki HA, Castle PE, Fetterman B, Wentzensen N et al (2014) Reassurance against future risk of precancer and cancer conferred by a negative human papillomavirus test. J Natl Cancer Inst 106, pii: dju153
12. Saslow D, Solomon D, Lawson HW, Killackey M, Kulasingam SL, Cain J et al (2012) American Cancer Society, American Society for Colposcopy and Cervical Pathology, and American Society for Clinical Pathology screening guidelines for the prevention and early detection of cervical cancer. CA Cancer J Clin 62:147–172
13. Maucort-Boulch D, Franceschi S, Plummer M, Group IHPSS (2008) International correlation between human papillomavirus prevalence and cervical cancer incidence. Cancer Epidemiol Biomarkers Prev 17:717–720
14. Munoz N, Bosch FX, de Sanjose S, Herrero R, Castellsague X, Shah KV et al (2003) Epidemiologic classification of human papillomavirus types associated with cervical cancer. N Engl J Med 348:518–527
15. Chen HC, Schiffman M, Lin CY, Pan MH, You SL, Chuang LC et al (2011) Persistence of type-specific human papillomavirus infection and increased long-term risk of cervical cancer. J Natl Cancer Inst 103:1387–1396
16. Cornet I, Gheit T, Franceschi S, Vignat J, Burk RD, Sylla BS et al (2012) Human papillomavirus type 16 genetic variants: phylogeny and classification based on E6 and LCR. J Virol 86:6855–6861
17. Yamada T, Manos MM, Peto J, Greer CE, Munoz N, Bosch FX et al (1997) Human papillomavirus type 16 sequence variation in cervical cancers: a worldwide perspective. J Virol 71:2463–2472
18. Quint KD, de Koning MN, van Doorn LJ, Quint WG, Pirog EC (2010) HPV genotyping and HPV16 variant analysis in glandular and squamous neoplastic lesions of the uterine cervix. Gynecol Oncol 117:297–301
19. Xi LF, Koutsky LA, Hildesheim A, Galloway DA, Wheeler CM, Winer RL et al (2007) Risk for high-grade cervical intraepithelial neoplasia associated with variants of human papillomavirus types 16 and 18. Cancer Epidemiol Biomarkers Prev 16:4–10
20. Cornet I, Gheit T, Iannacone MR, Vignat J, Sylla BS, Del Mistro A et al (2013) HPV16 genetic variation and the development of cervical cancer worldwide. Br J Cancer 108:240–244
21. Zehbe I, Richard C, DeCarlo CA, Shai A, Lambert PF, Lichtig H et al (2009) Human papillomavirus 16 E6 variants differ in their dysregulation of human keratinocyte differentiation and apoptosis. Virology 383:69–77
22. Niccoli S, Abraham S, Richard C, Zehbe I (2012) The Asian-American E6 variant protein of human papillomavirus 16 alone is sufficient to promote immortalization, transformation, and migration of primary human foreskin keratinocytes. J Virol 86:12384–12396

23. Jackson R, Togtema M, Lambert PF, Zehbe I (2014) Tumourigenesis driven by the human papillomavirus type 16 Asian-American e6 variant in a three-dimensional keratinocyte model. PLoS One 9, e101540
24. Burk RD, Terai M, Gravitt PE, Brinton LA, Kurman RJ, Barnes WA et al (2003) Distribution of human papillomavirus types 16 and 18 variants in squamous cell carcinomas and adenocarcinomas of the cervix. Cancer Res 63:7215–7220
25. Bruni L, Barrionuevo-Rosas L, Albero G, et al. ICO Information Centre on HPV and Cancer (HPV Information Center). Summary Report 2015;2015-03-24. Accessed 19 May 2015.
26. Vaccarella S, Franceschi S, Clifford GM, Touze A, Hsu CC, de Sanjose S et al (2010) Seroprevalence of antibodies against human papillomavirus (HPV) types 16 and 18 in four continents: the International Agency for Research on Cancer HPV Prevalence Surveys. Cancer Epidemiol Biomarkers Prev 19:2379–2388
27. Le GM, Gomez SL, Clarke CA, Glaser SL, West DW (2002) Cancer incidence patterns among Vietnamese in the United States and Ha Noi, Vietnam. Int J Cancer 102:412–417
28. Shi JF, Canfell K, Lew JB, Qiao YL (2012) The burden of cervical cancer in China: synthesis of the evidence. Int J Cancer 130:641–652
29. Javanbakht M, Gorbach PM, Amani B, Walker S, Cranston RD, Datta SD et al (2010) Concurrency, sex partner risk, and high-risk human papillomavirus infection among African American, Asian, and Hispanic women. Sex Transm Dis 37:68–74
30. Pham TH, Nguyen TH, Herrero R, Vaccarella S, Smith JS, Nguyen Thuy TT et al (2003) Human papillomavirus infection among women in South and North Vietnam. Int J Cancer 104:213–220
31. International Collaboration of Epidemiological Studies of Cervical Cancer (2006) Cervical carcinoma and reproductive factors: collaborative reanalysis of individual data on 16,563 women with cervical carcinoma and 33,542 women without cervical carcinoma from 25 epidemiological studies. Int J Cancer 119:1108–1124
32. Castellsague X, Diaz M, de Sanjose S, Munoz N, Herrero R, Franceschi S et al (2006) Worldwide human papillomavirus etiology of cervical adenocarcinoma and its cofactors: implications for screening and prevention. J Natl Cancer Inst 98:303–315
33. International Collaboration of Epidemiological Studies of Cervical Cancer, Appleby P, Beral V, de Gonzalez Berrington A, Colin D, Franceschi S et al (2007) Cervical cancer and hormonal contraceptives: collaborative reanalysis of individual data for 16,573 women with cervical cancer and 35,509 women without cervical cancer from 24 epidemiological studies. Lancet 370:1609–1621
34. International Collaboration of Epidemiological Studies of Cervical Cancer, Appleby P, Beral V, de Gonzalez Berrington A, Colin D, Franceschi S et al (2006) Carcinoma of the cervix and tobacco smoking: collaborative reanalysis of individual data on 13,541 women with carcinoma of the cervix and 23,017 women without carcinoma of the cervix from 23 epidemiological studies. Int J Cancer 118:1481–1495
35. Smith JS, Herrero R, Bosetti C, Munoz N, Bosch FX, Eluf-Neto J et al (2002) Herpes simplex virus-2 as a human papillomavirus cofactor in the etiology of invasive cervical cancer. J Natl Cancer Inst 94:1604–1613
36. Smith JS, Bosetti C, Munoz N, Herrero R, Bosch FX, Eluf-Neto J et al (2004) Chlamydia trachomatis and invasive cervical cancer: a pooled analysis of the IARC multicentric case–control study. Int J Cancer 111:431–439
37. Arnheim Dahlstrom L, Andersson K, Luostarinen T, Thoresen S, Ogmundsdottir H, Tryggvadottir L et al (2011) Prospective seroepidemiologic study of human papillomavirus and other risk factors in cervical cancer. Cancer Epidemiol Biomarkers Prev 20:2541–2550
38. Castellsague X, Pawlita M, Roura E, Margall N, Waterboer T, Bosch FX et al (2014) Prospective seroepidemiologic study on the role of Human Papillomavirus and other infections in cervical carcinogenesis: evidence from the EPIC cohort. Int J Cancer 135:440–452
39. Ries LA, Eisner MP, Kosary CL, et al. SEER Cancer Statistics Review, 1975–2000. http://seer.cancer.gov/csr/1975_2000/2003

40. (USPSTF) USPSTF (2012). Screening for Cervical Cancer, Topic Page. http://www.uspreventiveservicestaskforce.org/uspset/uspscerv.htm
41. Kim K, Yu ES, Chen EH, Kim J, Kaufman M, Purkiss J (1999) Cervical cancer screening knowledge and practices among Korean-American women. Cancer Nurs 22:297–302
42. McPhee SJ, Bird JA, Davis T, Ha NT, Jenkins CN, Le B (1997) Barriers to breast and cervical cancer screening among Vietnamese-American women. Am J Prev Med 13:205–213
43. McPhee SJ, Stewart S, Brock KC, Bird JA, Jenkins CN, Pham GQ (1997) Factors associated with breast and cervical cancer screening practices among Vietnamese American women. Cancer Detect Prev 21:510–521
44. Taylor VM, Yasui Y, Burke N, Nguyen T, Acorda E, Thai H et al (2004) Pap testing adherence among Vietnamese American women. Cancer Epidemiol Biomarkers Prev 13:613–619
45. Ma GX, Toubbeh JI, Wang MQ, Shive SE, Cooper L, Pham A (2009) Factors associated with cervical cancer screening compliance and noncompliance among Chinese, Korean, Vietnamese, and Cambodian women. J Natl Med Assoc 101:541–551
46. Fang CY, Ma GX, Tan Y, Chi N (2007) A multifaceted intervention to increase cervical cancer screening among underserved Korean women. Cancer Epidemiol Biomarkers Prev 16:1298–1302
47. Ma GX, Gao W, Fang CY, Tan Y, Feng Z, Ge S et al (2013) Health beliefs associated with cervical cancer screening among Vietnamese Americans. J Womens Health (Larchmt) 22:276–288
48. Ma GX, Shive SE, Wang MQ, Tan Y (2009) Cancer screening behaviors and barriers in Asian Americans. Am J Health Behav 33:650–660
49. Ma GX, Fang CY, Feng Z, Tan Y, Gao W, Ge S et al (2012) Correlates of cervical cancer screening among Vietnamese American women. Infect Dis Obstet Gynecol 2012:617234
50. American Cancer Society (2012) Cancer prevention and early detection: facts and figures. American Cancer Society, Atlanta, GA. http://www.cancer.org/acs/groups/content/@epidemiologysurveilance/documents/document/acspc-033423.pdf.
51. (ODPHP) OoDPaP (2012) Healthy People 2020. http://www.healthypeople.gov.
52. Juon HS, Seung-Lee C, Klassen AC (2003) Predictors of regular Pap smears among Korean-American women. Prev Med 37:585–592
53. Coughlin SS, Uhler RJ (2000) Breast and cervical cancer screening practices among Asian and Pacific Islander women in the United States, 1994–1997. Cancer Epidemiol Biomarkers Prev 9:597–603
54. Kim HLK, Lee SO, Kim S (2004) Cervical cancer screening in Korean American women: findings from focus group intervention. Taehan Kanho Hakhoe Chi 34:617–624
55. Lee EE, Tripp-Reimer T, Miller AM, Sadler GR, Lee SY (2007) Korean American women's beliefs about breast and cervical cancer and associated symbolic meanings. Oncol Nurs Forum 34:713–720
56. Jenkins CN, McPhee SJ, Bird JA, Pham GQ, Nguyen BH, Nguyen T et al (1999) Effect of a media-led education campaign on breast and cervical cancer screening among Vietnamese-American women. Prev Med 28:395–406
57. Ma GX, Fang C, Tan Y, Feng Z, Ge S, Nguyen C (2015) Increasing cervical cancer screening among Vietnamese Americans: a community-based intervention trial. J Health Care Poor Underserved 26:36–52
58. Mock J, McPhee SJ, Nguyen T, Wong C, Doan H, Lai KQ et al (2007) Effective lay health worker outreach and media-based education for promoting cervical cancer screening among Vietnamese American women. Am J Public Health 97:1693–1700
59. Nguyen TT, McPhee SJ, Gildengorin G, Nguyen T, Wong C, Lai KQ et al (2006) Papanicolaou testing among Vietnamese Americans: results of a multifaceted intervention. Am J Prev Med 31:1–9
60. Ma GX, Tan Y, Toubbeh JI, Edwards RL, Shive SE, Siu P et al (2006) Asian Tobacco Education and Cancer Awareness Research Special Population Network. A model for reducing Asian American cancer health disparities. Cancer 107:1995–2005

61. Taylor VM, Hislop TG, Jackson JC, Tu SP, Yasui Y, Schwartz SM et al (2002) A randomized controlled trial of interventions to promote cervical cancer screening among Chinese women in North America. J Natl Cancer Inst 94:670–677
62. Wang X, Fang C, Tan Y, Liu A, Ma GX (2010) Evidence-based intervention to reduce access barriers to cervical cancer screening among underserved Chinese American women. J Womens Health (Larchmt) 19:463–469
63. Lee MC (2000) Knowledge, barriers, and motivators related to cervical cancer screening among Korean-American women. A focus group approach. Cancer Nurs 23:168–175
64. Organization WH. (2011) United Nations Population Fund (2006) Preparing for the Introduction of HPV vaccines: policy and programming guidance for countries. Available at: http://whqlibdoc.who.int/hq/2006/WHO.RHR_06-11/eng.pdf. Assessed 16 May 2011.
65. (CDC) USCfDC (2007) Quadrivalent human papillomavirus vaccine: recommendation of the Advisory Committee on Immunization Practices (ACIP). MMWR.56 (No. RR-2).
66. (CDC) USCfDC. FDA licensure of bivalent human papillomavirus vaccine (HPV2, Cervarix) for use in females and update HPV vaccination recommendations from the Advisory Committee on Immunization Practices (ACIP). MMWR 2010;59L626-9.
67. Control USCfD (2010) FDA licensure of quadrivalent human papillomavirus vaccine (HPV4, Gardasil) for use in males and guidance from the Advisory Committee on Immunization Practices (ACIP). MMWR 59: 630–2.
68. Bastani R, Glenn BA, Tsui J, Chang LC, Marchand EJ, Taylor VM et al (2011) Understanding suboptimal human papillomavirus vaccine uptake among ethnic minority girls. Cancer Epidemiol Biomarkers Prev 20:1463–1472
69. Yi JK, Anderson KO, Le YC, Escobar-Chaves SL, Reyes-Gibby CC (2013) English proficiency, knowledge, and receipt of HPV vaccine in Vietnamese-American women. J Community Health 38:805–811

68. [illegible]

Index

A

Adenocarcinomas, 110, 219, 250, 277
Age-standardized incidence rates (ASR), 5, 166
Alcohol, 11, 13, 38, 39, 68, 73, 121, 143, 145, 147, 148, 151, 176, 187, 190, 198, 207, 226, 237–239, 241, 254–255
Alpha-fetoprotein (AFP), 244
American Association for the Study of Liver Diseases (AASLD), 242–244
American Institute for Cancer Research (AICR), 143, 145, 172–174, 198
Anaplastic lymphoma kinase (ALK), 112
Androgens, 168–169, 195, 204, 205, 223
Annual Percent Change (APC) in cancer incidence rates, 53, 57, 58, 61, 66, 68, 69, 73
Asian Americans and Pacific Islanders (AAPIs), 6, 8, 9, 11, 20, 22, 108–111, 114, 141, 187
Asian/Pacific Islander (API), 250, 251
Asian-Americans
- birthplace, 14
- cancer incidence and mortality, 5–6
- case-control study, 12–13
- case-only study, 11–12
- cohort study, 13–14
- cross-sectional study, 7, 11
- environmental and lifestyle risk factors, 1
- ethnic subgroups, 2
- foreign-born Asians, 3
- geographic distribution, 4
- immigration, 2
- lifestyle and environmental factors, 14
- migrant populations, 5
- migration, 1, 7
- US Census, 1–4, 10, 15, 48, 50, 51, 233
- 2010 US population, 2, 3
- Worldwide cancer rates, 5

B

Barcelona Clinic Liver Cancer (BCLC), 239–241
Behavioral Risk Factor Surveillance System (BRFSS), 11, 141
Benign prostate hyperplasia (BPH), 162
Bladder Cancer, 48, 73–74
Body mass index (BMI), 11, 13, 70, 119, 143, 166, 190, 191, 199, 203, 226, 239
Breast cancer, 35, 66–68, 191–202
- active and passive smoking, 202–203
- age, 188–189
- anthropometric measures
  - adult body size and postmenopausal women risks, 196
  - adult body size and premenopausal women risks, 195–196
  - birth weight, 196–197
- Asian-Americans, 191
- CA-HW study, 191
- diabetes, 197–198
- dietary factors
  - alcohol, 198
  - dietary patterns, 198, 201, 207
  - fat, 198, 199
  - green and black tea, 202
  - meat, red meat and processed meat, 199–200
  - plant foods—fruit and vegetable, 200
  - soy products, 200–201

A.H. Wu, D.O. Stram (eds.), *Cancer Epidemiology in Asian Americans*,
DOI 10.1007/978-3-319-41118-7

Breast cancer (*cont.*)
endogenous hormones, 204–205
exogenous hormones
hormone replacement therapy, 194–195
oral contraceptives, 194
family history, 203–204
genetic susceptibility, 203–204
incidence rates, 188
Los Angeles County (LAC), 191
mammographic density and screening, 205–207
menstrual and reproductive factors
age at first birth, 192
age at menarche, 191–192
breastfeeding, 193
menopause, 193
nulliparity, 192
physical activity, 197
screening, 86
staging and tumor characteristics, 189–190
survival, 190–191

C
California Breast Cancer Survivorship Consortium (CBCSC), 190
California Cancer Registry (CCR), 6, 8, 9, 109, 110, 188, 189, 251, 252
California Health Interview Survey (CHIS), 68, 69, 71, 84, 86, 87, 164
Cancer incidence and mortality, 20–28, 33–39, 49–61, 65–74
Chinese Americans
AAIRs, 34
AAPI, 20
age-specific incidence rates, 28, 33
breast cancer, 35
colorectal cancer, 37
counts and age, 27–28
data sources and methods, 22–28
gallbladder cancer, 39
liver cancer, 37–38
Los Angeles Cancer Surveillance Program (LACSP), 21, 22, 25, 28
lung cancer, 36
nasopharyngealcancer (NPC), 34, 38, 39
population size, 21
prostate cancer, 35
racial discrimination, 20
SEER, 21, 22, 24, 25, 27, 28, 34
sex, 22–24
sex-site-specific rate ratios, 34
stomach cancer, 37
Filipino Americans
annual counts and distributions, 52
bladder cancer, 73
breast cancer, 66–68
cancer sites and trends, 53–61
cervical cancer, 69
colorectal cancer, 68
corpus and uteri cancer, 70
kidney and renal pelvis cancer, 71
leukemia, 73
liver cancer, 71
lung cancer, 68–69
NHL, 72
ovarian cancer, 72
pancreatic cancer, 74
prostate cancer, 61
sociodemographic characteristics, 49
statistical analysis, 53
thyroid cancer, 70
trends in mortality, 65
U.S. Cancer Incidence Data, 50
U.S. Mortality Data, 50
U.S. Population Data, 51–52
Cancer Incidence in Five Continents (CI5), 5, 21, 22, 25, 28, 52
Cancer screening tests
American Cancer Society, 82
Asian ethnic groups, 82
cancer control intervention, 100
cervical cancer screening, 86–87
colorectal cancer screening, 87–88
community surveys, 84, 85
electronic health records, 85
estimation, 84
ethnicity and acculturation, 100
HBV testing, 82
health-care systems, 100
hepatitis B testing, 88–90
HPV testing, 82
mammograms, 82
mammography screening, 85–86
population-based surveys, 84
precancerous abnormal tissue, 82
quasi-experimental studies, 100
Cancer Surveillance Program (CSP), 6, 8, 21, 22, 25, 28, 251
Centers for Disease Control and Prevention's (CDC), 89, 242, 243, 250, 280
Cervical cancer
community-based approaches, 280
cumulative risks, 275
disparities, 280, 281
factors, 279
HPV, 274–278, 280

HPV test, 279
HR-HPV genotypes and worldwide attributable fraction, CxCa, 273, 274
incidence rates, 272
interventions, 280
knowledge, attitudinal, cultural and access barriers, 280
mortality rates, 273
Pap test, 279
race/ethnic groups, 273
risk factors, 278–279
screening, 86–87
screening rate, 279
SEER registries, 272
shyness and cultural beliefs, 279
squamous cell and adenocarcinoma, 272
Chemotherapy, 110, 258–261
Chinese Exclusion Act, 20
Cigarette smoking, 69, 71, 73, 74, 107, 144, 148, 225–226, 249, 271
Client-directed interventions, 93
Colorectal cancer (CRC), 37, 68, 145–147
age-adjusted incidence rates, 139
candidate genes, 150–151
characteristics, 139–140
comparisons, 138
diabetes, 144
diet and alcohol
calcium, 145, 147, 148, 151
dietary fiber, 145, 146, 148, 151
fruits and vegetables, 146
green tea, 147, 148
isothiocyanates, 146, 151
non-fiber carbohydrate, 146
polyunsaturated fatty acids, 146
pyridoxal-5′-phosphate, (PLP), 147
red meat, 146, 148, 153
serum cholesterol levels, 147
family history, 150
genetics, 149
genome-wide association studies (GWAS), 151–153
lifestyle, 148–149
male, 138
medications, 149
menopausal hormone therapy (MHT), 146
migrants, 140–141
obesity, 143–144
physical activity, 148
screening, 87–88
screening rates, 141–143
smoking, 144–145
Corpus and uteri cancer, 57, 70
Correlates of screening
cancer screening, 92
cross-sectional research design, 91
demographic factors, acculturation and health-care coverage, 91
Health Behavior Framework, 90
individual variables, 91–92
provider and health-care system factors, 92
Cytotoxin-associated gene A (CagA), 252–254

D
Diabetes, 38, 39, 74, 143, 166
breast cancer, 190, 197–198, 207
colorectal cancer (CRC), 144, 152
endometrial cancer, 222, 225, 226
liver, 229
prostate cancer, 171–172

E
Ecological study design
AAPI populations, 8
birthplace, 9
cancer rates, 9
case ascertainment (numerator), 7
CSP, 6, 8, 21, 22, 25, 28
denominator data, 8
ecologic comparisons, 10
incidence rates, 10
menopausal hormones, 9
migrant and nonmigrant groups, 10
numerator and denominator data, 9
risk factors, cancer, 7
SEER program, 8
US born *vs.* foreign born, 10
Endometrial cancer
age-adjusted incidence rates, 220, 221
characteristics, 221–222
cigarette smoking, 225–226
description, 219–220
diabetes, 225
dietary factors, 226
family history and genetic susceptibility, 227
female reproductive organs, 220
menstrual and reproductive factors, 224
metabolic syndrome, 222
obesity, 222–224
physical activity, 225
survivorship, 227–228
women emigrating, 221
Endoscopic mucosal resection (EMR), 259
Endoscopic submucosal dissection (ESD), 259

Epidermal growth factor receptor (EGFR), 110, 112
Estrogen–progestin therapy (EPT), 194, 195
Exogenous hormones, 194, 224

F
Fecal occult blood testing (FOBT), 87, 95–98, 141
Filipino American population, 47–49, 51, 52, 87
Filipino-Americans, 87

G
Gallbladder cancer, 19, 23, 24, 27, 28, 31–34, 39
Gastric cancer, 255–257
  adenocarcinomas, 250
  adjuvant and neo-adjuvant therapies, 260–261
  alcohol, 254–255
  cardia and non-cardia, 249
  chemoradiation, 261
  chemotherapy, 260
  diagnosis, 257–258
  dietary factors
    fruits and vegetables, 256–257
    salt, 257
    total meat and processed meat, 255–256
  East–West differences, 258–259
  EMR/ESD, 259
  epidemiology and risk factors, 262
  H. pylori, 253
  incidence patterns, 250–251
  jaundice, 257
  malignancies, 250
  mortality patterns, 251
  palliative treatments, 261–262
  pathology, 251–252
  screening and prevention, 262
  symptoms, 257
  tobacco smoking, 254
  treatment, 259
  tumor, node, metastasis (TNM), 258
Genome-wide association studies (GWAS), 204, 227
  Asian Colorectal Cancer Consortium, 152
  Chinese population, 153
  CRC, 151–153
  ethnic/racial groups, 152
  European-ancestry populations, 151
  fine-mapping, 153
  heredity, 151
  lung cancer, 123–125
  prostate cancer, 168
  SNPs, 152, 153

H
Hazard ratio (HR), 110, 139, 194, 237, 251
Health Behavior Framework, 90
Helicobacter pylori (*H. pylori*), 253
Hepatitis B immune globulin (HBIG), 242
Hepatitis B testing, 82, 88–90
Hepatitis B virus (HBV), 38
  antiviral therapy, 243
  HCC, 238–239
  screening, 242
  vaccination, 242
Hepatitis C virus (HCV)
  antiviral therapy, 243
  HCC, 238–239
  screening, 242–243
Hepatocellular carcinoma (HCC)
  age-adjusted incidence, 234–236
  hepatitis B and C, 238–239
  mortality rate, 236–239
  non-viral etiologies, 239
  risk factors, 237–238, 244
  surveillance, 244
Hereditary non-polyposis colorectal cancer (HNPCC), 227
Hmong, 84, 97, 100
Hormone replacement therapy (HRT), 119, 195
Hormone therapy (HT), 194
Human carcinogens, 172
Human papillomavirus (HPV), 69
  adenocarcinomas, 277
  carcinogenicity, 276
  cervical cancer rates and HPV16/18 prevalence, 277
  heterogeneity, 277
  intratypic variation, 276
  invasive and preinvasive cervical cancer, 275
  normal cervical cytology and invasive cervical cancer, geographic region, 276
  sexual activity, 278
  testing, 82
  type-specific prevalence, 276, 277

I
Insulin-like growth factors (IGF), 168–169
International Agency for Research on Cancer (IARC), 5, 25, 144, 253
International Association for Cancer Registries (IACR), 5, 25, 52, 165
International Cancer Databases, 25–28
Interventions to promote cancer screening
  cancer control interventions, 93
  community-based group education, 98

community-level interventions, 99
experimental designs, 93
health-care settings, 97
lay health worker (LHW), 93, 95–97
one-on-one education and small media, 98–99
quasi-experimental designs, 93
Isoflavones, 175, 226

J
Japan Public Health Center (JPHC), 148, 192, 198–200, 220
Japanese-Americans, 87

K
Kidney and Renal Pelvis Cancer, 71
Korean-Americans, 86, 87, 100

L
Lay health worker (LHW), 37–38, 71, 93, 97
Liver cancer, 234–235
epidemiology, 234
HBV, 242
HCC (*see* Hepatocellular carcinoma (HCC))
HCV, 242–243
treatment, 239–241
viral hepatitis and HCC, 241
Liver ultrasonography, 244
Los Angeles Cancer Surveillance Program (LACSP), 6, 8, 21, 22, 25, 28, 251
Lung cancer, 36, 68–69, 119–125
active smoking, 113–114
Asian American, 109
body size, 119
diet
alcohol, 121
antioxidant micronutrients, 120
dietary factors, 122
fruit and vegetables, 119–120
genetic susceptibility, 122–125
soy foods, 121
tea, 122
DNA Repair Genes, 124
EGFR gene mutations, 112
GWAS, 123
histopathology, 111
household coal combustion and cooking oils, 116
HPV infection, 118
incidence rates, 108
incidence rates, 108
indoor air pollution, 115–116
infectious disease, 118
mortality and survival rates, 110
occupational exposures, 117
outdoor air pollution, 116–117
P53 tumor suppressor mutations, 112
passive smoking, 115
reproductive history and hormone exposure, 119
screening, 125–126
SEER data, 111
smoking cessation, 114
somatic mutations, 111–112
stage of disease, 110
Lynch syndrome, 227

M
Mammography screening, 85–86
Menopausal hormone therapy (MHT), 145
Multiethnic Cohort Study (MEC), 14, 113, 144–150, 152, 153, 167–169, 171–177, 191–194, 196, 198–203, 205–207, 222–224, 226, 252, 254, 257

N
Nasopharyngeal cancer (NPC), 34, 38, 39
National Cancer Institute (NCI), 21
National Health and Nutrition Examination Survey (NHANES), 11, 254
National Health Interview Survey (NHIS), 11
National Immunization Survey, 280
National Lung Screening Trial (NLST), 125
N-nitroso compounds (NOCs), 256
Non-Hodgkin Lymphomas (NHL), 48, 53, 59–60, 62, 64, 66, 72
Non-small cell lung cancers (NSCLCs), 109
Nonsteroidal anti-inflammatory drugs (NSAIDs), 149
North American Association of Central Cancer Registries (NAACCR), 140

O
Oral cavity and pharyngeal cancers, 73
Oral contraceptives (OCs), 72, 149, 194, 222, 224, 278
Ovarian cancer, 72

P
Pancreatic cancer, 48, 60, 74
Polyunsaturated fatty acids (PUFA), 199

Prostate cancer, 35, 61, 174–176
age, 167
age-standardized incidence rates, 165, 166
androgens and insulin-like growth factors, 168–169
Asian Americans, 177
body size and obesity, 170–171
BPH, 162
carcinogenesis, 167
diabetes, 171–172
diagnosis, 177
dietary factors, 167
dairy products, 176
fat, 174
fruits/vegetables, 175
green tea, 176
isoflavones, 175
micronutrients, 176
processed and red meat, 174–175
soy, 175–176
family history, 168
genetic susceptibility, 168
heterogeneity, 163–164
incidence rates, 162–163
infection/inflammation, 169–170
migrant, 165–166
mortality, 163
physical activity, 172
PSA screening, 164, 165
race/ethnicity, 167
risk factors, 167
screening, 82
smoking, 172–173
TURP/PSA testing, 162
Prostate, Lung, Colorectal, and Ovarian (PLCO), 118
Prostatitis, 169
Pyridoxal-5′-phosphate (PLP), 147

R
Radon, 115
Ramucirumab, 262

S
Sex hormone binding globulin (SHBG), 204
Sexually transmitted infections (STIs), 169, 278, 281
Smoking, 11, 36, 38, 39, 48, 68, 69, 71, 73, 74, 83, 107, 109, 111–119, 121–126, 144, 145, 148, 151, 153, 161, 171, 172, 177, 190, 193, 202, 203, 225, 226, 249, 254, 255, 278
Socioeconomic status (SES), 1, 82, 109, 142, 278
Soy, 13, 36, 114, 121, 146, 148, 161, 175, 177, 198, 200, 201, 203, 207, 226–228
Stomach cancer, 37
Stomach cancer screening, 82
Surveillance Epidemiology and End Results (SEER), 6, 51, 108, 139, 234
Systematically collected in the USA until 1973 by the Surveillance, 21

T
Tea, 36, 122, 147, 148, 161, 176, 177, 202, 226
Telomerase reverse transcriptase (TERT), 123
Thyroid cancer, 70
Transurethral resection of the prostate (TURP), 162
Trastuzumab, 262

U
United Network for Organ Sharing (UNOS), 238
US Preventive Services Task Force (USPSTF), 82, 83, 164, 242

V
Vietnamese-Americans, 86, 87, 91, 100

W
Waist circumference (WC), 1, 143, 152, 170, 223, 224
Waist-to-hip ratio (WHR), 143, 170, 195, 223
Women's Contraceptive and Reproductive Experiences (CARE), 192
World Cancer Research Fund/American Institute for Cancer Research (WCRF/AICR), 143, 145, 171–173, 176, 198

X
Xenobiotic Metabolic Genes, 120, 122, 124